Ultrasound in Assisted Reproduction and Early Pre

Ultrasound in Assisted Reproduction and Early Pregnancy

Edited by

Arianna D'Angelo, MD, Associate MRCOG
Consultant in Assisted Reproduction, Wales Fertility Institute,
Swansea Bay University Health Board
Senior Clinical Lecturer in Obstetrics and Gynaecology, Cardiff University
Consultant Gynaecologist, University Hospital of Wales, Cardiff

Nazar N. Amso, MB ChB, FHEA, FRCOG, PhD (London University)
Emeritus Professor in Obstetrics and Gynecology
Former Head of the Academic Department of Obstetrics and Gynecology,
School of Medicine, Cardiff University
Honorary Consultant Obstetrician and Gynecologist,
University Hospital of Wales
Consultant Gynaecological Surgeon
Spire Cardiff Hospital, Cardiff

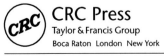

CRC Press
Taylor & Francis Group
Boca Raton London New York

CRC Press is an imprint of the
Taylor & Francis Group, an **informa** business

First edition published 2021
by CRC Press
6000 Broken Sound Parkway NW, Suite 300, Boca Raton, FL 33487-2742

and by CRC Press
2 Park Square, Milton Park, Abingdon, Oxon, OX14 4RN

ISBN: 978-1-138-48617-1 (hbk)
ISBN: 978-1-138-48585-3 (pbk)
ISBN: 978-1-351-04623-7 (ebk)

Typeset in Times LT Std
by Nova Techset Private Limited, Bengaluru & Chennai, India

Contents

Preface

Ultrasound has played a pivotal role in the investigation of patients with infertility since 1978 when Joachim Hackeloer, working in Glasgow, Scotland, published his classic paper on the tracking of ovarian follicular growth and showed a correlation between follicular size and serum estradiol. With the introduction of assisted reproduction treatments (ARTs) in the late 1970s, coupled with the innovative development of transvaginal sonography (TVS) technology, its role became more embedded in the assessment and management of patients undergoing these treatments—for preassessment, during monitoring of controlled ovarian stimulation, ovum pick-up, embryo transfer, or confirmation of early pregnancy and its location. It truly can be described as indispensable.

The European Society of Human Reproduction and Embryology (ESHRE) workshop that was held on November 16–17, 2017, in Cardiff, United Kingdom, sought to address the role of ultrasound in the broader context, to include connected topics in addition to the diagnostic and treatment-related applications.

In this book, we examine the physiology of implantation, the role of ultrasound in assessing implantation potential, and the factors that may affect it adversely in women undergoing ART. In Chapter 14, early embryonic and fetal development are described in detail, and readers are offered clear and beautiful two- and three-dimensional and ultrasound images and short video clips that are truly informative of sonoembryology. Maternal and fetal consequences of multiple pregnancies and the widely recognized and evidence-based benefits from single embryo transfer in ART are articulated. Other chapters address quality of service and key performance indicators related to the use of ultrasound in ART, infection control and safety protocols necessary for the use of ultrasound systems in clinical practice, ultrasound training and the role of simulation, and the need for credentialing and certification as quality assurance measures for ultrasound practitioners in ART units.

The chapters in this book are not meant to be the definitive reviews of ultrasound in ART and early pregnancy. They are merely intended to succinctly present readers with our current understanding of ultrasound applications in clinical ART practice accompanied by a large collection of ultrasound images and short video clips, which may help those working in the field to appreciate the full potential of ultrasound and serve as useful teaching aids for those in training.

Arianna D'Angelo
Nazar N. Amso

Acknowledgments

The editors are indebted to all of the contributing authors, without whom this book would not have been possible.

We are especially grateful to the patients who agreed for their ultrasound images and video clips to be published.

We are also grateful to all the organizations and publishers acknowledged in the figure and table captions who gave permission to use their material, particularly to Dr. Veronika Frisova for allowing us to use the image on the book's front cover.

Finally, we thank our families for their unfailing support and patience.

Arianna D'Angelo
Nazar N. Amso

Contributors

Arianna D'Angelo
Consultant in Assisted Reproduction
Wales Fertility Institute
Swansea Bay University Health Board
Wales, United Kingdom

and

Senior Clinical Lecturer in Obstetrics and
  Gynaecology
Cardiff University
and
Consultant Gynaecologist
University Hospital of Wales
Cardiff, United Kingdom

Nazar N. Amso
Emeritus Professor in Obstetrics and
  Gynecology
Former Head of the Academic Department of
  Obstetrics and Gynecology
School of Medicine
Cardiff University
and
Honorary Consultant Obstetrician and
  Gynecologist
University Hospital of Wales
and
Consultant Gynaecological Surgeon
Spire Cardiff Hospital
Cardiff, United Kingdom

Thoraya Ammar
Department of Radiology
King's College Hospital
London, United Kingdom

Candice Cheung
Shrewsbury and Telford Hospital NHS Trust
and
Keele University School of Medicine
Staffordshire, United Kingdom

Veronika Frisova
Profema Fetal Medicine Centre
Prague, Czech Republic

and

Department of Obstetrics and Gynecology
Faculty Hospital
Palacky University
Olomouc, Czech Republic

Rudaina Hassan
Department of Obstetrics and Gynaecology
Sidra Medicine
Doha, Qatar

Dean C.Y. Huang
Department of Radiology
King's College Hospital
London, United Kingdom

Rezan A. Kadir
The Royal Free NHS Hospital and University
  College
London, United Kingdom

Yacoub Khalaf
Assisted Conception Unit
Guy's and St. Thomas' Hospital NHS Foundation
  Trust
London, United Kingdom

Jure Knez
Department of Obstetrics and Gynaecology
University Medical Centre
Maribor, Slovenia

Julia Kopeika
Assisted Conception Unit
Guy's and St. Thomas' Hospital NHS Foundation
  Trust
London, United Kingdom

Roberto Marci
Department of Morphology
Surgery and Experimental Medicine
University of Ferrara
Ferrara, Italy

Dimitrios Mavrelos
Department of Obstetrics and Gynecology
University College London Hospital
London, United Kingdom

Henriette Svarre Nielsen
Fertility Department
Juliane Marie Centre
Rigshospitalet
Copenhagen, Denmark

Costas Panayotidis
Freelance Consultant Obstetrician Gynaecologist
United Kingdom

Neil D. Pugh
School of Engineering
Cardiff University
Cardiff, United Kingdom

Kuhan Rajah
Department of Obstetrics and Gynecology
University College London Hospital
London, United Kingdom

Ghada Salman
Gynaecology Diagnostic and Treatment Unit
University College London Hospital
London, United Kingdom

Ippokratis Sarris
King's Fertility
King's College Hospital
London, United Kingdom

Paul S. Sidhu
Department of Radiology
King's College Hospital
London, United Kingdom

Andrew Sizer
Department of Reproductive Medicine and
    Surgery
Shrewsbury and Telford Hospital NHS Trust
and
Senior Lecturer
Keele University School of Medicine
Staffordshire, United Kingdom

Ilaria Soave
Department of Surgical and Clinical Sciences and
    Translational Medicine
S. Andrea Hospital "Sapienza" University
    of Rome
Rome, Italy

Karin Sundberg
Department of Obstetrics and Gynecology
Juliane Marie Centre
Rigshospitalet
Copenhagen, Denmark

Caryl Thomas
Department of Obstetrics and Gynaecology
University Hospital of Wales
Cardiff, United Kingdom

Kelly Tilleman
Department for Reproductive Medicine
Ghent University Hospital
Ghent, Belgium

Martin G. Tolsgaard
Copenhagen Academy for Medical Education
    and Simulation
Copenhagen, Denmark

Zdravka Veleva
Department of Obstetrics and Gynecology
Helsinki University and Helsinki University
    Central Hospital
Helsinki, Finland

Kugajeevan Vigneswaran
King's Fertility
King's College Hospital
London, United Kingdom

Veljko Vlaisavljević
IVF Adria Consulting
Maribor, Slovenia

C. Jason Wilkins
Department of Radiology
King's College Hospital
London, United Kingdom

1

Ultrasound in Assisted Reproductive Technology: Anatomy and Core Examination Skills

Nazar N. Amso

Introduction

Ultrasound imaging has extensive applications in medicine, and these continue to evolve [1]. Its influence on gynecological practice has been transformational. The practice has become more office and ambulatory based for several reasons, namely, a more efficient and cost-effective service associated with higher patient satisfaction. Although both transabdominal sonography (TAS) and transvaginal or endovaginal sonography (TVS) have been available for many decades [2], it is the transvaginal route that has by far been the most influential on practice. This is due to (1) the higher frequency of the transvaginal transducer in comparison with the transabdominal one (6–8 MHz versus 2–6 MHz) resulting in better image resolution, (2) proximity of the ultrasound emitting tip of the probe to the region of interest, i.e., the pelvis, and (3) the ability to undertake many procedures through the vaginal route under direct ultrasound guidance without the need for general anesthesia.

Hence, ultrasound, as a noninvasive tool, is now the modality of choice for the assessment of normal and abnormal pelvic anatomy. It is ideal to image the uterine morphology and dimensions, ovaries, urinary bladder, adnexa, anal sphincter, and retroperitoneal space. At present, TAS and TVS are used in a variety of settings, e.g., in early pregnancy assessment, outpatient and reproductive health clinics, gynecologic oncology, adolescent gynecology, urogynecology, infertility, and postmenopausal gynecology [4]. The introduction of three-dimensional (3D) ultrasound has further increased the diagnostic role of TVS for uterine malformations. Many of these applications are explored in detail in other chapters of this book.

The acceptability of TVS was previously reported [3,4]. Most women undergoing TVS dating scans described no or mild discomfort (52% and 47.5%, respectively), while 0.7% experienced marked discomfort. In the same study, 88% of women accepted TVS, and 95% said that they would have no concerns about another TVS in a future pregnancy [5]. These findings were confirmed by a more recent study [6].

Ultrasound remains very subjective and operator dependent. The increasing applications and greater availability of cheaper general-purpose portable ultrasound machines necessitate adequate training in the technique and interpretation of the acquired images before commencing independent practice. In this chapter, the author focuses on the TVS technique and the appearance of the normal pelvis, as it is the most relevant to infertility practice. Other chapters expand on abnormal findings in the nonpregnant and pregnant states.

Know Your Anatomy

There is need for clarity in describing the anatomical planes used to obtain images during TVS. The conventional anatomical planes nomenclature used in anatomy or radiology, namely, sagittal, transverse, and coronal, do not generally correspond closely with the anatomical planes in TVS. Several factors should be considered; the transducer is inserted into the vagina, which runs in a downward and posterior direction, and the pelvis is tilted at an angle 30° to the long axis of the body; the vaginal walls and vaginal vault limit the depth and range of hand movement employed to obtain the images; and limitations imposed by the angle of view, transducer position, and image magnification lead to incomplete assessment of a pelvic plane in one image [8]. Hence, the transducer is continually manipulated in various directions to assist the operator in acquiring relevant information to form a virtual 3D image of the pelvis.

The sagittal plane, also referred to as median or longitudinal, runs along the long axis of the body dividing it into right and left halves and is at right angles to both the coronal, also called frontal, and transverse planes. These respectively divide the body into front and back parts and upper and lower parts (Figure 1.1) [7].

However, during TVS, it is not possible to obtain these views in most instances. When the transducer is held in a manner whereby the ultrasound beam is directed in plane running from the anterior abdominal to the posterior abdominal wall, usually referred to as sagittal or longitudinal view, a true sagittal plane is only obtained when the transducer is positioned in the midline. When the beam is angled to the right or left without changing its direction, it cannot be called sagittal or parasagittal but is at an oblique angle to the midline (Figure 1.2).

Similarly, when the transducer is held in a manner whereby the beam is directed in the plane running from the right to the left side of the patient, a coronal view is only obtained when the beam is parallel to the anterior or posterior abdominal walls along the long axis of the body (Figure 1.3). When it is angled either anteriorly toward the abdominal wall or posteriorly toward the rectum, it becomes angled at an oblique angle. The term *transverse plane* is often used interchangeably with the term *coronal plane*. This, in principle, is both inaccurate and misleading, as an anatomical transverse plane bisects the body into superior and inferior portions, which clearly does not happen during TVS [7].

It has been proposed that better descriptors for the TVS planes should be *anteroposterior pelvic plane* or *AP pelvic plane* and *transpelvic plane*, referring to the ultrasound beam being across the pelvis [7]. These descriptors are accurate and do not contradict the anatomical or radiological planes. During TVS the probe is swept from the right to the left side of the patient in the AP plane and from the anterior to the posterior abdominal walls in the transpelvic plane to examine the pelvic structures comprehensively.

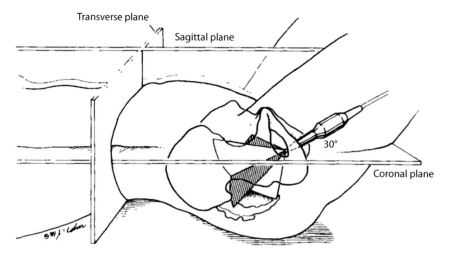

FIGURE 1.1   The three anatomical planes of the human body and their relationship to the ultrasound beam during transvaginal scanning. The transverse plane is at right angles to the long axis of the body; the coronal plane is at right angles to the median plane in the longitudinal axis passing through the coronal sutures (and generally includes planes parallel to the planes passing through the coronal sutures); and the sagittal plan is parallel to the median plane passing through the sagittal sutures (planes parallel to the sagittal plane but not in the midline are often referred to as parasagittal planes). (From Dodson MG and Deter RL, Definition of anatomical planes for use in transvaginal sonography, *J Clin Ultrasound* 1990; 18:239–42, with permission.)

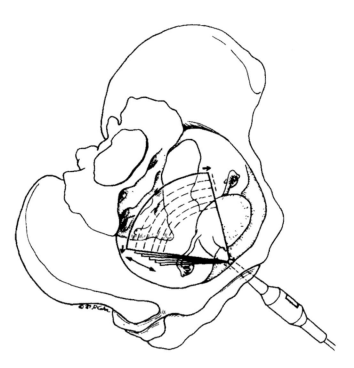

FIGURE 1.2 The ultrasound beam is directed from the anterior abdominal to the posterior abdominal wall. As the probe is directed to the right and left side, it becomes oblique to the midline. (From Dodson MG and Deter RL, Definition of anatomical planes for use in transvaginal sonography, *J Clin Ultrasound* 1990; 18:239–42, with permission.)

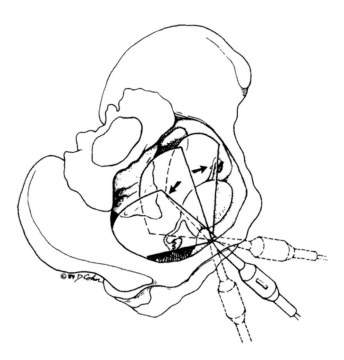

FIGURE 1.3 The ultrasound beam is directed in the plane running from the right to the left side of the body. As the probe is directed to the anterior to the posterior abdominal walls, it becomes oblique to the true coronal plane running parallel to the abdominal walls. (From Dodson MG and Deter RL, Definition of anatomical planes for use in transvaginal sonography, *J Clin Ultrasound* 1990; 18:239–42, with permission.)

It is this understanding of the commonly used descriptors' inaccuracies that should assist the novices to comprehend the confusing terminology and learn the basics of TVS technique. Despite these pitfalls, the terms *sagittal*, *coronal*, and *transverse* remain predominantly in use.

Prerequisites

The sonographer should be familiar with the following skills through a structured training program, as outlined in Chapter 20, before independently undertaking a scan on a patient:

- Patient-related skills and general scanning conventions
- Machine-related skills
- Image acquisition and optimization skills
- Systematic approach to the examination technique

Patient-Related Skills and General Scanning Conventions

TVS is an intimate examination, and as such, patient-related skills are of utmost importance.

Prescan preparations include giving an information leaflet on TVS before or on arrival for the scan appointment. This would give the patient an opportunity to consider having TVS or TAS or clarify elements of the examination. The patient should also empty her bladder before coming to the scan room. TVS should always be undertaken in the presence of a female chaperone, and this must be documented in the notes. The date of the last menstrual period should be documented, and the ultrasound transducer cleaned and disinfected as described in Chapter 19. The sonographer should wear gloves on both hands. The sonographer should also exclude latex allergy to avoid its serious consequences. Latex-free probe covers and gloves should be available in the clinic. Sachets of sterile gel should be used for the outside of the cover. Aprons or personal protective devices might be used for infection control.

Consent is generally verbal but must be documented in the records. It should be obtained by the person who is undertaking the scan. The procedure should be explained in full, and the patient is given the opportunity to ask questions.

Enhancing patient experience during TVS is paramount. A study utilizing "critical incident technique" reported on the personal experiences of sonographers performing TVS and provided viewpoints of their practices and their evaluation of patient experiences. Distinct themes that impacted patient experience overall were identified: patient comfort, chaperones and companions, sonographer gender, patient privacy, language and culture, communication, patient empowerment, sonographer advocacy for the patient, and previous experiences or preconceptions [9]. Communication at several levels will help to minimize patient anxiety. The sonographer, if he or she deems it appropriate, may "narrate" the steps of the procedure and point out the various structures to the patient as the scan is underway. This helps to distract the patient's attention from transducer manipulation in the vagina and build rapport with the patient. Should right or left iliac fossa pressure be required, the patient herself could undertake that.

Communication of results after the scan must be done in a sensitive manner, especially if there is bad news. Depending on the experience of the sonographer, the findings may be explained in detail or the patient is referred to the most experienced member of the team for full explanation.

Patient positioning on the examination table is very important to ensure successful assessment of the pelvis. Ideally, the examination couch should be like that used for colposcopy (Figure 1.4) so the patient can bring her buttocks to the edge and the feet or knees are supported. In this way, the sonographer has ample space to maneuver the transducer in various directions. This is particularly useful for visualization of the ovaries when their position is such that it requires excessive anterior angulation of the transducer.

The scanning table and chair should be height adjustable. Sonographers should scan from the foot of the table sitting centrally or to the right in relation to the patient, with the ultrasound machine placed laterally. This ensures that the scanning arm is not extended and reduces the risk of repetitive strain injury (RSI).

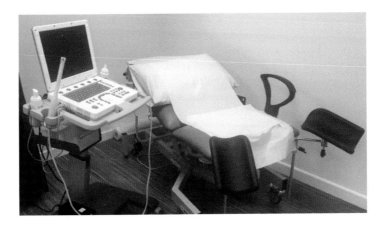

FIGURE 1.4   The general layout of the scanning area where the patient lies on the couch with her buttocks right at the edge and the legs are supported below the knees. This allows maximum space for manipulation of the transvaginal transducer. The operator sits either in the middle or to the right of the couch. An ultrasound machine on a trolly is shown to the right of the patient.

Machine-Related Skills

Knowing the intricacies of the ultrasound machine is frequently termed *knobology*. The sonographer must be familiar with the machine she or he is using, its capabilities, settings including the use of Doppler, and how to adjust the various controls to acquire and optimize the image. As different systems have their unique configurations, discussion of which is beyond the scope of this chapter, the reader is advised to consult the user manual of their system or the manufacturer's technical team.

Image Acquisition and Optimization Skills

Understanding Anatomical Landmarks

Anatomical structures in the pelvis and their relation to each other provide the sonographer with important markers during the examination. Thus, knowledge of their location is of immense value during scanning.

Some landmarks, such as the bladder and the iliac vessels, have a permanent location, the former in the center anteriorly and the latter on the pelvic side walls. This should enable the sonographer to refer to them whenever other pelvic structures cannot be found.

Female pelvic anatomy varies considerably at different stages of the menstrual cycle and between patients. Morphological changes at different stages of the menstrual cycle are described in the next section. The presence or absence of the uterus and its position, anteverted, axial, or retroverted, are dependent on many factors. The position and appearance of the ovaries are also variable and influenced by age, stage of the menstrual cycle, menopausal status, and history of infection or previous surgery. Equally, the appearance and content of the pouch of Douglas have similar variations.

Video 1.1 teaches skills to identify key anatomical structures of the female pelvis.

VIDEO 1.1
Identification of key anatomical structures of the female pelvis. (https://youtu.be/OihrTQbqfCk)

Ultrasound image orientation and its correlation with the woman's pelvic anatomy are pivotal to accurate diagnosis. As the sonographer is facing the patient, the ultrasound image on the screen must correspond in its orientation to the woman's anatomy. The woman's right ovary will be seen on the left-hand side of the sonographer and conversely for the opposite side. It is crucial that the sonographer maintain the right and left orientations on the screen with those of the woman. The sonographer should check that transducer and image orientation on the screen are in agreement before starting the scan. During the scan, agreement between probe and image orientation must be maintained whether the examination is in the sagittal (AP pelvic) or coronal (transpelvic) planes. When the transducer is angled from one side to the other, it must not be rotated along its axis, as this will change its orientation and become discordant with the screen orientation. This is explained further in Video 1.2.

Image optimization of the region of interest ensures that the sonographer acquires an optimal diagnostic image for interpretation of the findings and reaching a diagnosis. The points that follow summarize the key parameters of image optimization and together with video should give the reader a toolkit for scanning. The background physical principles pertinent to image optimization are further explained in chapter 2.

VIDEO 1.2
Principles of image orientation. (https://youtu.be/3X4zx6SR6Xs)

- A—**A**djust the frequency and power settings to reflect the type of scan and patient characteristics
- B—**B**eware of artifacts and ultrasound safety issues, i.e., mechanical and thermal indices, and comply with the ALARA (as low as reasonably achievable) principle
- C—**C**entralize the "region of interest" (ROI) in the middle of the field of view (FOV)
- D—Adjust the **D**epth of the FOV to sufficiently magnify the whole ROI within the FOV
- E—**E**nlarge or zoom the image so the ROI is magnified within the FOV (D and E complement each other)
- F—Adjust the **F**ocal zone(s) to optimize the lateral resolution at or just below the ROI
- G—Adjust **G**ain and time gain compensation (TGC); adjust to have shades of gray rather than too bright or dark an image
- H—**H**armonics and their impact on image quality must be understood and applied appropriately

Video 1.3 explains in detail the key steps taken to ensure that images are optimized during transvaginal scanning.

VIDEO 1.3
Steps taken to optimize the image during scanning. (https://youtu.be/jhLTCoE-qkA)

Systematic Approach to the Examination Technique

The merits of TVS and thorough assessment of pelvic structures were highlighted many years ago [11]. Later, an ultrasound protocol for systematic assessment of the pelvis was developed in the context of a clinical trial and became established in clinical practice [10]. In this section, key steps of the examination technique are outlined, and the accompanying videos demonstrate the procedure.

Examination of the Uterus in the Sagittal Plane

In Video 1.4, the following key skills are demonstrated:

- Identify the uterus and cervix and optimize the image.
- In the sagittal plane, examine the uterus from one edge to the other.

- Demonstrate the endometrium and cervical canal in the sagittal plane.
- Optimize the view and enlarge the image if the endometrium is very thin.
- Examine the endometrium/endometrial cavity from right to left.
- Freeze at plane of maximum endometrial thickness in the upper uterine body and then measure.
- Endometrial thickness is measured from the one endometrial-myometrial interface to the one opposite, maintaining a perpendicular (90°) angle to the midline interface.

VIDEO 1.4
Full examination of the uterus in the sagittal plane. (https://youtu.be/7rTEdGFW1qs)

Examination of the Uterus in the Coronal Plane

In Video 1.5, the following key skills are demonstrated:

- Rotate the probe 90° toward the bladder to maintain the right-left orientation.
- In the coronal plane, examine the uterus from the cervix to the outer serosa of the fundus.

VIDEO 1.5
Full examination of the uterus in the coronal plane. (https://youtu.be/4heXDG_4k1s)

Optimal Demonstration of the Right Ovary and Adnexa

In Video 1.6, the following key skills are demonstrated:

- In the first instance, the ovary is best identified in the coronal plane.
- Rotate the probe to the coronal plane, and at the level of the uterine fundus, follow the ovarian ligament by tilting the probe laterally.
- In a split screen mode, remain in the coronal plane and move the probe up and down the pelvic side wall until you identify the ovary. Optimize the image, and then remaining in coronal plane, examine the ovary fully.
- Freeze the image when the ovary is at maximum dimensions.
- Press the split screen again, then reorient the probe into the sagittal plane, optimize the image, and examine the ovary fully.
- Freeze the image when the ovary is at maximum dimensions.
- Take maximum measurements in three orthogonal diameters (A, B, and C): (A) right to left direction in the coronal plane, (B) caudocephalic, and (C) anteroposterior directions in the sagittal plane.
- The ultrasound machine normally calculates the ovarian volume automatically.
- Alternatively, apply the multiplication formula for calculating the volume of an ellipsoid: 0.523ABC.

VIDEO 1.6
Optimal demonstration of the right ovary and adnexa. (https://youtu.be/_xtkHTm8gac)

Optimal Demonstration of the Left Ovary and Adnexa

In Video 1.7, the following key skills are be demonstrated:

- After examining and taking measurements of the right ovary, return to the midline and remain in the coronal view. Do not rotate the probe 180°.
- Tilt the probe toward the left adnexa.
- Repeat this procedure to identify the left ovary on the pelvic side wall using the split screen approach. Ensure your measurements are correct.

VIDEO 1.7
Optimal demonstration of the left ovary and adnexa. (https://youtu.be/Vt8_ZcFZAvg)

Examination of the Pouch of Douglas

Finally, to conclude the examination, the pouch of Douglas (cul-de-sac) is examined by noting the following:

- Identify the pouch of Douglas or the rectouterine pouch, an extension of the peritoneal cavity between the rectum and back wall of the uterus, cervix, and upper vagina.
- Examine fully from one side of the pelvis to the other.
- Note any fluid collection, adhesions, endometriotic deposits, loops of bowel, or any other solid or cystic masses. A small amount of fluid is normally present around the time of ovulation and not infrequently.

Tips and Tricks during the Procedure

- Abdominal pressure and/or instructing the patient to take a deep breath and hold momentarily help to bring a high ovary down into the FOV. As the ovary moves down, it becomes more distinct from the surrounding peristalsing loops of bowel. The patient should be able to exert pressure herself and surprisingly does not manifest the experience of significant pain.
- Pressure from below with the probe has a similar effect but from the opposite direction and results in moderate discomfort. A combination of abdominal and vaginal pressure may be occasionally required.
- Observing ovarian and adnexal mass mobility is important, as sliding freely against the pelvic side wall or the uterus strongly suggests the absence of significant adhesions.
- Excessive bowel peristalsing motility in the pelvis should point the sonographer to the possibility of an associated bowel problem, especially in patients with pelvic pain.
- The ovary(ies) may not be visualized or only partially seen, especially in postmenopausal women. In this instance, the sonographer needs to demonstrate a good view of the iliac vessel and measure between 3 and 5 cm of its length. Ideally, the vessels should have a clear outline with

a central anechoic lumen. An image of this view should be recorded and correctly annotated. If the iliac vessels cannot be seen clearly, this should be recorded in the report.

- TVS provides a more limited field of view than TAS. If a mass is lying outside the field of view of the TVS transducer, a TAS should be performed. A full bladder is not necessary, as such a mass will be sufficient in size to be seen transabdominally, even if the bladder is empty [11].
- A patient experiencing moderate or severe pain during TVS may have acute or chronic pelvic pathology such as pelvic inflammatory disease or endometriosis.
- Beware of unusual findings that you may encounter, such as an unusually positioned pelvic kidney.

Sonographic Changes of the Pelvic Organs

The normal sonographic appearance of the pelvic organs depends on knowledge of the menstrual cycle and its influence on the pelvic structures.

- *The menstrual cycle*: Hormonal changes during the menstrual cycle are well documented (Figure 1.5) and detailed in Chapters 3 and 4. Uterine and endometrial morphological changes

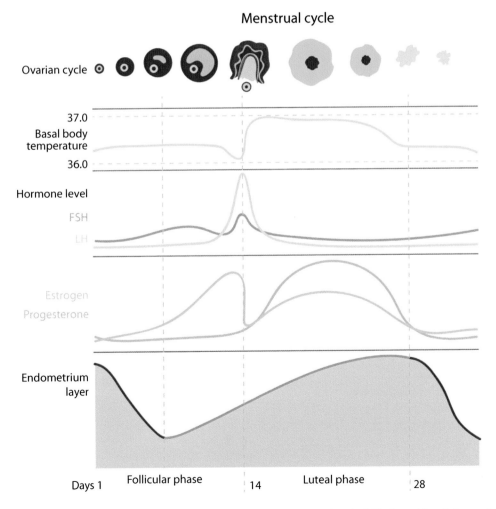

FIGURE 1.5 Hormonal (FSH, LH, Estrogen, and Progesterone) changes during the follicular and luteal phases of the menstrual cycle and their respective ovarian and endometrial morphological changes are shown.

during the menstrual cycle and their sonographic appearances are reported in Chapter 3 and are not discussed further here. Similarly, ovarian changes and follicular development during the menstrual cycle and their sonographic appearances are elaborated on in Chapter 4 and are not discussed further here.

The uterus and ovaries undergo changes at the various stages of the menstrual cycle:

- Cyclical changes
  - Menstrual phase
    - Uterus
    - Ovary(ies)
  - Follicular phase
    - Uterus
    - Ovary(ies)
  - Peri-ovulatory phase
    - Uterus
    - Ovary(ies)
  - Luteal phase
    - Uterus
    - Ovary(ies)

Discipline-Specific Professional Skills

- *Required images and annotation*: The required views of the uterus and ovaries/adnexa are outlined as follows. The images should be appropriately labeled with the examination date and patient ID number and should be correctly annotated.

  For each examination, the required images, as a minimum, should include:
  - A good sagittal view of the uterus or vaginal vault, if previous hysterectomy.
  - Endometrial thickness; any endometrial pathology, if present, should be correctly measured.
  - Both ovaries in sagittal and coronal planes with measurements in three diameters, preferably using split screen feature; if the ovary(ies) not seen, a good view of iliac vessel(s) with measurements.
  - Ovarian and adnexal pathology, correctly described and measured.
  - Color Doppler applied and documented where appropriate.
- *Accuracy of measurements*: Endometrial thickness (ET) should be measured at its widest point from the anterior to the posterior wall in the sagittal plane of the uterus. Calipers should be placed perpendicular to the outer edges of the endometrium or midline echo. If fluid is present in the uterine cavity, the ET should be measured as described earlier, including the cavity fluid and the double endometrial stripe, then subtract the fluid diameter at the same point.

  Polyps should be measured separately from the endometrium in two dimensions at 90° in the sagittal plane of the uterus but should be confirmed by visualizing in two planes of the uterus and color Doppler applied to look for feeder vessels.

  Fibroids should be measured. Where possible, their relationship to the endometrium and cavity, myometrium, and serosal surface as well as any degenerative changes should be documented.

  The position of the ovary in the pelvis is subject to wide variation; hence, the ovarian longest axis could be either in the caudocephalic (inferior-superior) or anteroposterior direction. In the sagittal plane, measure two diameters starting with the longest axis of the ovary and then the second being the widest measurement at 90° to the first. One of the two diameters in the sagittal plane will generally correspond to an axis that starts from the tip of the probe located in the vagina (caudal end of the body) in the direction of the patient's head (cephalic end), and the second axis is in the direction of anterior to posterior abdominal walls, which is often referred to as depth (CC and AP directions, respectively). In the coronal plane, measure the maximum width diameter (w) in the direction from the patient's right to left. The volume of an ovary follows the formula for an ellipsoid by multiplying the three perpendicular diameters by a factor $\times 0.5233$. Most ultrasound machines calculate the volume automatically. These directions are explained in the video "orientation in the sagittal and coronal planes" (Video 1.2).

The general convention is to measure the whole ovary including any cysts to calculate the overall volume. Ovarian cysts should also be measured separately to calculate a mean diameter. All measurements should be recorded in the ultrasound report form in millimeters and to one decimal place, e.g., $26.1 \times 17.8 \times 12.6$ mm.

- *Documentation and archiving*: The report should describe uterine and ovarian/adnexal appearance accurately. The presence of any pathology should be documented as well. Where abnormal ovarian morphology is present, it should be clearly described in accordance with internationally agreed upon terminology [12]. Details of such descriptors are beyond the scope of this chapter. Images should be archived in digital format, or thermal prints are filed in the patient's records.
- Suggested reporting template (Table 1.1). In addition to the findings, the report should also include the clinical indication for the scan.

TABLE 1.1

Sample Standard Record and Reporting of Transvaginal Scanning

Date of Scan	Date of Last Menstrual Period:	Latex Allergy: Y/N
Uterus		
Position		
Size, shape		
Myometrial appearance		
Cavity		
Endometrium		
Describe appearance and measure		
Correlation with menstrual cycle if appropriate		
Ovaries and adnexa		
Right-position; mobility; accessibility; appearance; antral follicle count		
Measurement in three planes; size		
Left-position; mobility; accessibility appearance; antral follicle count		
Measurement in three planes; size		
Pouch of Douglas		
Fluid present/no fluid present		
And if present measure		
Any pathology seen? If so, describe appearance		
Chaperone name:	Verbal consent: Y|N	Disinfection method:
Name and position:		Signature:

Acknowledgment

Videos demonstrating the TVS examining technique were kindly provided by Intelligent Ultrasound plc from their ScanTrainer simulator educational material.

REFERENCES

1. Kurjak A. Ultrasound scanning—Prof. Ian Donald (1910–1987). *Eur J Obstet Gynecol Reprod Biol.* 2000;90(2):187–9.
2. Schwimer SA and Lebovic J. Transvaginal pelvic ultrasonography. *J Ultrasound Med.* 1984;3:381.
3. Absi C, Reddy K, and Amso N. Patients' perception of transvaginal ultrasound scanning (TVS). *Int J Gynecol Obstet.* 2000;70(Suppl 3):C149–50 (D).
4. Amso NN and Griffiths A. The role and applications of ultrasound in ambulatory gynaecology. *Best Pract Res Clin Obstet Gynaecol.* 2005;19(5):693–71 (C) ISI IF-1.512.
5. Braithwaite JM and Economides DL. Acceptability by patients of transvaginal sonography in the elective assessment of the first trimester fetus. *Ultrasound Obstet Gynecol.* 1997;9(2):91–3.
6. Deed K, Childs J, and Thoirs K. What are the perceptions of women towards transvaginal sonographic examinations? *Sonography.* 2014;1:33–8.
7. Dorland's Illustrated Medical Dictionary. 24th ed. Philadelphia, PA: WB Saunders, 1967, pp. 1166–1167.
8. Dodson MG and Deter RL. Definition of anatomical planes for use in transvaginal sonography. *J Clin Ultrasound.* 1990;18:239–42.
9. Thoirs K, Deed K, and Childs J. 2017 Transvaginal sonography: Sonographer reflections on patient experience using a critical incident technique. *Sonography.* 2017;4:55–62, https://doi.org/10.1002/sono.12104
10. Sharma A, Burnell M, Gentry-Maharaj A et al. Quality assurance and its impact on ovarian visualisation rates in the multicentre United Kingdom Collaborative Trial of Ovarian Cancer Screening (UKCTOCS). *Ultrasound Obstet Gynecol.* 2015;47(2):228–35.
11. Lyons EA, Gratton D, and Harrington C. Transvaginal sonography of normal pelvic anatomy. *Radiol Clin North Am.* 1992;30:663–75.
12. Timmerman D, Valentin L, Bourne TH, Collins WP, Verrelst H, and Vergote I. Terms, definitions and measurements to describe thee sonographic features of adnexal tumors: A consensus opinion from the International Ovarian Tumor Analysis (IOTA) group. *Ultrasound Obstet Gynecol.* 2000;16:500–5.

2

Basic and Technical Aspects of Ultrasound

Neil D. Pugh

Introduction

Ultrasound has found many uses in medicine, from diagnosis to therapy in a wide range of specialties. Ultrasound is particularly useful in the field of reproductive medicine; it has advantages over other imaging modalities in that it is quick, inexpensive, noninvasive, and importantly, does not use ionizing radiation. Hence, ultrasound is perfectly suited to reproductive medicine where the risk of teratogenic effects needs to be avoided at all costs.

The purpose of this chapter is to discuss the principles and technical aspects of ultrasound, so that users are equipped with the appropriate knowledge to enable them to "drive" an ultrasound machine in such a way as to perform a competent ultrasound scan. To this end, this chapter covers the following topics:

- The basic principles of sound
- The generation of ultrasound
- The interactions of ultrasound with tissue
- Real-time B-mode imaging
- The basic principles of Doppler ultrasound
- Machine controls and image optimization
- Safety of ultrasound

Basic Principles of Sound

Sound is a pressure wave, that is a mechanical disturbance of a medium, which passes through the medium at a fixed speed. Sound travels through the medium as a series of molecular vibrations, and the speed at which sound travels through the medium depends on the nature of the medium (solid, liquid, or gas). As the position of the molecules can be fixed, particularly in solids, the molecular vibrations travel as a "wave" through the medium, away from the vibrating source. In other words, sound is a variation in pressure, with regions of increased pressure known as the compression part of the wave and regions of decreased pressure known as the rarefaction portion of the wave. In addition, sound is a longitudinal wave, which means that disturbance is in the same direction as that of the propagation of the wave.

As sound is a pressure wave, it can be characterized by a number of parameters, such as frequency, amplitude, wavelength, speed, and phase.

There are three main categories of sound defined by their frequency, as shown in Figure 2.1a. Frequency is the number of cycles per second, and the SI unit of frequency is the Hertz (Hz). Audible sound is in the range of 20 Hz–20 kHz. As can be seen, any sound above 20 kHz is ultrasound, and medical ultrasound is in the low megahertz range, from about 1 to 24 MHz (Figure 2.1b). This gives an optimum balance of resolution and penetration, as discussed later.

Amplitude is another important parameter, which is a measure of the amount of energy in the sound wave. For audio sound, this would be the loudness of the sound. For ultrasound, it is the power of the

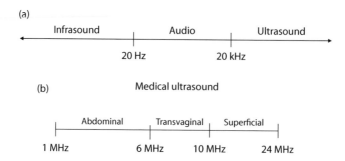

FIGURE 2.1   (a) Categories of sound. (b) Categories of ultrasound.

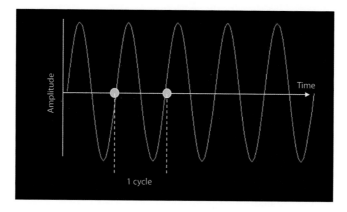

FIGURE 2.2   Defining a sound wave. A wave can be defined by amplitude (intensity or power); frequency (cycles per second – Hz); equation relating wavelength to frequency $c = f$ (where c = velocity of sound, f = frequency of sound, λ = wavelength of sound).

wave. This has implications for penetration of ultrasound and the safety of ultrasound, as discussed later. Figure 2.2 shows the relationship between these two parameters.

The speed of sound depends on the medium through which it is propagating. It is generally affected by two main things, namely, density and compressibility. Sound generally travels faster in solids and liquids than in gas. The speed of sound is faster in materials that have some rigidity and slower in softer materials. Knowing the speed of ultrasound in various tissues is important because:

- It gives the ability to convert echo return time into depth
- The velocity can be used to calculate the acoustic impedance
- Refraction occurs
- Velocity must be known to calculate Doppler shift

We have seen the relationship between wavelength, frequency, and speed of sound in Figure 2.2. Finally, phase is also important in the way in which the ultrasound beam is formed, but this is beyond the scope of this chapter.

Generation of Ultrasound

To produce ultrasound, a pressure wave needs to be generated. This is achieved by use of a piezoelectric crystal that is placed just beneath the front face of an ultrasound transducer or probe. The piezoelectric crystal is made to oscillate at a given frequency or range of frequencies by the application of an electrical voltage. The transducer is then placed in contact with the tissue under investigation, and the ultrasound pressure wave is transmitted through the tissue, where it undergoes various interactions that are discussed later.

Two types of ultrasound can be generated, namely, pulsed-wave or continuous-wave ultrasound, but for the purpose of medical imaging, only pulsed-wave ultrasound is used. With pulsed-wave ultrasound, spatial resolution is possible, and positional information can be obtained. Therefore, imaging is possible.

The piezoelectric crystal can be incorporated in a range of transducers, and the type of transducer used depends on the application and the frequency requirement. Generally, in assisted reproduction, two types of transducers are required. Low-frequency ultrasound transducers are used for transcutaneous abdominal or pelvic imaging. This requires a wide field of view, curvilinear transducer. More commonly, transvaginal transducers are used for monitoring and oocyte retrieval. These require a higher frequency and narrow transducer head with a wide field of view.

Interactions of Ultrasound with Tissue

To produce an ultrasound image, the ultrasound wave needs to interact with the tissue under investigation and return to the transducer, where it is converted from a pressure wave to an electrical signal that can be processed by the ultrasound scanner. There are three principle interactions of ultrasound with tissue, namely:

- Reflection
- Scatter
- Absorption

Reflection occurs at interfaces between tissues with different characteristics. The tissue property responsible for the amount of reflection that occurs is called the *acoustic impedance* and is designated by the symbol Z. The Z is related to the density (ρ) of a particular tissue and the velocity (c) of ultrasound in that particular tissue by the following equation:

$$Z = \rho c$$

The greater the difference in acoustic impedance between the two different tissues, the greater is the degree of reflection. The amounts of reflection at some typical interfaces are as follows:

- Water/soft tissue 5%
- Skull bone/brain 65%
- Soft tissue/air 99.95%

Scatter occurs when ultrasound interacts with structures whose dimensions are similar to or less than the wavelength of the ultrasound wave. This is known as Rayleigh scattering, and the resultant wave is scattered in all directions (360° scattering). Rayleigh scattering is the principal interaction of ultrasound with small structures such as blood cells or parenchyma. The intensity of the scattered wave depends primarily on the dimensions of the target and the wavelength of the ultrasound. Generally, the intensity of scattered ultrasound increases very rapidly with frequency, and this contributes to an upper limit on the frequency of ultrasound that can be used in clinical practice.

Clearly, it follows that some echoes generated from reflections at tissue boundaries and scattering within tissues and organs will return to the ultrasound transducer, and these signals will give rise to a complex "echo train" from which the diagnostic information is derived.

There is a third interaction of ultrasound with tissue that does not contribute to the signals returning to the ultrasound transducer but is nevertheless important—that is, absorption. Absorption is basically the conversion of ultrasound (mechanical) energy into another form of energy due to the interaction of the pressure wave with tissue. The most common conversion of ultrasound energy is into internal molecular energy or heat. In diagnostic ultrasound, heating is undesirable, as it can lead to detrimental bioeffects, particularly in sensitive tissues. This is covered at a later point. In addition, absorption leads to energy loss from the ultrasound beam, which reduces the penetration of the beam. As absorption increases with frequency, this effectively also contributes to the upper limit of ultrasound frequency possible. In general terms, diagnostic ultrasound rarely exceeds 20–24 MHz.

Real-Time B-Mode (Brightness-Mode) Imaging

To produce an ultrasound image, a narrow ultrasound beam needs to be "swept" rapidly and repetitively through a section of tissue and the resulting echoes converted into an array of grayscale pixels to produce a resultant B-mode image (Figure 2.3). Typically, up to 200 effective ultrasound beams are required to produce an ultrasound image.

The basic components of a real-time scanner consist of:

- The ultrasound transducer
- A beam former
- A signal processor
- An image processor
- A display

The ultrasound transducer houses the piezoelectric crystal, as discussed earlier. Almost all transducers used in common practice are sequential array transducers, where the ultrasound beam is formed by sequentially firing a small group of elements across the face of the transducer.

In recent years, the range of frequencies available has widened. Generally, transvaginal transducers run in a frequency range of about 5–8 MHz. Being an endocavity probe, the design of the probe is such that it has a narrow footprint for ease of insertion but a wide field of view (Figure 2.4a). Historically, abdominal

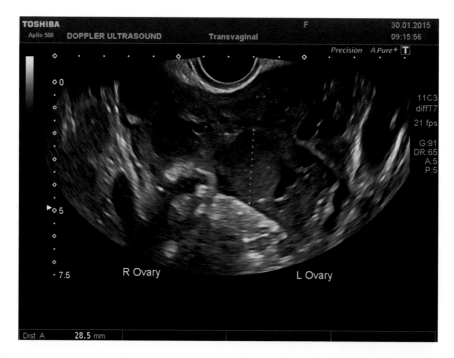

FIGURE 2.3　A typical high-resolution B-mode transvaginal ultrasound scan showing a small endometrioma.

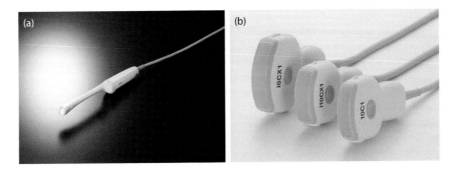

FIGURE 2.4 (a) Typical transvaginal ultrasound transducer showing its suitability for endocavity scanning. (b) A typical range of curvilinear abdominal transducers, from the classic low-frequency large footprint transducers on the left of the image to the smaller, higher-frequency transducers middle and right. (Image courtesy of Canon Medical Systems.)

probes were of low frequency, also with a wide field of view, typically 1–5 MHz, but now smaller, higher-frequency curvilinear transducers operating at about 5–10 MHz are also available for use on slimmer patients, giving better resolution (Figure 2.4b). It is important to remember that all transducers are now broadband transducers, which allows the operator to select the frequencies within the bandwidth of the piezoelectric crystal. Generally, three frequencies are available on most ultrasound machines and often these are labeled resolution (highest frequency), general, and penetration (lowest frequency).

The primary function of the beam former is to drive the transducer and convert the voltages from returning echoes into usable signals. It consists of a pulser that ensures all the sections of the instrument function at the correct time. It produces the electric voltages that generate regularly spaced ultrasound pulses and the pulse delays needed for complex sequencing and phasing of arrays. The beam former also amplifies the returning signal and converts the signal to a digital format in readiness for the signal processing.

The signal processor applies filtering and compression to the returning signal to produce a signal suitable for image production.

The image processor controls the way in which the image is presented. It basically converts the returning ultrasound signal to a grayscale image. It stores the information as an array of pixels representing the appropriate shade of gray for each region of the image and displays it on the screen.

The display is generally a flat screen monitor, although in recent years it has been possible to display ultrasound images on tablets or even mobile phones.

Basic Principles of Doppler Ultrasound

When there is relative motion between moving objects, a change in frequency occurs. This was first described by Christian Andreas Doppler in 1842 when he realized that the wavelength recorded by an observer depends on the movement of a source and observer relative to one another. This was henceforth known as the Doppler effect.

This change in frequency (the Doppler shift frequency) can be used in ultrasound to give us two useful pieces of information, namely:

- The speed at which a target is moving
- The direction of motion

It is particularly useful in medicine for assessing blood flow.
The Doppler equation is as follows:

$$f_d = \frac{2f_t v \cos\theta}{c}$$

In practical terms, stand-alone Doppler machines are very limited, with no imaging capabilities and are used simply to detect pulses or the fetal heart. In modern practice, Doppler is combined with imaging systems, and the main instrument now available is the real-time color flow scanner that combines a real-time B-mode image with pulsed-wave and color Doppler capabilities. Color flow scanners provide a way of displaying directional and velocity information pictorially. The directional information is color coded (usually red and blue to indicate flow to or away from the direction of the transducer), with turbulence sometimes represented as green or a mosaic of colors. The hue of the color is used to represent mean velocity, which is usually indicated by a scale bar on the side of the image. Most scanners can operate in triplex mode, which displays color-flow, B-mode, and spectral Doppler simultaneously.

Although color Doppler imaging is the mainstay of diagnosis, over the years a number of different imaging techniques have been developed, from power Doppler imaging to newer techniques such as B-flow imaging (GE Medical Systems), advanced dynamic flow (ADF), and superb microvascular imaging (SMI), both by Canon Medical Systems.

Machine Controls and Image Optimization

A typical top of the range ultrasound scanner is shown in Figure 2.5. An ultrasound image needs to represent the true anatomical and physiological situation so that the best medical assessment can be made. The image can be affected by:

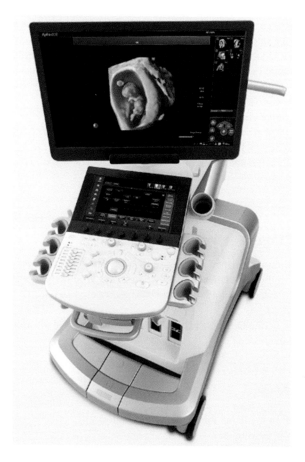

FIGURE 2.5   A typical top of the range ultrasound scanner showing a typical flat screen monitor, a touch control panel, and the main control panel where the most common functions are located. (Image courtesy of Canon Medical Systems.)

- Suboptimal scanner settings producing a poor image
- Ultrasound artifacts producing misleading features on an image
- Condition and performance of equipment

In order to produce the best image, the operator needs to be able to "drive" the ultrasound machine. Many of the functions discussed in the previous section can be adjusted, either by the operator or by the ultrasound manufacturers, generally the applications specialist within the companies. There are several controls the operator needs to be familiar with, as these will be used in day-to-day practice to optimize the image.

The quality of an ultrasound image depends on two main factors, namely:

- Signal strength (penetration)
- Resolution (the minimum separation of two surfaces that gives rise to two identifiable echo signals)

Resolution is frequency dependent. Higher-frequency ultrasound gives better resolution due to its shorter pulse length. Therefore, high-frequency ultrasound is preferable, particularly for looking at small structures or making fine measurements. However, it is attenuated much more than low-frequency ultrasound. Improvement in resolution will often reduce penetration, and vice versa; therefore, a balance has to be found, which is appropriate for the particular scan, patient, and structure of interest.

If we first consider the signal strength that is responsible for the penetration, this can be controlled by:

- Adjusting acoustic power
- Adjusting gain (and time gain compensation [TGC])
- Adjusting focal position
- Accounting for attenuation (which is controlled by adjusting the frequency of ultrasound used)

If we consider first the acoustic power, this determines the amplitude of the ultrasound pulse generated, in other words, how much energy is put into the body. The more energy used, the greater is the penetration. However, using greater energy has implications for safety (heating and cavitation). It is possible for the operator to select the acoustic power used, but within the limits of the investigations undertaken.

The gain and TGC determine the amplitude of the ultrasound displayed. This is very much like a volume control on an audio device. It amplifies the signals that have returned to the scanner. There is, however, an upper limit above which increasing the gain will not improve the image (as it simply increases the background noise). The TGC can help. It varies the amplitude of the displayed ultrasound signal strength at different depths. However, once again, there is an upper limit above which increasing the gain will not improve the image.

The focal position or focusing will concentrate the signal strength in a particular region (called the focal zone). This improves the signal strength and therefore increases penetration. The focus is a very important control and should be utilized whenever scanning.

As discussed previously, attenuation is very frequency dependent. Greater penetration is achieved with lower frequency (less attenuation). This improves the signal strength and therefore increases penetration, but at a cost to resolution.

In summary, the penetration can be improved by thinking of its effects in transmission and reception. It is improved in transmission by using the:

- Highest acoustic power for given investigation
- Correct focal position
- Lower frequency (last resort)

It is improved in reception by using the:

- Correct overall gain
- Optimal TGC

Resolution determines how well the fine detail within an image can be seen. It is the minimum separating distance of two surfaces that give rise to two identifiable echo signals from which two separate pixels can be displayed. As an ultrasound beam is three-dimensional; there are three separate resolutions, namely, the axial and lateral resolutions and the slice thickness. In sequential array transducers, the slice thickness is fixed by the use of a focusing lens on the front face of the transducer, and there is nothing the operator can do to change it. However, the operator is able to improve both the axial and lateral resolutions of an image.

The axial resolution is the minimum separating distance along the beam axis at which two objects can be seen as independent objects. It is determined by pulse length, which is shorter at higher frequencies (indeed the axial resolution is half the pulse length). Higher frequencies therefore give better axial resolution. This is, however, only half the story. There is also a resolution that is the minimum separating distance at the same range. This is known as the lateral resolution and is determined by beam width with a narrower beam, giving better lateral resolution. The beam width can be made narrower by focusing the beam at the point of interest. This is because focusing reduces the effective beam width and increases the amplitude of the signal at that point.

To summarize, an optimal image is achieved when the balance resolution and penetration are achieved by the judicious use of the ultrasound machine.

Safety of Ultrasound

Diagnostic and interventional ultrasound have been used for many years without any documented ill effects in humans. However, ultrasound is increasingly used for a wider range of investigations, using a broader range of ultrasound intensities and frequencies and an increased use of Doppler with its concomitant higher intensities.

Although ultrasound has an excellent safety record, we have already seen that ultrasound energy is deposited within the body as a result of relaxation processes converting one form of energy to another. The two main interactions of ultrasound with tissue are heating and cavitation.

Heating occurs as a result of absorption. Heating is likely to occur at sites where absorption is higher. This generally occurs around bone, and consequently, the surrounding soft tissue can experience secondary heating as a result of conduction. Heating needs to be considered during routine fetal scans, but heating also occurs in soft tissues and is particularly hazardous to sensitive organs and the developing embryo. Consequently, thermal indices have been developed to account for potential bioeffects as a result of heating. The main indices for routine scanning are the thermal index in soft tissue (TIS) and the thermal index in bone (TIB), which are continually displayed on screen.

Cavitation is a mechanical effect that occurs in tissue due to the passage of the mechanical ultrasound wave. This effect is not as a result of heating but due to the presence of gas-filled microbubbles or cavities in the exposed tissue, which can oscillate or collapse under the pressure of the ultrasound beam. This can produce high shear forces or pressures as well as heat, which can damage cell membranes or produce highly reactive free radicles. Once again, an index has been developed in an attempt to account for the effects of cavitation, and this is known as the mechanical index (MI).

The British Medical Ultrasound Society (BMUS) and other international ultrasound societies and safety bodies have made a series of recommendations regarding the safe and judicious use of medical ultrasound. These include, but are not limited to the following:

* Ultrasound should only be used for medical diagnosis.
* The equipment should only be used by people who are fully trained in its safe and proper operation.
* The scan operator is responsible for controlling the output of the ultrasound equipment. This requires a good knowledge of scanner settings and an understanding of their effect on potential thermal and mechanical bioeffects.

The BMUS states that "A fundamental approach to the safe use of diagnostic ultrasound is to use the lowest output power and the shortest scan time consistent with acquiring the required diagnostic information. This is the ALARA principle (i.e., as low as reasonably achievable)."

As there are a number of recommendations and guidelines for the safe use of ultrasound, which are changing when new information becomes available, it is prudent to check these at regular intervals. Good reviews of current guidelines and current safety limits can always be found on the society and organization websites, a list of which is given in the references.

FURTHER READING
General Physics and Instrumentation

Gibbs V, Cole D, and Sassano A. *Ultrasound Physics and Technology. How, When and Why*. London, UK: Churchill Livingstone; 2009.
Hoskins PR, Martin K, and Thrush A. *Diagnostic Ultrasound. Physics and Instrumentation*. 3rd ed. Cambridge, UK: Cambridge University Press; 2019.
Kremkau FW. *Sonography Principles and Instruments*. 9th ed. St. Louis, MO: Elsevier; 2015.

Safety

The British Medical Ultrasound Society. Guidelines for the safe use of diagnostic ultrasound equipment. http://www.bmus.org/static/uploads/resources/BMUS-Safety-Guidelines-2009-revision-FINAL-Nov-2009.pdf
The British Medical Ultrasound Society. Policies, statements and guidelines. Safety statements. https://www.bmus.org/policies-statements-guidelines/safety-statements
ter Haar G (ed). *The Safe Use of Ultrasound in Medical Diagnosis*. 3rd ed. 2012. London, UK: British Institute of Radiology. https://issuu.com/efsumb/docs/safe_use_of_ultrasound?viewMode=magazine&mode=embed
WFUMB policy and statements on safety of ultrasound. *Ultrasound in Med & Biol*. 2013;39(5):926–9.

3

The Uterus

Jure Knez and Veljko Vlaisavljević

Introduction

Pelvic ultrasound is a key investigation in the evaluation of the female reproductive system. Recent improvements in ultrasound technology have significantly enhanced our knowledge of normal uterine physiology. With the development of high-resolution transvaginal ultrasound (TVUS) transducers, we can today monitor subtle changes in the morphology of the uterus and the endometrium. Ultrasound has enabled us to noninvasively diagnose uterine abnormalities that just a decade ago could only be seen with more invasive diagnostic methods. This chapter covers some of the common uterine pathologies that need to be evaluated when assessing women with reproductive problems.

Basics of Uterine Examination

Due to its central location, relatively large size, and distinct shape, the uterus is usually the landmark in the ultrasound examination of the female pelvis. Anatomically, the uterus can be divided into the uterine fundus, which extends laterally into the interstitial parts of the fallopian tubes. These can rarely present the site of unusual ectopic pregnancy implantation, and to the inexperienced observer, it can sometimes be difficult to differentiate this from intrauterine pregnancy that is implanted high in the cavity. Inferior to the fundus is the uterine corpus, and the lowermost part presents the isthmus. The isthmus forms the lower extension part of the uterus in pregnancy. This is usually the site for incision at cesarean section; hence, the cesarean section scar can be seen in this area in women after cesarean delivery. The cervix extends inferiorly, and the uterosacral ligaments attach it to the upper vagina. In contrast, the upper part of the uterus is normally largely mobile. This means that it is usually anteverted and anteflexed, which can be visualized on ultrasound. In some women, the uterus projects toward the rectum (retroversion), and this has clinical implications when performing intrauterine procedures. In cases of adhesion formation in the pelvis, this can have consequences on the position of the uterus and may result in loss of mobility.

The uterine wall consists of several layers. These are the serosa, myometrium, junctional zone, and endometrium. The serosa is a peritoneal covering of the uterus and is seen on ultrasound as a hyperechoic outline. The myometrium is composed of smooth muscle and uterine blood vessels. On ultrasound it is normally seen as a layer of low-level echogenicity. The junctional zone has only recently been recognized as a separate histological and embryological entity. The endometrium represents the innermost part of the uterus. It is the hormone responsive tissue that varies in appearance depending on the menstrual cycle. In the following text, we cover some of the most common pathologies that can affect different parts of the uterus and can influence the reproductive potential of women.

Myometrium

The basic examination of the uterus starts with the assessment of uterine morphology and the myometrium. The myometrium is the thick, mainly muscular layer of the uterine wall. It also contains supporting stromal and vascular tissue. It is formed of three distinct layers: outer longitudinal smooth muscle layer, middle layer of crossing muscle fibers, and inner circular fibers. The inner part of the myometrium appears to be developmentally distinct from the outer two layers and develops from the Müllerian ducts, while the outer two layers are of nonmüllerian origin. This is called the junctional zone and is capable of peristaltic activity, which has an important role in embryo implantation and parturition.

Uterine Fibroids

Uterine fibroids are benign tumors of the smooth muscle and are the most common benign pathology of the uterus. They are present in up to 40% of women aged over 40 years and in about 25% of women in the general population. The incidence of fibroids is dependent on ethnicity and is typically two- to threefold higher in black women compared to white women. Clinically, they are most often associated with heavy menstrual bleeding and dysmenorrhea. Rarely, they may also cause pressure symptoms on surrounding structures or may cause infertility in women. Fibroids' clinical implications are most often related to their anatomical location. They can arise underneath the endometrium (submucous), in the wall of the uterus (intramural), or below the serosa of the uterus (subserous). The submucous fibroids often result in menstrual problems, usually menorrhagia, but subserous fibroids often remain asymptomatic. An enlarged fibroid uterus can result in pressure symptoms on the bladder, or in the case of a retroverted uterus, also rectal symptoms. A markedly enlarged uterus can rarely also cause acute urinary retention. Fibroids are usually categorized according to their location, since this correlates with their clinical significance. There are several classifications of fibroids according to their location, the most recent and most commonly used is the classification of the International Federation of Gynecology and Obstetrics (FIGO) [1]. According to the FIGO classification, fibroids are categorized into nine categories based on their location in the uterus. Categories 0 through 2 represent submucous fibroids. Type 0 fibroid is located completely within the uterine cavity, while type 2 is greater than 50% intramural. Categories 3 through 8 characterize fibroids outside of the endometrial cavity and include intramural, subserous, and fibroids in other locations (e.g., cervical, parasitic). This classification has its implications when considering surgical management of fibroids. The precise impact of fibroids on fertility is today still largely unknown. Although it is widely accepted for submucous fibroids to be surgically treated in the presence of infertility, there is no good quality evidence to support such practice. There are several mechanisms by which fibroids could interfere with normal fertility. They can present an obstruction to tubal ostia in the uterus [2]. Besides presenting a physical obstacle for successful conception, fibroids can also interfere with normal reproductive function with altered uterine contractions, cytokine factors, and genetic aspects of uterine receptivity [3]. However, the clinical evidence of fibroids' effect on fertility and reproductive outcomes is weak and mostly inconclusive. Even for submucous fibroids, there is no conclusive evidence on their clinical importance [4]. There is even less clinical evidence showing a potential benefit of treatment of intramural or subserous fibroids.

The ultrasound appearance of fibroids varies, but most commonly they present as well-defined, echo-dense, single or multiple uterine tumors (Figure 3.1). This is consequent to the fact that the smooth-muscle fibers are arranged in dense concentric rings that are well demarcated from the surrounding normal endometrium. Occasionally they may undergo degeneration and may contain calcified, hyperechoic foci. Pregnancy has various effects on fibroids; however, most often fibroids remain unchanged in size. Occasionally, increased levels of estrogens in pregnancy may stimulate fibroids to undergo a period of rapid growth. This may cause fibroids to overgrow their blood supply, and areas of necrosis may be seen. The "red degeneration" of fibroids may cause significant pain in pregnancy. More importantly, the unusual appearance of such fibroids may seem alarming and may be mistaken for more serious pathology, such as sarcoma or ovarian mass. Because fibroids are hormone dependent, they generally occur well after the onset of puberty. Their incidence increases with age until menopause. Following menopause, they often but not always regress in size. The hormone dependency of fibroids yields the possibility of medical management, such as treatment with gonadotropin-releasing hormone agonists or selective progesterone receptor modulators.

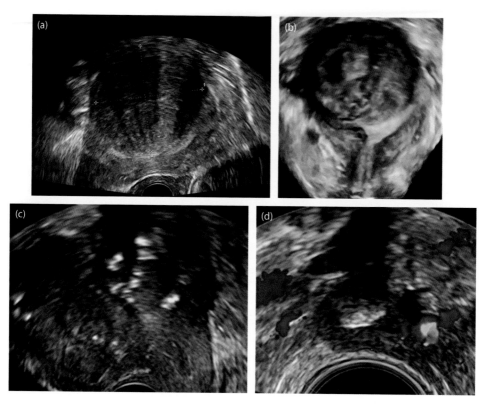

FIGURE 3.1   Ultrasound of fibroids. (a) A large intramural fibroid of homogeneous appearance. (b) On three-dimensional image, distortion of the uterine cavity by the large intramural fibroid can be seen. (c) Fibroids with calcified appearance. (d) A fibroid with central calcified area.

Adenomyosis

Adenomyosis is a benign condition of the uterus characterized by the presence of endometrial glands and stroma within the myometrium. Historically, the diagnosis could only be made by histological examination, but today we can diagnose this condition reliably with ultrasound. The prevalence in the general population has been estimated to be around 20%, which makes it one of the most common acquired uterine abnormalities [5]. The prevalence increases with age and reaches a peak at 40–49 years of age. Clinically, adenomyosis is most often associated with heavy and prolonged periods and menstrual pain. Although the correlation with fertility problems is less clear, recent clinical studies show that especially severe forms of adenomyosis can have an influence on reproductive function in women [6].

By using ultrasound, adenomyosis is diagnosed based on visualization of a number of different features characterizing the disease. As seen on two-dimensional ultrasound, these include asymmetrical myometrial thickening (not caused by fibroids), the presence of myometrial cysts, linear striations, parallel shadowing, hyperechoic islands, globular configuration of myometrium, heterogeneous myometrium, disruptions of the endometrial-myometrial junction, and the presence of adenomyoma [5,7] (Figure 3.2). Still, the diagnostic accuracy of these parameters varies, and there are no universally accepted criteria. If looking at specific ultrasound features, globular configuration of the myometrium has the highest diagnostic accuracy of 80% (sensitivity 86.4%, specificity 69.2%) followed by myometrial cysts (diagnostic accuracy 74.3%, sensitivity 61.5%, specificity 81.8%) and subendometrial linear striations (diagnostic accuracy 71.4%, sensitivity 30.8%, specificity 95.5%) [7]. Endometrial implants can be interspersed within the myometrium as multiple isolated ectopic islands of glandular and stromal endometrial tissue, which can be seen as a diffuse form of adenomyosis. Ectopic endometrial tissue can be organized in a

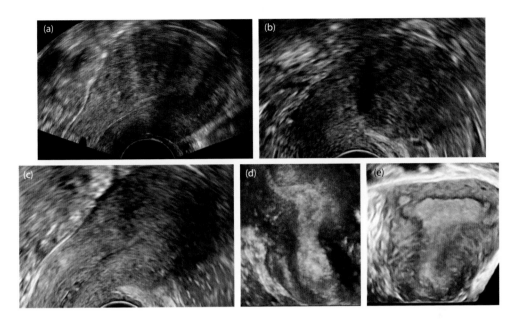

FIGURE 3.2 Sonographic features of adenomyosis. (a) Asymmetrically thickened and irregular myometrium that is typical in adenomyosis. Parallel striations can also be seen. (b) The endometrial-myometrial junction can be disrupted in adenomyosis, which can make visualization of the endometrium difficult. (c) Irregular and thickened myometrium in adenomyosis. (d) Irregular endometrial-myometrial junction. (e) Hyperechoic islands.

well-circumscribed nodular lesion, which can be visualized as "focal" disease. Overall, it is most likely that different imaging characteristics of adenomyosis are related to different manifestations of the disease.

The development of three-dimensional (3D) ultrasound techniques has allowed for better visualization of the junctional zone. Two-dimensional sonographic assessment of the junctional zone is often imprecise and difficult, even with high-resolution ultrasound probes. The endometrial-myometrial junctional zone is best visualized by 3D ultrasound, and this also allows for the best visualization of endometrial protrusion into the myometrium. This is further enhanced by the use of additional image postprocessing tools. The junctional zone is best visualized on the rendered image of the coronal plane of the uterus and appears as a hypoechoic zone around the endometrium. Hence, there have been propositions that the measurement of the junctional zone thickness could be diagnostic of adenomyosis [8]. Subjective evaluation of infiltration and disruption of the junctional zone by endometrial tissue appears to be an accurate marker of adenomyosis that can be used in clinical practice [5,9]. Today, it is believed that the junctional zone is a separate anatomical entity, embryologically distinct from the endometrium or the myometrium, and this may be a common initiating region for the development of adenomyosis.

Assessment of vascularity is also beneficial in the diagnosis of adenomyosis. Color Doppler can be used to discriminate myometrial cysts from blood vessels. The use of color Doppler may also help in differentiating adenomyomas from fibroids, which represent another commonly acquired uterine anomaly, with similar clinical symptoms and signs. This is especially important when planning possible surgical treatment of fibroids. If an adenomyoma is misdiagnosed for a fibroid, this can lead to complications at surgery due to nonexistent clear cleavage planes. The presence of "central vascularity" and "ill-defined junctional zone on 3D ultrasound" seems to have high sensitivity and specificity in distinguishing adenomyomas from fibroids [10].

Congenital Uterine Anomalies

The female reproductive system develops in the embryo from the urogenital sinus and two paramesonephric (or Müllerian) ducts. These two entities are conjoined in the sinus tubercle. In the course of embryo development, the paramesonephric ducts are formed lateral to the mesonephric ducts.

In a female fetus, the caudal parts of the paramesonephric ducts fuse into a uterovaginal primordium before flowing into the dorsal aspect of the urogenital sinus. These parts of the paramesonephric ducts form the uterus, cervix, and superior part of the vagina. The cranial parts remain separate and form the fallopian tubes. This takes place from the third or fourth week of gestation and is finalized in the second trimester of pregnancy. Interruption of this process most commonly results in incomplete fusion, and incomplete development of one or both ducts can result in anomalies of the reproductive tract. Uterine anomalies are common, with a prevalence of 5.3%–12% in the population of infertile women and even higher in women with histories of miscarriage [11]. These anomalies arise embryologically from failure of Müllerian duct formation, canalization, fusion, or absorption of different parts of the ducts. Different anomalies have been associated with reduced fertility, miscarriage, preterm birth, and other adverse fetal outcomes. However, given the variation in diagnostic techniques and classification of the anomalies, the true impact of congenital uterine anomalies on the reproductive function remains uncertain [12]. Today, there is still no uniform classification system for these anomalies. It is out of the scope of this chapter to provide a detailed overview of all congenital uterine anomalies, but most often these are defined according to the modified American Society of Reproductive Medicine (ASRM) [13] classification system or according to the European Society of Human Reproduction and Embryology (ESHRE)/European Society for Gynaecological Endoscopy (ESGE) classification system [14]. All of these systems have their advantages and drawbacks, and none has gained universal clinical acceptance [15]. Moreover, different diagnostic methods used in the process add to the confusion. Historically, invasive methods, such as laparoscopy and hysteroscopy, have represented the reference in diagnosis of female genital tract anomalies. In recent years, however, ultrasound, especially 3D ultrasound, is being increasingly recognized as a diagnostic method of choice, since it is relatively affordable, accessible, and allows for accurate visualization of uterine morphology [16]. The 3D ultrasound technique overcomes anatomical limitations that restrict the number and orientation of the scanning planes on transvaginal sonography.

The Endometrium

The endometrium is a key factor in the process of embryo implantation. It is also a part of the uterus that is very easily visualized by transvaginal ultrasound. Endometrial development resulting in endometrial receptivity during the window of implantation requires subtle collaboration of an extremely large number of different factors [17]. Morphological characteristics of endometrium depend on the circulating levels of estrogen and progesterone. Transvaginal ultrasonography can provide insight to the state and development of the endometrium and its capacity to be receptive for embryos. Anterior and posterior myometrial-endometrial interfaces are easily recognized at all phases of the menstrual cycle. It is important to remember that the endometrium is a 3D structure and needs to be scanned fully by angling the transducer from left to right in longitudinal view and from cervix to fundus in the transverse section. At the end of the menstrual phase, the endometrium appears as a thin, hyperechoic line. During the proliferative phase, it becomes thicker (double-layer endometrial thickness is normally 5–12 mm) and less echogenic (Figure 3.3). As early as day 6 and as late as 1 day before the luteinizing hormone peak, the sonographic picture of the endometrium changes to the "triple stripe" pattern. This is seen as a hypoechoic area compared to the myometrium, surrounded by a prominent, highly reflective echo. At the time of ovulation, the endometrium thickens is approximately 10–16 mm. After ovulation, in the secretory phase of the menstrual cycle, the characteristic "triple stripe" pattern disappears as the consequence of progesterone influence. The endometrium becomes homogenous and hyperechoic in comparison to the myometrium, but its thickness increases only slightly. Just before menstrual bleed, the endometrium appears as a homogeneous, hyperechoic structure. During menstrual bleed it is possible to visualize the endometrial cavity separated by low-level echoes, representing blood and mucus. When evaluating the endometrium, the sonographer should be well acquainted with normal menstrual physiology and interrelationships between reproductive organs controlling the menstrual cycle. When assessing the endometrium, the ovaries should always be examined, and their appearance in relation to the menstrual cycle and the endometrium should be assessed.

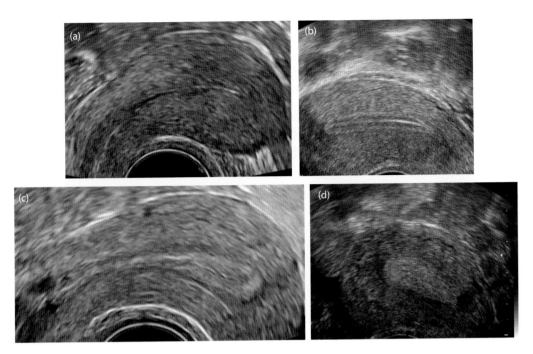

FIGURE 3.3 Sonography of the endometrium. (a) Endometrium in the early proliferative phase appears as a thin, hyperechoic line. (b) Through the proliferative phase, the endometrium becomes thicker and less echogenic. (c) Due to progesterone action, the endometrium becomes homogeneous and hyperechoic in the secretory phase of the menstrual cycle. (d) Endometrium in the secretory phase.

Evaluating Endometrial Receptivity

Endometrial thickness is defined as the distance between the anterior and posterior stratum basalis layers [18]. Its measurement should be performed in the midsagittal plane of the uterus from one endometrial-myometrial interface to the other (outer to outer). Normal endometrial thickness is the sign of normal physiological function and was hence one of the first suggested sonographic markers of endometrial receptivity. It is an essential part of the evaluation of patients with fertility problems, and several studies have investigated the value of this marker to predict a pregnancy [19]. In the luteal phase of an unstimulated cycle, the endometrium does seem to be thicker in conception compared to nonconception cycles, and in normal pregnancy compared to abnormal pregnancy. However, endometrial thickness or volume does not have the necessary discriminatory capacity to be useful in differentiating between early normal and abnormal pregnancy [20]. Although multiple studies have investigated the predictive value of endometrial thickness and sonographic appearance in assisted reproduction cycles, conclusions remain controversial. A recent systematic review has shown that although the frequently used cut-off endometrial thickness of 7 mm is related to lower chances of pregnancy, the discriminatory capacity of this thickness in the prediction of pregnancy is virtually absent [21]. There are also other sonographic aspects of the endometrium, such as homogenous appearance on the day of human chorionic gonadotropin (hCG) administration, that were associated with poor results of a stimulated *in vitro* fertilization (IVF)/intracytoplasmic sperm injection (ICSI) cycle [22–24]. While some investigators suggested that excessive endometrial growth (greater than 14 mm) was also shown to be a poor prognostic indicator [25], others refuted this conclusion [26,27].

During a normal menstrual cycle, spontaneous uterine contractions may occur, and this may influence the accuracy of endometrial measurement [28,29]. Although not commonly used in routine clinical practice, it was proposed that the endometrium should be measured before, during, and after these wave-like contractions, and the mean value should be used as the most accurate thickness [30]. The normal peristalsis is toward the cervix during menstrual bleed and toward the uterine cavity in midcycle. These contractions are more frequent at the time of ovulation, but they are slow and are most easily visualized by cine-loop video recordings of the endometrium. They are thought to have a function in both sperm transport and implantation. Abnormal contractions of the endometrium and subendometrial region have been suggested to impair the receptivity for embryo implantation or increase the chance of embryo translocation to the fallopian tube. Difficult embryo transfers and use of tenaculum during embryo transfer have also been associated with lower chances of pregnancy, and this may be due to an increase in endometrial contractions. The endometrial contractions have been recorded and quantified in women undergoing embryo transfer following IVF, and it would appear that clinical and ongoing pregnancy rates are significantly lower with increasing rates of contractions [31].

Blood Flow

Blood supply to the uterus and ovaries fluctuates throughout the menstrual cycle. These changes in perfusion can be monitored by Doppler ultrasound. The endometrium exhibits angiogenesis during the course of the normal menstrual cycle, and these low resistance vessels can be quantitatively examined with Doppler ultrasound. However, the main blood vessels feeding the uterus are the uterine arteries, which are positioned just lateral to the cervix. They can be more easily monitored with ultrasound, with more reproducible waveforms compared to the smaller, low-velocity arcuate branches that have much lower velocities and tend to have poorly defined envelopes, making the measurements prone to error.

In the normal menstrual cycle, the resistance of the uterine artery is at its highest 1–2 days after ovulation and at its lowest during the mid- to late-luteal phase. This is believed to formulate the optimal setting for embryo implantation. There are certain factors that have been documented to influence the resistance indices. A lower resistance index has been seen in women on hormone replacement therapy, taking tamoxifen, and in the presence of uterine fibroids. Malignant diseases of the uterus have also been related to lower uterine artery resistance. Uterine artery resistance increases with age but has also been associated with infertility, tubal damage, and endometriosis.

Clinical studies evaluating the importance of Doppler angiographic indices as tools for the evaluation of endometrial receptivity have been published, but the predictive value of resistance indices is limited [32,33].

Based on these relatively disappointing predictive capabilities of blood flow evaluation, there is more focus toward the molecular aspects of endometrial receptivity. These are currently a subject of extensive research; however, there are no clinically validated markers of endometrial receptivity available. Until such determinants are discovered and made clinically applicable and reliable, caution should be used in applying treatment decisions based on assessment of individual markers of endometrial receptivity [34,35].

Focal Intracavitary Lesions

A common finding when evaluating the endometrium is the observation of a focal intracavitary lesion that most commonly represents an endometrial polyp. These are hyperplastic masses that can be located in the uterine cavity or the cervix. They consist of fibrous tissue (stroma), blood vessels, and hyperplastic endometrial epithelium. They can present as pedunculated masses in the uterine cavity or may occur as sessile structures with large flat bases. They are a common gynecologic finding, and especially in the case of smaller polyps, their influence on reproductive function is unknown [36]. If they arise close to the fallopian tubes ostia, they could cause an obstruction in the path of the fertilized egg. They have also been associated with an increased chance of miscarriage. They often cause no symptoms but may be associated with heavy menstrual bleeding or irregular vaginal bleeding. This means that small polyps are commonly diagnosed as incidental findings when performing transvaginal ultrasound for other indications. They are usually benign structures. It is difficult to predict the growth pattern of polyps when managed expectantly. Especially in some premenopausal women, they can also regress spontaneously [37]. The vast majority of endometrial polyps are benign. A systematic review including a large number of women concluded that the incidence of malignant or hyperplastic histological result was significantly higher in postmenopausal

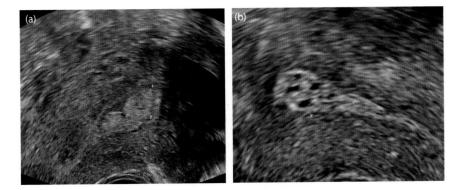

FIGURE 3.4 Endometrial polyp. (a) Hyperechoic, well-delineated structure disturbing the midline echo, typical of endometrial polyp. (b) Cystic appearances of the endometrial polyp.

compared with premenopausal women (5.4% versus 1.7%) [38]. It seems that larger polyps, especially those greater in size than 15 mm are more often associated with malignancy [39,40]. On ultrasound, polyps most commonly appear as well-defined lesions of increased echogenicity. Sometimes, cystic changes may be seen within a polyp, and typical single-vessel vascularity may be observed (Figures 3.4 and 3.5). The differential diagnosis of endometrial polyp includes other focal intracavitary lesions, most often intracavitary fibroids. In contrast to polyps, these usually appear on ultrasound as solid structures, and less commonly, a typical single-vessel vascularization is seen [41].

Ultrasound of Uterus after Cesarean Section

Cesarean section rates are increasing worldwide. The scar that forms in the isthmic part of the uterus after cesarean incision has been associated with several complications. These include abnormal uterine bleeding, dysmenorrhea, obstetric complications in subsequent pregnancies, and infertility [42]. Hence, when performing ultrasound examination of the uterus, it is also important to assess the area where the cesarean section incision is located on the uterus. This is commonly referred to as a cesarean section scar, "isthmocele," or "niche." This can be heterogenous in morphological appearance and involve defects in the myometrium of different degrees. There is currently little data showing the clinical importance of different sonographic characteristics of cesarean section scars. However, according to the recent consensus, cesarean section scars can be systematically evaluated, and this could improve our understanding of their clinical importance in the future [42]. When scanning pregnant women after previous cesarean section in the first trimester, it should be considered mandatory for the location of the pregnancy to be evaluated and recorded in relation to the cesarean section scar. The pregnancy can implant in the cesarean section

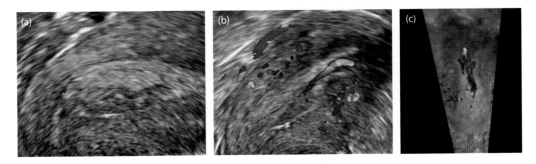

FIGURE 3.5 Endometrial polyp. (a) Large endometrial polyp filling the endometrial cavity. (b) Typical single feeder vessel seen in the presence of an endometrial polyp. (c) Three-dimensionally rendered image showing vascularity of an endometrial polyp.

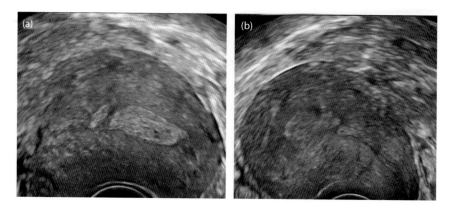

FIGURE 3.6   Intrauterine adhesions. (a and b) Bands of myometrial tissue traversing the endometrial cavity typical of intrauterine adhesions and connecting the opposing uterine walls.

scar, the condition known as cesarean scar ectopic pregnancy, and this can result in severe complications if left untreated or misdiagnosed [43]. It is generally also becoming accepted that the pregnancy implanted in the cesarean section scar is a precursor for morbidly adherent placenta [44].

Intrauterine Adhesions

In comparison to other uterine pathologies, uterine adhesions are relatively rare, and our understanding of their clinical significance is sparse. The incidence of intrauterine adhesions is reported to be between 0.3% and 21.5% with incidence differing between different regions in the world [45]. Women with multiple previous miscarriages have a higher risk of developing intrauterine adhesions [46]. Although hysteroscopy is today considered to be the "gold standard" for diagnosis of intrauterine adhesions, high-resolution ultrasound has in recent years largely replaced diagnostic hysteroscopy as the primary tool for assessment of the uterine cavity. Ultrasound allows us to assess the integrity of the endometrium and the possible disruptions in the endometrial-myometrial junction. The proposed diagnostic algorithm of diagnosing intrauterine adhesions using ultrasound also includes 3D ultrasound and the use of saline infusion sonography [45]. Two-dimensional (2D) ultrasound is a sensitive method of diagnosing intrauterine adhesions and should be the first method employed. In women with concomitant uterine pathology, the visualization may be difficult, and in these cases saline infusion sonography may improve the diagnostic accuracy. In diagnosing intrauterine adhesions, 3D ultrasound is also of significant benefit and should be offered to women with suspected intrauterine adhesions. This allows for better assessment of location and extent of intrauterine adhesions. On ultrasound, adhesions are seen as bands of myometrial tissue traversing the endometrial cavity and connecting the opposing uterine walls (Figure 3.6). The echogenicity of the bands is usually similar to the adjacent myometrium. Complete or even partial obstruction of the uterine cavity can also result in the accumulation of blood in the cavity, which can be visualized on ultrasound. It is important not to confuse intrauterine adhesions with subendometrial fibrosis. This typically appears as echogenic foci in the basal endometrial layer with no loss of functional endometrium. The reported sensitivity of 2D ultrasound in detecting adhesions varies significantly between 0% and 97% and is highly dependent on the experience of the operator [47,48].

Conclusion

The uterus is the landmark of pelvic ultrasound examination. In reproductive medicine, careful examination of the uterus and endometrium is the cornerstone of diagnostics. With modern ultrasound technology, an experienced operator can reliably diagnose most clinically important uterine pathologies that would require treatment. There are different aspects of uterine physiology that can be monitored with ultrasound, although most sonographic markers of endometrial receptivity have not been shown to be of significant clinical value. Recent developments in ultrasound technology, such as developments in Doppler analysis and 3D ultrasound, warrant further investigations in this field. It is of utmost importance to offer women with reproductive problems a high-quality ultrasound examination, since this can reduce the burden and costs related to the use of more invasive diagnostic methods.

REFERENCES

1. Munro MG, Critchley HOD, Broder MS, and Fraser IS. FIGO classification system (PALM-COEIN) for causes of abnormal uterine bleeding in nongravid women of reproductive age. *Int J Gynecol Obstet.* 2011;113:3–13.
2. Pritts EA, Parker WH, and Olive DL. Fibroids and infertility: An updated systematic review of the evidence. *Fertil Steril.* 2009;91(4):1215–23.
3. Purohit P, and Vigneswaran K. Fibroids and infertility. *Curr Obstet Gynecol Rep.* 2016;5:81–8.
4. Metwally M, Cheoung YC, and Horne AW. Surgical treatment of fibroids for subfertility. *Cochrane Database Syst Rev.* 2012;(11):CD003857.
5. Naftalin J, Hoo W, Pateman K, Mavrelos D, Holland T, and Jurkovic D. How common is adenomyosis? A prospective study of prevalence using transvaginal ultrasound in a gynaecology clinic. *Hum Reprod.* 2012;27(12):3432–9.
6. Mavrelos D, Holland TK, O'Donovan O et al. The impact of adenomyosis on the outcome of IVF–embryo transfer. *Reprod Biomed Online.* 2017;35(5):549–54.
7. Kepkep K, Tuncay YA, Goynumer G, and Tutal E. Transvaginal sonography in the diagnosis of adenomyosis: Which findings are most accurate? *Ultrasound Gynecol Obstet.* 2007;30:341–5.
8. Exacoustus C, Manganaro L, and Zupi E. Imaging for the evaluation of endometriosis and adenomyosis. *Best Pract Res Clin.* 2014;28(5):655–81.
9. Luciano DE, Exacoustos C, Albrecht L et al. Three-dimensional ultrasound in diagnosis of adenomyosis: Histologic correlation with ultrasound targeted biopsies of the uterus. *J Minim Invasive Gynecol.* 2013;20:803–10.
10. Sharma K, Bora MK, Venkatesh BP et al. Role of 3D ultrasound and Doppler in differentiating clinically suspected cases of leiomyoma and adenomyosis of uterus. *J Clin Diagn Res.* 2015;9:QC08–12.
11. Chan YY, Jayaprakasan K, Zamora J, Thornton JG, Raine-Fenning N, and Coomarasamy A. The prevalence of congenital uterine anomalies in unselected and high-risk populations: A systematic review. *Hum Reprod Update.* 2011;17:761–71.
12. Prior M, Richardson A, Asif S et al. Reproductive outcome of women with congenital uterine anomalies after assisted reproduction: A prospective observational study. *Ultrasound Obstet Gynecol.* 2017;51(1). doi: 10.1002/uog.18935.
13. Gibbons W, Buttram VC Jr, Jan Behrman S, Jones H, and Rock J (American Fertility Society; Committee for Mullerian Anomalies). The American Fertility Society classifications of adnexal adhesions, distal tubal occlusion, tubal occlusion secondary to tubal ligation, tubal pregnancies, Mullerian anomalies and intrauterine adhesions. *Fertil Steril.* 1988;49:944–55.
14. Grimbizis GF, Gordts S, Di Spiezio Sardo A et al. The ESHRE/ESGE consensus on the classification of female genital tract congenital anomalies. *Hum Reprod.* 2013;28:2032–44.
15. Knez J, Saridogan E, Van Den Bosch T, Mavrelos D, Ambler G, and Jurkovic D. ESHRE/ESGE female genital tract anomalies classification system—The potential impact of discarding arcuate uterus on clinical practice. *Hum Reprod.* 2018;33(4):600–6.
16. Grimbizis GF, Di Spiezio Sardo A, Saravelos SH, Gordts S, Exacoustos C, and Van Schoubroeck D. The Thessaloniki ESHRE/ESGE consensus on diagnosis of female genital anomalies. *Hum Reprod.* 2016;31:2–7.
17. Knez J, and Blockeel C. Endometrial receptivity. In: Tandulwadkar, Sunita R (ed.) *The Art and Science of Assisted Reproductive Technology.* New Delhi: Jaypee Brothers Medical Publishers; 2015, pp. 297–304.
18. Persadie R. Ultrasonographic assessment of the endometrial thickness: A review. *J Obstet Gynecol Can.* 2002;24:131–6.
19. Friedler S, Schenker JG, Herman A, and Lewin A. The role of ultrasonography in the evaluation of endometrial receptivity following assisted reproductive treatments: A critical review. *Hum Reprod Update.* 1996;2:323–35.

20. Dmitrovic R, and Simunic V. Will endometrial volume measurements add something new to the diagnosis of early pregnancy? *Curr Wom Health Rev.* 2009;5:24–8.

21. Kasius A, Smit JG, Torrance HL et al. Endometrial thickness and pregnancy rates after IVF: A systematic review and meta-analysis. *Hum Reprod Update.* 2014;20(4):530–41.

22. Ueno J, Oehninger S, Bryzski RG, Acosta AA, Philput B, and Muasher SJ. Ultrasonographic appearance of the endometrium in natural and stimulated *in vitro* fertilization cycles and its correlation with outcome. *Hum Reprod.* 1991;6:901.

23. Check JH, Nowroozi K, Choe J, Lurie D, and Dietterich C. The effect of endometrial thickness and echo pattern on *in vitro* fertilization outcome in donor oocyte-embryo transfer cycle. *Fertil Steril.* 1993;59:72.

24. Oliveira JB, Baruffi RL, Mauri AL et al. Endometrial ultrasonography as a predictor of pregnancy in an *in vitro* fertilization programme after ovarian stimulation and gonadotropin-releasing hormone and gonadotropins. *Hum Reprod.* 1997;12:2515.

25. Weissman A, Gotlieb L, and Casper RF. The detrimental effect of increased endometrial thickness on implantation and pregnancy rates and outcome in an *in vitro* fertilization program. *Fertil Steril.* 1999;71:147.

26. Dietterich C, Check JH, Choe JK et al. Increased endometrial thickness on the day of human chorionic gonadotropin injection does not adversely affect pregnancy or implantation rates following *in vitro* fertilization-embryo transfer. *Fertil Steril.* 2002;77:781.

27. Yakin K, Akarsu C, and Kahraman S. Cycle lumping or 'sampling a witches' brew? *Fertil Steril.* 2000;73:175.

28. De Vries K, Lyons EA, Ballard G et al. Contractions of the inner third of the myometrium. *Am J Obstet Gynecol.* 1990;162:679–82.

29. Aguilar HN, and Mitchell BF. Physiological pathways and molecular mechanisms regulating uterine contractility. *Hum Reprod Update.* 2010;16(6):725–44.

30. Dastidar KG, and Dastidar SG. Dynamics of endometrial thickness over time: A reappraisal to standardize ultrasonographic measurements in an infertility program. *Fertil Steril.* 2003;80:213–5.

31. Fanchin R, Righini C, Olivennes F, Taylor S, de Ziegler D, and Frydman R. Uterine contractions at the time of embryo transfer alter pregnancy rates after in-vitro fertilization. *Hum Reprod.* 1998;13(7):1968–74.

32. Steer CV, Campbell S, Tan SL et al. The use of transvaginal color flow imaging after *in vitro* fertilization to identify optimum uterine conditions before embryo transfer. *Fertil Steril.* 1992;57:371–6.

33. Steer CV, Tan SL, Dillon D et al. Vaginal color Doppler assessment of uterine artery impedance correlates with immunohistochemical markers of endometrial receptivity for the implantation of an embryo. *Fertil Steril.* 1995;63:101–8.

34. Fanchin R, Righini C, Ayoubi JM et al. New look at endometrial echogenicity objective computer-assisted measurements predict endometrial receptivity in *in vitro* fertilization-embryo transfer. *Fertil Steril.* 2000;74:274.

35. Quigley MM. *In vitro* fertilization 1986: New procedures and new questions. *Invest Radiol.* 1986;21:503–10.

36. Jayaprakasan K, Polanski L, Sahu B, Thornton JG, and Raine-Fenning N. Surgical intervention versus expectant management for endometrial polyps in subfertile women. *Cochrane Database Syst Rev.* 2014;(8):CD009592.

37. Wong M, Crnobrnja B, Liberale V, Dharmarajah K, Windschwendter M, and Jurkovic D. *Hum Reprod.* 2017;32:340–5.

38. Lee SC, Kaunitz AM, Sanchez-Ramos L, and Rhatigan RM. The oncogenic potential of endometrial polyps: A systematic review and meta-analysis. *Obstet Gynecol.* 2010;116(5):1197.

39. Ben-Arie A, Goldchmit C, Laviv Y et al. The malignant potential of endometrial polyps. *Eur J Obstet Gynecol Reprod Biol.* 2004;115:206.

40. Ferrazzi E, Zupi E, Leone FP et al. How often are endometrial polyps malignant in asymptomatic postmenopausal women? A multicenter study. *Am J Obstet Gynecol.* 2009;200(3):235.

41. Cil AP, Tulunay G, Kose MF, and Haberal A. Power Doppler properties of endometrial polyps and submucosal fibroids: A preliminary observational study in women with known intracavitary lesions. *Ultrasound Obstet Gynecol.* 2010;35:233–7.

42. Jordans IPM, de Leeuw R, Stegwee SI et al. A practical guideline for examining a uterine niche using ultrasonography in non-pregnant women: A modified Delphi method amongst European experts. *Ultrasound Obstet Gynecol.* 2019;53(1):107–15.

43. Jurkovic D, Knez J, Appiah A, Farahani L, Mavrelos D, and Ross JA. Surgical treatment of Caesarean scar ectopic pregnancy: Efficacy and safety of ultrasound-guided suction currettage. *Ultrasound Obstet Gynecol*. 2016;47(4):511–7.

44. Timor-Tritsch IE, Monteagudo A, Cali G et al. Cesarean scar pregnancy is a precursor of morbidly adherent placenta. *Ultrasound Obstet Gynecol*. 2014;44(3):346–53.

45. Amin TN, Saridogan E, and Jurkovic D. Ultrasound and intrauterine adhesions: A novel structured approach to diagnosis and management. *Ultrasound Obstet Gynecol*. 2015;46(2):131–9.

46. Hooker AB, Lemmers M, Thurkow AL et al. Systematic review and meta-analysis of intrauterine adhesions after miscarriage: Prevalence, risk factors and long-term reproductive outcome. *Hum Reprod Update*. 2014;20(2):262–78.

47. Fedele L, Bianchi S, Dorta M, and Vignali M. Intrauterine adhesions: Detection with transvaginal US. *Radiology*. 1996;199:757–9.

48. Soares SR, Barbosa dos Reis MM, and Camargos AF. Diagnostic accuracy of sonohysterography, transvaginal sonography, and hysterosalpingography in patients with uterine cavity diseases. *Fertil Steril*. 2000;73:406–11.

4

The Ovaries and the Adnexa

Kuhan Rajah and Dimitrios Mavrelos

Introduction

Pelvic ultrasound is the imaging modality of choice for women suffering from subfertility. With a high-quality transvaginal ultrasound examination, we can evaluate the ovaries for their physiological function as well as identify ovarian pathology that may contribute to difficulty with conception. In this chapter, we review the physiological function of the ovary as well as ovarian and adnexal pathology commonly encountered in the subfertile woman.

Normal Physiology

During the menstrual cycle, the ovary undergoes a series of ultrasound-visible changes that reflect its function. With respect to the ovary, the cycle is commonly divided into two principal phases: follicular and luteal, the transition demarcated by ovulation. In a 28-day cycle, each phase lasts approximately 14 days with day 1 being the first day of full menstrual flow. In our practice, by convention, if full flow occurs after midday, day 1 is the next calendar day.

In the beginning of the follicular phase, during days 2–5 of the cycle, the ovary is quiescent with a wealth of ultrasound-visible follicles between 2 and 5 mm in diameter called antral (Figure 4.1). These reflect the presence of follicles that have completed the first stages of follicular recruitment and have transitioned from primordial, primary and secondary follicles to become available for follicle-stimulating hormone (FSH) induced maturation and potential ovulation [1]. There have been differing theories on how pre-antral follicles develop into antral follicles. Some studies have proposed that antral follicles develop continuously during the menstrual cycle, while others have proposed the idea of cyclic "waves" during the menstrual cycle [2]. In the next few days of the cycle (days 6–9), antral follicles undergo a common growth phase until one follicle begins to diverge and become dominant, reaching a diameter of over 10 mm, while the rest, now termed "subordinate," will eventually become atretic (Figure 4.2). This process is called *selection* [3]. The dominant follicle continues to grow by 1–4 mm/day during the late follicular phase (days 10–14) to reach a preovulatory diameter of 16–29 mm (Figure 4.3). The oocyte remains microscopic during this whole process. Increased production of estradiol 17ß from this now preovulatory follicle triggers a positive feedback loop from the hypothalamus and anterior pituitary gland leading to the surge of luteinizing hormone (LH) which in turns triggers ovulation 34–36 hours later. Ovulation describes either the point of maximum follicular growth or the process of rupture of the dominant follicle and release of the oocyte [4]. There are a few sonographic changes that can be detected around the time of ovulation: a sudden decrease in size or disappearance of the dominant follicle following follicle rupture is the most frequently observed with a sensitivity of over 80% in detecting ovulation [5]. Less sensitive signs include an increase in echogenicity within the dominant follicle, irregularity in follicle walls, as well as the appearance or increase of anechoic free fluid in the pouch of Douglas. The definitive sign of ovulation is the transformation of the dominant follicle into the corpus luteum [6]. The corpus luteum can adopt a variety of ultrasonic appearances, including solid, cystic, and hemorrhagic. It is the most vascular organ in the human body by surface area with this extensive vascularity visible on ultrasound as a characteristic "ring

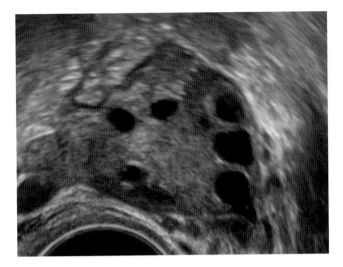

FIGURE 4.1   Ovary in the early follicular phase.

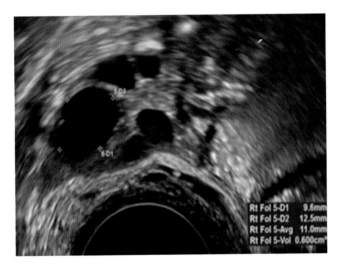

Rt Fol 5-D1	9.6mm
Rt Fol 5-D2	12.5mm
Rt Fol 5-Avg	11.0mm
Rt Fol 5-Vol	0.600cm³

FIGURE 4.2   Dominant follicle following "selection."

of fire," which allows it to fulfill its endocrine function of progesterone production (Figure 4.4). Rupture of the corpus luteum commonly leads to formation of a hemorrhagic cyst. When seen on ultrasound, a hemorrhagic corpus luteum is 3–5 cm in diameter, regular in outline, and typically contains thin strands that represent fibrin deposition (Figure 4.5). These appearances are associated with acute pain, which is mostly self-limiting but may require strong analgesia. The appearance of the corpus luteum signposts the luteal phase of the menstrual cycle (days 14–28), which ends with the withdrawal of anterior pituitary LH support. In the absence of pregnancy, the corpus luteum degenerates, ovarian steroid hormone production declines, and menstruation ensues, leading another follicular wave to start the next cycle.

Antral Follicle Count

As discussed earlier, at the beginning of the menstrual cycle, the ovaries contain a wealth of antral follicles seen on transvaginal ultrasound as simple sac-like pockets that contain anechoic fluid between 2 and 10 mm arranged at the periphery of the ovary. Quantification of these follicles is a direct assessment

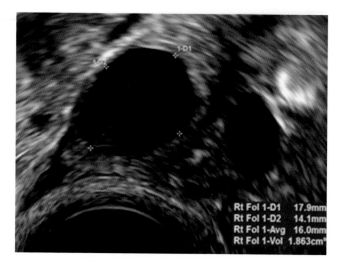

Rt Fol 1-D1   17.9mm
Rt Fol 1-D2   14.1mm
Rt Fol 1-Avg   16.0mm
Rt Fol 1-Vol   1.863cm³

FIGURE 4.3   Dominant follicle at the start of the preovulatory phase.

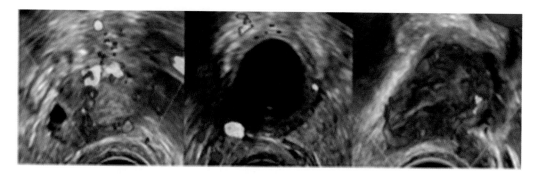

FIGURE 4.4   Corpus luteum with characteristic "ring of fire"—solid (left), cystic (center), and hemorrhagic (right).

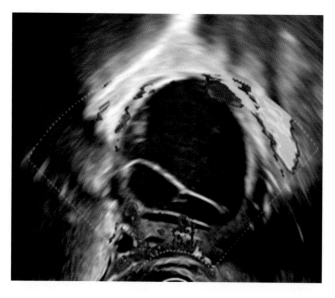

FIGURE 4.5   Hemorrhagic functional cyst.

of a woman's ovarian reserve as the number of antral follicles that emerge will reflect the number of primordial follicles available to start the journey of maturation approximately 180 days earlier [9]. The subpopulation of antral follicles that best correlates with ovarian reserve includes those between 4 and 6 mm [10]. Counting smaller ones is likely to include atretic follicles and therefore be an overestimate. However, to avoid the time-consuming process of measuring each follicle individually, by convention, all follicles measuring 2–10 mm are included in antral follicle counts (AFCs) [11].

AFC assessment is typically performed in the early follicular phase (days 2–5) but can be carried out at any time in the natural menstrual cycle [12]. It is thought to be easier to assess antral follicles at the start of the menstrual cycle prior to the development of a dominant follicle or corpus luteum [11,13]. Studies have shown that despite there being intracycle variation in the AFC, this does not alter the planning and outcome of *in vitro* fertilization (IVF) treatment, as women are largely categorized as having low, normal, or high AFCs or ovarian reserve [14,15]. There is also evidence of intercycle variation of the AFC of up to 30% despite the assessment being performed on the same day of the cycle by the same operator using the same machine [10].

Both two-dimensional (2D) and three-dimensional (3D) transvaginal ultrasound may be employed to assess AFC. Real-time 2D ultrasound, cine-loop 2D ultrasound, 3D manual mode, and SonoAVC are different methods used to count antral follicles. There is currently no strong evidence in favor of one particular method; therefore, an operator should employ a method based on availability as well as personal skill and preference [16]. Antral follicles appear as sonolucent structures on ultrasound and are typically round or oval in shape. Practically, to perform an AFC assessment in real-time 2D ultrasound, we start by scanning either the right or left ovary in both the longitudinal and transverse planes to determine the boundaries of the ovary, exclude any abnormalities within the ovary, and determine the plane that provides the clearest image of the ovary. We then perform a sweep to identify the largest follicle. We measure the largest follicle in two orthogonal diameters to confirm it is under 10 mm in mean diameter and ensure no follicles over 10 mm are included in the count. We then systematically scan the ovary from one end to the other, maintaining the standard plane, and count all follicles between 2 and 10 mm to provide the AFC for that ovary. Operators should take care to not include fimbrial or paraovarian cysts or parametrial blood vessels. Application of gentle pressure on the ovary will help delineate ovarian margins and avoid overestimation. Operators should be mindful that such pressure may be uncomfortable for the patient. Color Doppler can also be used to exclude blood vessels. The process is then repeated on the other ovary. A total AFC refers to the total number of antral follicles measured in both ovaries, while the "follicle number per ovary" describes the number of follicles in the ovary.

Interpretation of an AFC needs careful consideration. Normal ranges have been published both in healthy volunteers and women presenting with subfertility [17] and can be helpful to explain a woman's relative position on this scale. However, care should be taken to explain that an AFC is not a measure of natural fertility—that is, even at low counts of under 5, the possibility of spontaneous conception remains as long as the woman continues to have ovulatory cycles. In contrast, as becomes clear from the brief description of ovarian physiology presented earlier, AFC is a reflection of selectable follicles [18] and can be used to anticipate responsiveness to ovarian stimulation in IVF, and thus select an appropriate treatment protocol and stimulation dose [19]. The AFC can also be used to counsel the woman regarding the outcome of an IVF cycle, with lower counts associated with reduced probability of live birth, which is most likely due to a lower number of embryos available to choose from for transfer or even having no embryos to transfer at all [12]. At the other end of the spectrum, an AFC over 16 is associated with an increased risk of ovarian hyperstimulation syndrome following ovarian stimulation, and this threshold can be used for due precautions to be put in place [20]. Besides its use in IVF, an AFC also provides an assessment of the impact of gonadotoxic cancer treatment on ovarian reserve [21].

Common Ovarian Pathology and Impact on Fertility

Functional Cysts

On occasion, the process of ovulation "malfunctions," leading to the formation of a luteinized unruptured follicle (LUF), which is seen on ultrasound as a simple ovarian cyst (Figure 4.6). The formation of LUFs can be a subtle cause of subfertility, as these women do not have normal ovulation but continue

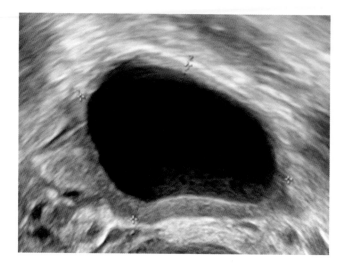

FIGURE 4.6   Luteinized unruptured follicle.

having cycles [4]. LUFs have been associated with a number of conditions, including in patients taking nonsteroidal anti-inflammatory drugs (NSAIDs) [7]. The mechanism through which LUFs occur remains unclear, a possibility being NSAID-mediated inhibition of prostaglandin synthesis necessary for ovulation [8]. This property has been exploited in natural IVF cycles that use indomethacin, an NSAID to delay ovulation and reduce the risk of premature ovulation before transvaginal egg collection [9].

Polycystic Ovary

Following the Rotterdam consensus in 2003, the definition of a polycystic ovary has been an ovary containing more than 12 antral follicles or with a volume exceeding 10 cm^3 [12]. More recently this definition has been found not to be fit for purpose, as the availability of higher-definition ultrasound machines in the last few years has meant that a large proportion of ovulatory women would be diagnosed with polycystic ovaries. The recent international consensus guideline raised the threshold for characterizing polycystic ovarian morphology (PCOM) to a follicle number per ovary of 20 or greater, while maintaining a volume threshold of 10 cm^3 (Figure 4.7) [22]. PCOM needs to be combined with irregular menstrual cycles and clinical or biochemical hyperandrogenism in order to make the diagnosis

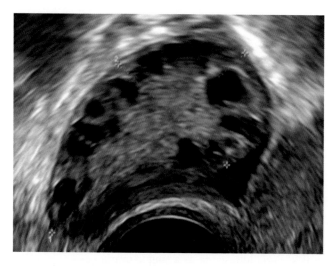

FIGURE 4.7   Polycystic ovary (with an antral follicle count of 25).

of polycystic ovary syndrome (PCOS). The diagnosis of PCOS can also be made in the absence of PCOM, when both irregular menstrual cycles and hyperandrogenism are present.

Endometriomas

Endometriosis is a common condition in women of reproductive age and is associated with difficulty in conception. High-quality pelvic ultrasound can assist in the diagnosis of pelvic endometriosis in infertile women but cannot be used to exclude mild or minimal disease. In contrast, moderate or severe disease and endometriotic ovarian cysts are readily seen on pelvic ultrasound, and the diagnosis can be highly accurate [23]. Endometriomas have a typical appearance. They are regular cystic structures with ground glass appearance typically between 10 and 70 mm, poorly vascularized on Doppler examination, and can have multiple cysts in a single ovary (Figure 4.8). Endometriosis may result in the formation of pelvic adhesions, and so inevitably the pathophysiology of the ovary is affected. An endometrioma may be adherent to the pelvic side wall, or possibly the back or side of the uterus medially and less commonly to the contralateral ovary posterior to the uterus, forming "kissing ovaries" (Figure 4.9). Endometriomas can adopt more bizarre appearances, particularly if there has been a fresh bleed into them.

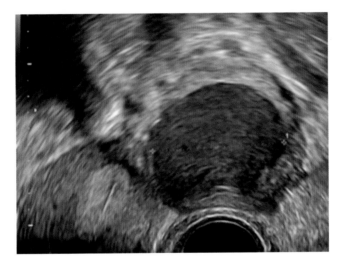

FIGURE 4.8 Endometrioma with typical "ground glass" appearance (adherent to lateral aspect of uterus).

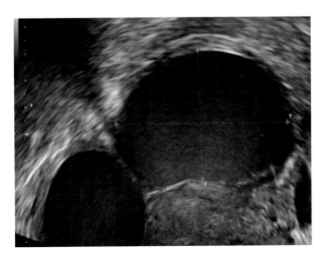

FIGURE 4.9 "Kissing ovaries"—right and left ovary containing an endometrioma each adherent to each other.

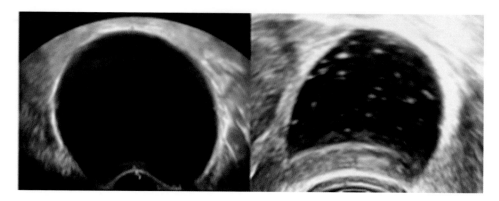

FIGURE 4.10 Serous cystadenoma (left) and mucinous cystadenoma (right).

Despite pelvic endometriosis appearing to be more prevalent in couples with subfertility, it is not an absolute cause of infertility. Recent studies following up women diagnosed with an endometrioma before attempting conception showed that up to 50% of these women conceived spontaneously despite the presence of the endometrioma [24]. Nevertheless, the presence of an ovarian endometrioma is not without consequence, as affected ovaries have been found to be less responsive to ovarian stimulation compared to the contralateral normal ovary [25]. However, surgical removal of an endometrioma has been associated with a reduction in ovarian reserve, as it is inevitable that some healthy ovarian tissue is removed during removal of the cyst. Surgeons should proceed with care, especially in women with previous ovarian surgery [26].

Cystadenomas

Cystadenomas are regular cystic structures found within the ovary and surrounded by healthy ovarian tissue. They can be serous or mucinous (Figure 4.10). The former have anechoic content, reach 50–80 mm in mean diameter, and are bilateral in 15% of cases. The latter have low-level echogenic contents that represent their mucin content and are usually unilateral [27]. These tumors are not typically thought to affect fertility but can cause diagnostic confusion, as the differential diagnosis of a serous cystadenoma is a functional ovarian cyst, while a mucinous cystadenoma can appear similar to an endometrioma. Interval scans are useful to make the differential diagnosis, as serous cystadenomas are persistent while functional cysts are transient. We do not routinely use tumor markers as an adjunct to diagnosis but rely on simple rules classification, as this has been shown to be a more effective method [28,29]. As previously discussed, endometriomas tend to render the ovary less mobile through the development of adhesions, while an ovary containing a mucinous cystadenoma is likely to be mobile on gentle pressure with the ultrasound probe.

Recent studies have suggested that surgical removal of nonendometriotic cysts also has an impact on ovarian reserve [30], which should be kept in mind when discussing treatment options of these benign conditions.

Dermoid Cysts/Mature Teratomas

These are cystic-solid tumors that are usually unilocular and have the characteristic appearance of mixed echogenicity that represents their components of fat, bone, hair, and sebaceous fluid [31]. Dermoid cysts often cast extensive shadowing, further adding to their typical appearances. Transvaginal ultrasound is highly sensitive and specific for these tumors, but they require a degree of vigilance, as the mixed echogenicity can blend into the background bowel making the ovarian limits difficult to fully delineate (Figure 4.11).

The presence of ovarian dermoid cysts is associated with an increased risk of ovarian torsion, which may be compounded by ovarian stimulation and pregnancy [32]. Patients should be informed of the risk and asked to report any relevant symptoms immediately.

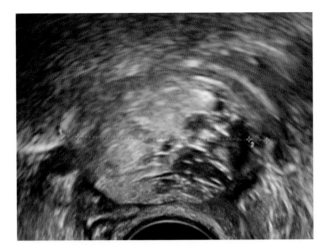

FIGURE 4.11   Dermoid cyst with mixed echogenicity and shadowing.

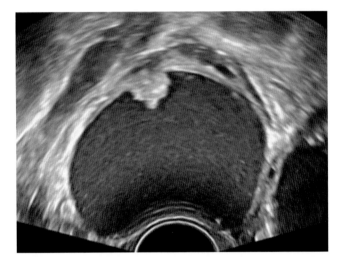

FIGURE 4.12   Serous borderline tumor with papillary projections.

Borderline Ovarian Tumors

Borderline ovarian tumors are an entity separate from benign and invasive ovarian tumors, are more prevalent in women of childbearing age and can therefore be incidentally found in women presenting with subfertility [33]. Ovarian borderline tumors are usually unilocular with a positive ovarian crescent sign with either extensive papillary projections arising from the cyst wall (serous or mucinous endocervical type) (Figure 4.12) or with a well-defined multilocular or honeycomb nodule (mucinous gastrointestinal type) (Figure 4.13) [34]. Such appearances should prompt an urgent referral to a gynecological oncologist for further management, and this should allow fertility-sparing surgery to be performed [35].

Adnexal Pathology

Fallopian Tube Disorder

The fallopian tube is not commonly visible on transvaginal ultrasound unless it is enhanced using echogenic dye during a hysterosalpingo-contrast sonography (HyCoSy). However, occlusion of the

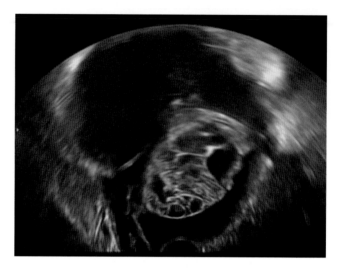

FIGURE 4.13   Mucinous borderline tumor with characteristic "honeycomb" nodule.

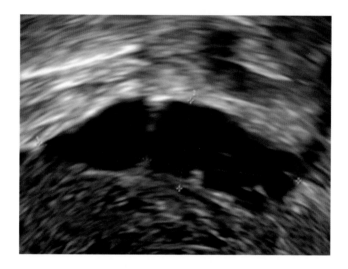

FIGURE 4.14   Hydrosalpinx with incomplete septations and anechoic fluid.

fallopian tube by a pathological process such as pelvic inflammatory disease (PID), endometriosis, or postoperative peritubal adhesions can lead to the formation of ultrasound visible hydrosalpinges.

A hydrosalpinx on transvaginal ultrasound scan has a characteristic appearance. It is a tubular cystic structure with incomplete septations located in the adnexa between uterus and ovary. The septations form a typical cog-wheel appearance on the cross-sectional plane as the fallopian tube serosa contains longitudinal striations (Figure 4.14). Care should be taken to differentiate a hydrosalpinx from a simple fimbrial cyst, which is typically small, located at the proximal end of the fallopian tube and unlikely to exhibit incomplete septations (Figure 4.15).

Variations of a hydrosalpinx include a pyosalpinx (Figure 4.16) and a hematosalpinx (Figure 4.17). The first can remain beyond the acute phase of inflammation due to PID and be sterile. The second is commonly seen during menstruation with reflux of menstrual blood into the occluded fallopian tube.

In the authors' experience, hydrosalpinges can be transient, and previously unseen hydrosalpinges may become visible during ovarian stimulation. A hydrosalpinx is susceptible to infection and transformation into an abscess, and for this reason we routinely carry out a 2D ultrasound before performing saline

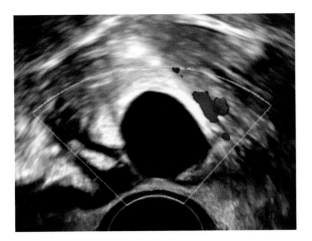

FIGURE 4.15   Fimbrial cyst.

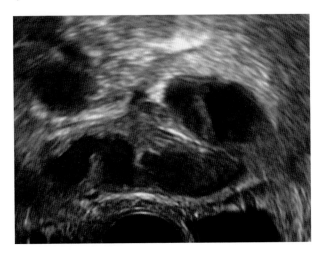

FIGURE 4.16   Pyosalpinx with incomplete septations and echogenic contents.

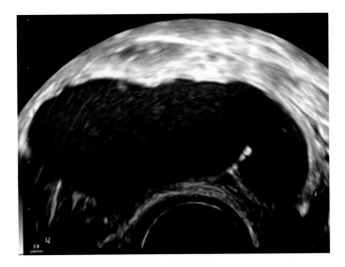

FIGURE 4.17   Hematosalpinx with incomplete septations and contents with low-level echoes (blood).

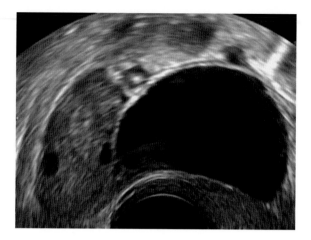

FIGURE 4.18   Paraovarian cyst with normal ovary adjacent and separate.

infusion sonohysterography and HyCoSy and would suggest a prolonged course of antibiotics if there is suspicion of a hydrosalpinx.

The detection of a hydrosalpinx on ultrasound, in a woman hoping to conceive, should prompt a discussion with a fertility specialist regarding the option of tubal surgery or IVF. It is now established that an untreated hydrosalpinx will reduce the chance of success with IVF be it through endometrial or embryonic effects [36,37] and will increase the risk of ectopic pregnancy, hence bilateral salpingectomy or proximal tubal occlusion will restore the woman's chances of conception following embryo transfer [38].

Paraovarian Cysts

A paraovarian cyst is typically a simple cyst located in the adnexa adjacent to the ovary. An ipsilateral healthy ovary seen adjacent to the cyst is vital in making the diagnosis (Figure 4.18).

Peritoneal Pseudocysts

Peritoneal pseudocysts are frequently located in the pouch of Douglas and adnexa in women with pelvic adhesions secondary to previous surgery, pelvic infection, and endometriosis. Peritoneal pseudocysts have a bizarre star-like shape with blurred and indefinite margins and multiple thin septa that undulate under pressure from the ultrasound probe (Figure 4.19) [39].

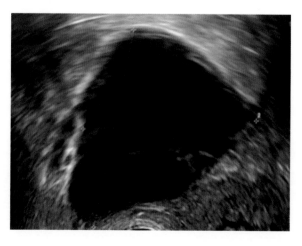

FIGURE 4.19   Peritoneal pseudocyst with indefinite margins.

REFERENCES

1. Fauser CM. Intraovarian control of early folliculogenesis. *Endocr Rev.* 2015;36(1):1–24.
2. Baerwald AR, Adams GP, and Pierson RA. Characterization of ovarian follicular wave dynamics in women. *Biol Reprod.* 2003;69(3):1023–31.
3. Baerwald AR, Adams GP, and Pierson RA. Ovarian antral folliculogenesis during the human menstrual cycle: A review. *Hum Reprod Update.* 2012;18(1):73–91.
4. Pearlstone A, and Surrey E. The temporal relation between the urine LH surge and sonographic evidence of ovulation: Determinants and clinical significance. *Obstet Gynecol.* 1994;83(2):184–8.
5. Ecochard R, Marret H, Rabilloud M et al. Sensitivity and specificity of ultrasound indices of ovulation in spontaneous cycles. *Eur J Obstet Gynecol Reprod Biol.* 2000;91(1):59–64.
6. Duggavathi R, and Murphy BD. Ovulation signals. *Science.* 2009;324(5929):890–1.
7. Qublan H, Amarin Z, Nawasreh M et al. Luteinized unruptured follicle syndrome: Incidence and recurrence rate in infertile women with unexplained infertility undergoing intrauterine insemination. *Hum Reprod.* 2006;21(8):2110–3.
8. Rijken-Zijlstra TM, Haadsma ML, Hammer C et al. Effectiveness of Indometacin to prevent ovulation in modified natural-cycle IVF: A randomized controlled trial. *Reprod Biomed Online.* 2013;27(3):297–304.
9. Gougeon A. Dynamics of follicular growth in the human: A model from preliminary results. *Hum Reprod Oxf Engl.* 1986;1(2):81–7.
10. Haadsma ML, Bukman A, Groen H et al. The number of small antral follicles (2–6 mm) determines the outcome of endocrine ovarian reserve tests in a subfertile population. *Hum Reprod.* 2007;22(7):1925–31.
11. Broekmans FJ, de Ziegler D, Howles CM, Gougeon A, Trew G, and Olivennes F. The antral follicle count: Practical recommendations for better standardization. *Fertil Steril.* 2010;94(3):1044–51.
12. Jayaprakasan K, Chan Y, Islam R et al. Prediction of *in vitro* fertilization outcome at different antral follicle count thresholds in a prospective cohort of 1,012 women. *Fertil Steril.* 2012;98(3):657–63.
13. Rombauts L, Lambalk CB, Schultze-Mosgau A et al. Intercycle variability of the ovarian response in patients undergoing repeated stimulation with corifollitropin alfa in a gonadotropin-releasing hormone antagonist protocol. *Fertil Steril.* 2015;104(4):884–90.e2.
14. Mavrelos D, Chami A, Talaulikar V et al. Variation in antral follicle counts at different times in the menstrual cycle: Does it matter? *Reprod Biomed Online.* 2016;33(2):174–9.
15. van Disseldorp J, Lambalk C, Kwee J et al. Comparison of inter- and intra-cycle variability of anti-Mullerian hormone and antral follicle counts. *Hum Reprod (Oxf, Engl).* 2010;25(1):221–7.
16. Neto CM, Ludwin A, Borrell A et al. Counting ovarian antral follicles by ultrasound: A practical guide. *Ultrasound Obst Gynecol.* 2018;51(1):10–20.
17. Almog B, Shehata F, Shalom-Paz E, Tan SL, and Tulandi T. Age-related normogram for antral follicle count: McGill reference guide. *Fertil Steril.* 2011;95(2):663–6.
18. Jayaprakasan K, Hilwah N, Kendall NR et al. Does 3D ultrasound offer any advantage in the pretreatment assessment of ovarian reserve and prediction of outcome after assisted reproduction treatment? *Hum Reprod.* 2007;22(7):1932–41.
19. Olivennes F, Howles C, Borini A et al. Individualizing FSH dose for assisted reproduction using a novel algorithm: The CONSORT study. *Reprod Biomed Online.* 2009;18(2):195–204.
20. Marca A, and Sunkara S. Individualization of controlled ovarian stimulation in IVF using ovarian reserve markers: From theory to practice. *Hum Reprod Update.* 2014;20(1):124–40.
21. Gracia CR, Sammel MD, Freeman E et al. Impact of cancer therapies on ovarian reserve. *Fertil Steril.* 2012;97(1):134–140.e1.
22. Teede HJ, Misso ML, Costello MF et al. Recommendations from the international evidence-based guideline for the assessment and management of polycystic ovary syndrome. *Hum Reprod.* 2018;33(9):1602–18.
23. Holland T, Hoo W, Mavrelos D, Saridogan E, Cutner A, and Jurkovic D. Reproducibility of assessment of severity of pelvic endometriosis using transvaginal ultrasound. *Ultrasound Obstet Gynecol.* 2013;41(2):210–5.
24. Maggiore LU, Scala C, Venturini PL, Remorgida V, and Ferrero S. Endometriotic ovarian cysts do not negatively affect the rate of spontaneous ovulation. *Hum Reprod.* 2015;30(2):299–307.
25. Gupta S, Agarwal A, Agarwal R, and de Mola LJ. Impact of ovarian endometrioma on assisted reproduction outcomes. *Reprod Biomed Online.* 2006;13(3):349–60.

26. Dunselman G, Vermeulen N, Becker C et al. ESHRE guideline: Management of women with endometriosis. *Hum Reprod (Oxf Engl)*. 2014;29(3):400–12.
27. Sayasneh AH, Ekechi C, Ferrara L et al. The characteristic ultrasound features of specific types of ovarian pathology (Review). *Int J Oncol*. 2014;46(2):445–58.
28. Kaijser J, Sayasneh A, Hoorde VK et al. Presurgical diagnosis of adnexal tumours using mathematical models and scoring systems: A systematic review and meta-analysis. *Hum Reprod Update*. 2013;20(3):449–62.
29. Nunes N, Ambler G, Foo X et al. Comparison of two protocols for the management of asymptomatic postmenopausal women with adnexal tumours—A randomised controlled trial of RMI/RCOG vs Simple Rules. *Brit J Cancer*. 2017;116(5):584–91.
30. Salihoğlu KN, Dilbaz B, Cırık D, Ozelci R, Ozkaya E, and Mollamahmutoğlu L. Short-term impact of laparoscopic cystectomy on ovarian reserve tests in bilateral and unilateral endometriotic and nonendometriotic cysts. *J Minim Invas Gynecol*. 2016;23(5):719–25.
31. Ameye L, Timmerman D, Valentin L et al. Clinically oriented three-step strategy for assessment of adnexal pathology. *Ultrasound Obst Gynecol*. 2012;40(5):582–91.
32. Vloeberghs V, Peeraer K, Pexsters A, and D'Hooghe T. Ovarian hyperstimulation syndrome and complications of ART. *Best Pract Res Clin Obstet Gynaecol*. 2009;23(5):691–709.
33. Gotlieb WH, Chetrit A, Menczer J et al. Demographic and genetic characteristics of patients with borderline ovarian tumors as compared to early stage invasive ovarian cancer. *Gynecol Oncol*. 2005;97(3):780–3.
34. Yazbek J, Raju K, Ben-Nagi J, Holland T, Hillaby K, and Jurkovic D. Accuracy of ultrasound subjective "pattern recognition" for the diagnosis of borderline ovarian tumors. *Ultrasound Obstet Gynecol*. 2007;29(5):489–95.
35. Maneo A, Vignali M, Chiari S, Colombo A, Mangioni C, and Landoni F. Are borderline tumors of the ovary safely treated by laparoscopy? *Gynecol Oncol*. 2004;94(2):387392.
36. Daftary GS, and Taylor HS. Hydrosalpinx fluid diminishes endometrial cell HOXA10 expression. *Fertil Steril*. 2002;78(3):577580.
37. Beyler S, James K, Fritz M, and Meyer W. Hydrosalpingeal fluid inhibits in-vitro embryonic development in a murine model. *Hum Reprod*. 1997;12(12):2724–8.
38. Strandell A, Lindhard A, Waldenström U, Thorburn J, Janson PO, and Hamberger L. Hydrosalpinx and IVF outcome: A prospective, randomized multicentre trial in Scandinavia on salpingectomy prior to IVF. *Hum Reprod*. 1999;14(11):2762–9.
39. Savelli L, Iaco DP, Ghi T, Bovicelli L, Rosati F, and Cacciatore B. Transvaginal sonographic appearance of peritoneal pseudocysts. *Ultrasound Obst Gyn*. 2004;23(3):284–8.

5

Uterine Cavity Assessment (Saline Hysterosonography)

Zdravka Veleva

Introduction

Saline hysterosonography is an outpatient method to examine tubal patency and the uterine cavity with ultrasound, using saline to create contrast within the uterus and tubes. It is at least as powerful a diagnostic method as transcervical salpingography but it avoids the use of ionizing radiation and iodine contrast medium and can be performed in the gynecologist's office. Saline hysterography has many names:

- Hysterosonography
- Sonohysterography
- Hydrosonography
- Saline hysterosalpingography
- Saline contrast hysterosalpingography
- Saline infusion sonography
- Gel instillation sonography
- Foam hysterosalpingography

The latter names derive from the fact that apart from saline, gel and foam can also be used as contrast medium during the procedure. Regardless of the name, hysterosonography with or without tubal assessment is a diagnostic procedure [1].

The following abbreviations have also been used to describe the procedure:

- SIS—saline instillation (infusion) sonography
- Sono-TSSG—Sono-transvaginal salpingo-sonography
- HSG—hysterosalpingography
- HyCoSy—hysterosalpingo-contrast sonography
- GIS—gas-instillation sonography
- HyFoSy—hysterosalpingo-foam sonography

The examination can be divided into two parts: evaluation of the uterine cavity and evaluation of the fallopian tubes. This chapter focuses on the technique of hysterosonography and on the examination of the uterine cavity. For the evaluation of tubal patency, the term HyCoSy (hysterosalpingo-contrast sonography) is used and is described in the next chapter.

History

The assessment of the uterine cavity has traditionally been carried out as part of x-ray HSG, a method that involves the instillation of contrast iodine solution into the uterus and the fallopian tubes. After

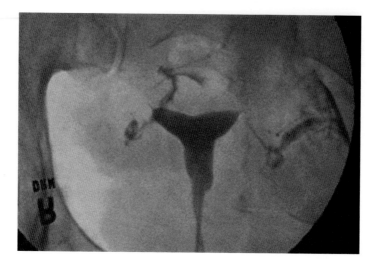

FIGURE 5.1   Hysterosalpingogram. Infusion of radiographic contrast into the uterus and fallopian tubes using fluoroscopic guidance. (Reproduced with permission from Saunders RD et al. *Fertil Steril.* 2011;95[7]:2171–9.)

this, a series of x-ray pictures are taken from the anterior-posterior and lateral aspects. Only the contrast medium is clearly visible in the pictures (Figure 5.1). Thus, the examiner can view the image of the uterine cavity and assess its size, shape, and any defects, and can determine the presence or absence of any pathology.

While ultrasound examinations have been used in gynecology since 1958 [3], the first practical endovaginal mechanical sector transducer was only produced in 1985 [4]. Thus, the first hysterosalpingographic investigation was performed by transabdominal ultrasound. The concept of intrauterine saline infusion was first described by Nannini et al. [5], who used the method to improve uterine cavity images. Shortly thereafter, the first report of assessment of uterine cavity and tubes by ultrasound was made [6]. Because of poor resolution, the method required the injection into the uterus of about 200 mL saline, which is about 10–20 times the amount of liquid used nowadays. By 1987, the method was already practiced with transvaginal transducers, as reported by a German group [7].

Today, saline hysterosonography is widely practiced, for example in the Nordic countries, where it is the most common method for evaluation of the uterine cavity and fallopian tubes.

An overview of indications and contraindications of saline hysterosonography are shown in Table 5.1.

TABLE 5.1

Indications and Contraindications of Saline Hysterosonography

Indications
- Abnormal uterine bleeding
- Suspected submucous or intramural uterine myomas or intracavitary focal lesions, e.g., polyps
- Suspected intracavitary synechiae or septum
- Focal or diffuse endometrial abnormality
- Suspected uterine structural abnormalities
- As part of routine investigation of subfertility and in patients with recurrent pregnancy loss
- Pre- and postoperative evaluation of uterine myomas and polyps
- In cases with suboptimal visualization of the endometrium in transvaginal ultrasonography, for example, in obese patients

Contraindications
- Pregnancy, whether confirmed or suspected
- Active infection or otherwise unexplained pelvic tenderness
- Menstruation or heavy bleeding
- Confirmed malignancy of the reproductive tract

Contrast Media

Different contrast media can be used in hysterosonography. They share some of the same properties: they are not toxic, they provide good ultrasonographic contrast, and they are eliminated by reabsorption into the abdominal cavity. As contrast media other than saline are more frequently used in HyCoSy, a list of commercially available preparations can be found in Chapter 6. In the early years of HSG, oil-soluble contrast media were used. This was, however, found to be associated with an increased risk of complications, such as granulomatous changes and fibrosis on the peritoneal surfaces [8]. More recently, oil-soluble media have been suggested to be as safe as water-based media; nevertheless, water-based contrast media are still by far the most popular [8].

Saline

Saline is nonallergenic and virtually harmless, except when administered in unusually high doses, in which cases it causes water and electrolyte disbalance. Hysterosonography with saline is the cheapest investigation of the uterus and/or the fallopian tubes. Its disadvantages include its rapid passage through the reproductive organs in case of patent fallopian tubes, and its rapid absorption through the peritoneum. In a typical procedure, 5–10 mL of saline is used [9].

Procedure

The necessary equipment includes, most importantly, an ultrasound machine with a transvaginal probe and good resolution capabilities. Transabdominal probes are not routinely used because of the proximity of the transvaginal probe to the pelvic organs. The use of Doppler imaging during the investigation of the uterus is seldom necessary. For review purposes, the examination can be recorded and reexamined as needed.

Before starting the procedure, it is important to be sure that the patient is not pregnant and that she is in the follicular phase of the menstrual cycle. Sonohysterography is not carried out later than cycle day 10 because of the possibility of flushing an ovulated and fertilized oocyte into the fallopian tubes or even in to the abdominal cavity. It is also recommended that the examination be performed after the cessation of menstrual bleeding.

Hysterosonography can be performed without premedication; however, in most centers, an NSAID (e.g., ibuprofen 600 mg orally) and/or different painkillers can be administered about 1 hour prior to the procedure. The administration of an NSAID has a double function: it provides pain relief and prevents tubal spasm.

The procedure is easier to perform after the patient has emptied her bladder. This results in better visualization of the uterus and is also more comfortable for the patient, who is placed into the lithotomy position on a gynecological examination chair or couch. A routine gynecological examination is performed to rule out infections or suspicious lesions. If purulent vaginal or cervical discharge, unusual pain, and lesions are observed, further investigation may be required before the procedure can be carried out. After the gynecological examination, detailed transvaginal ultrasound scan is performed in order to detect any abnormality in cervix, uterus, adnexa, and pelvic cavity. Since the focus of saline hysterosonography is the evaluation of the uterus and uterine cavity, the position and size of the uterus should be noted. The uterus is scanned in longitudinal and transverse section. Endometrial thickness is measured, and its sonographic appearance recorded. Pregnancy signs or signs of ovulation are also ruled out. In the pelvis, the amount of free fluid before the start of hysterosonography is also measured.

Necessary equipment for hysterosonography is shown in Figure 5.2. For investigations of the uterine cavity, saline infusion 5–10 mL [9] with or without air is the recommended and most used contrast medium. It is filled into a syringe before the start of the procedure.

The probe is removed, and the speculum is placed in the vagina to visualize the cervix. The external os is cleansed from vaginal discharge or mucus, if necessary. The catheter is then inserted into the cervical canal or into the uterine cavity in an aseptic manner. If necessary, the cervix is fixed with tenaculum and manipulated to align it with the uterus. The catheter can be fixed into position by an inflatable balloon.

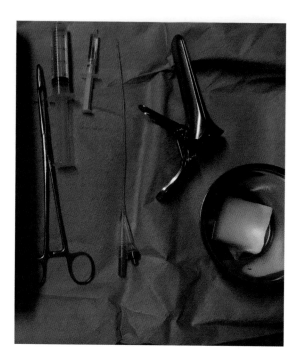

FIGURE 5.2 Typical equipment for saline hysterosonography includes a catheter, a syringe filled with saline or another contrast matter, a vaginal speculum, swabs moistened with saline used to wipe away any secretion in the cervical os and vagina, as well as an atraumatic instrument used for wiping and also for guiding the catheter into the cervical canal or uterine cavity. Occasionally a tenaculum might be necessary to facilitate difficult cannulations.

Different types of 6F-8F (French) catheters can be used, for example, neonatal urinary Foley catheters or intrauterine insemination catheters. The choice of catheter depends, among other findings, on uterine position with relation to the cervix and on the nature of the cervical canal. In case of a convoluted or very angular canal, an insemination catheter with guide can be of use. A cervical sound can also help distend an otherwise stenotic canal before a catheter is inserted. These problems are more common in postmenopausal women but are worth noting also as part of infertility workup. The rate of cervical stenosis has been reported to be 1.8%–6% [10,11].

The use of a balloon catheter was investigated by Dessole and colleagues who studied 610 women who underwent sonohysterography with six different catheter types [12]. They assessed the reliability, the physician's ease of use, the time requested for insertion of the catheter, the volume of contrast medium used, patient's tolerance, and cost of the catheters. No statistically significant differences were found in terms of procedure performance. Catheters without balloons were better tolerated by the patient but necessitated a higher infusion volume because of vaginal backflow of the saline infusion.

The catheter should be placed into the cervical canal at the internal os level even if a balloon catheter is used, as this diminishes patient discomfort and pain [13]. In addition, in case of intracervical placement, a lower volume of saline is required to complete the procedure. A balloon placed in the uterine cavity can also obscure the view from a pathologic structure (Figure 5.3).

Once the catheter is in position, either the investigator or the assistant slowly instills the contrast into the uterus. Using real-time ultrasound, the passage of saline into the uterine cavity and further into the tubes and pouch of Douglas is monitored, and pictures or videos are taken as needed. Regardless of whether the aim of hysterosonography is the diagnosis of tubal patency or not, the procedure always evaluates first the uterine cavity and endometrium, then fallopian tubes, and finally, the pelvis and pouch of Douglas. Imaging should also include the cervical canal.

In a normal saline hysterosonography, the endometrium appears symmetric, surrounding an anechoic, ovoid, saline-distended uterine cavity. At least the interstitial parts of the fallopian tubes are visible, and the passage of saline into the pelvic cavity can be visualized (Video 5.1).

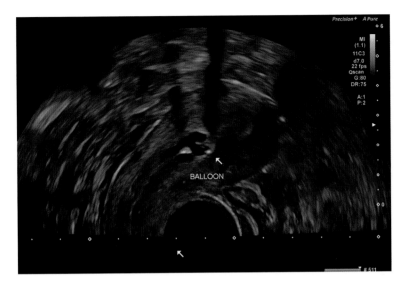

FIGURE 5.3 Intrauterine placement of catheter tip can obscure the view of a pathologic structure.

VIDEO 5.1
Normal saline hysterosonography. (https://youtu.be/90kfXya8dpU)

In two-dimensional (2D) hysterosonography, coronal and longitudinal scanning of the entire uterus must be performed. With three-dimensional (3D) hysterosonography, capture of the entire uterine cavity can be performed within a shorter time. The image can be reevaluated, especially in the coronal plane because of possible anomaly of the uterine cavity.

Learning Curve

The diagnostic accuracy of saline hysterosonography is operator dependent and could result in the reporting of false-negative or false-positive findings in the hands of a less-experienced operator [14]. Up to about 10–20 mL of saline and air mix is usually used in hysterosonography, but if a longer examination is necessary, even higher amounts can be used safely. This is important in case of an inexperienced operator and when nonballoon catheters are used, resulting in vaginal backflow of saline.

Hysterosonography is a relatively straightforward procedure, and experience greatly improves performance. In the study of Saunders and colleagues [15], one investigator performed 96 hysterosonographies during a 16-month period (a mean of six procedures per month). Less saline and air were utilized over time, and the mean amount diminished from 92 to 44 mL, while reported pain scores remained the same.

Pain and Tubal Spasm

Since saline sonohysterography is an outpatient procedure that causes some discomfort to the patient ranging from mild to severe vasovagal reaction, staff should be prepared to treat and prevent pain complications. Pain sensation is caused by the increased pressure in the cervical canal that stimulates nerve endings and uterine contractions. If the catheter's balloon is placed in the uterine cavity, resulting pressure also causes pain [12]; therefore, only a small amount of saline should be used to inflate the balloon. In addition to premedication, verbal anesthesia performed by an assistant during the procedure is very important. Although not sufficiently researched, verbal anesthesia is a potent tool in outpatient procedures [16]. It represents a continuous conversation with the patient with the aim of diversion of her attention to comfortable topics unrelated to medical treatment. When properly administered, verbal anesthesia has the potential of eliminating most pain, fear, and discomfort of the patient and ensures the smooth execution of the examination.

Overall, saline sonohysterography is well tolerated, especially if verbal anesthesia is used actively. Between 41% and 59% of patients do not experience pain [17,18]. In a study of 99 women, pain was about twice more frequently observed in postmenopausal women (71% versus 32% in premenopausal women), who more often felt sharp pain [15]. By contrast, premenopausal women more often experienced burning and/or cramping pain. Other studies have indicated that some cramping is experienced by 24%–73% of patients [18,19]. It is reassuring to know that only 6.5%–6.8% of patients have severe pain during the procedure [9,18].

The experience of pain does not depend on the volume of saline infused [20], and most likely it has a reflex component. However, pain is experienced more often in patients with tubal block and adhesions either in adnexa or in Asherman syndrome, as well as in cases where the uterus cannot distend, such as in adenomyosis, multiple myomas, and postmenopausal uterus.

The most severe complication during hysterosonography is vasovagal reaction, which is caused by a reflex. Vasovagal reaction occurs in about 4%–5% of patients [17,21] but usually resolves without the need of atropine administration [17].

Tubal spasm is another complication that can occur when the saline infusion comes into contact with the tubal epithelium. This is especially important when investigating tubal patency. Usually, tubal spasm resolves spontaneously over a couple of minutes. If the infusion of saline is not interrupted, tubal spasm can cause pain to the patient because the liquid accumulates in the uterus and distends it. This spasm can be prevented by the administration of an NSAID or spasmolytic medication before the procedure, and by gentle injection of the contrast media.

Use of Nonsteroidal Anti-inflammatory or Other Pain Relief Medication

Since uterine and tubal wall contractions are responsible for most pain sensations, medicated pain relief is administered to diminish the frequency and strength of these contractions. The prophylactic administration of ibuprofen 600 mg and paracetamol 1 g orally 1 hour prior to saline sonohysterography is therefore the treatment of choice. If necessary, in case of persistent pain, the patient can be given tramadol 50 mg orally, intravenously, or intramuscularly.

The effect of mefenamic acid and hyoscine for pain relief during saline sonohysterography was investigated in a double-blind randomized controlled trial [22]. Patients were randomized to 500 mg mefenamic acid, 10 mg of hyoscine, or placebo taken 30 minutes before the procedure. There was no difference in pain scores in the three arms of the study.

In another large study, 816 patients were randomized to receive 10 mg hyoscine-*N*-butylbromide or placebo [23]. Again, no differences in pain scores were observed, and the authors suspected that 10 mg might not be enough in the setting of hysterosonography. It is worth noting that 33% of patients experienced no pain during the procedure, and a further 40%–42% experienced mild pain that was equivalent to menstrual periods. In total, five patients (0.6%) had significant vasovagal reaction that necessitated resuscitation.

Other types of pain relief have been used, for example, a combination of paracetamol and codeine [24]. Several research units have attempted to use lidocaine solution instead of saline in hysterosonography; however, pain scores were similar to those in patients who received only saline [25,26].

Rest is an essential part of the procedure. While times for rest have not been clearly defined in the literature, practical advice is to ask the patient to remain in the outpatient clinic for at least half an hour and, if necessary, to provide her with bed rest during this time. This diminishes the chance of a late-onset vasovagal reaction after the patient has been discharged.

Postprocedure Infection

Hysterosonography is a very safe procedure, provided that active infection has been ruled out. Antibiotics in the contrast fluid are not routinely recommended. The use of antibiotic prophylaxis has been recommended on an individual basis [27]; however, if active infection is ruled out, there is hardly any reason for such a prophylaxis. In a review of 1153 procedures, the incidence of peritonitis and fever after sonohysterography was reported to be about 1% [12]. It is worth remembering that the procedure is not very safe in immunocompromised patients undergoing infertility investigation, as one case reported a patient with psoriatic arthritis treated with TNF-α who developed life-threatening sepsis caused by group A streptococci [21].

Uterine Abnormalities

Uterine abnormalities that can be detected by saline hysterosonography are

- Uterine polyps
- Submucosal myomas
- Intrauterine adhesions
- Endometrial hyperplasia
- Postoperative uterine niche (isthmocele)
- Uterine malformations

Uterine Polyps and Submucosal Myomas

Uterine polyps and submucosal myomas are the most common findings in saline hysterosonography (Figures 5.4–5.7) (Video 5.2). Polyps are typically elongated and appear hyperechoic, in contrast to the

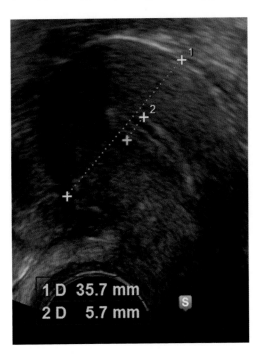

FIGURE 5.4   Normal endometrium.

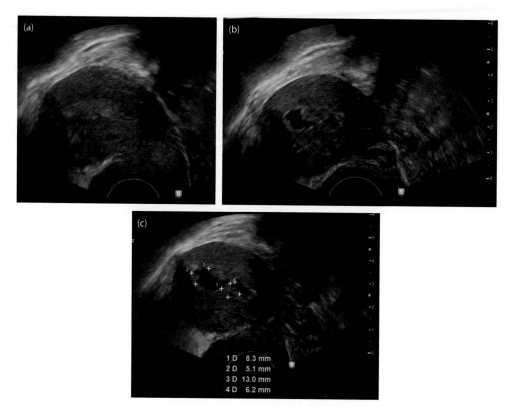

FIGURE 5.5 Ultrasound appearance of uterine polyposis (a) before hysterosonography, (b) at hysterosonography, and (c) with polyps measurements.

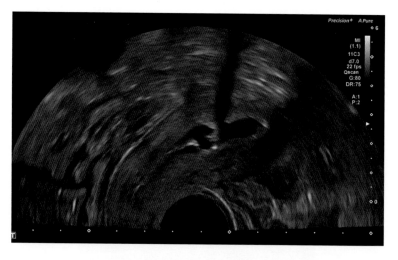

FIGURE 5.6 Ultrasound appearance of uterine polyp. (Courtesy of Arianna D'Angelo.)

hypoechoic spongy endometrium identified on transvaginal ultrasound during the proliferative phase of the menstrual cycle. Myomas are typically round and appear hypoechoic, isoechoic, or hyperechoic on transvaginal scans. In most cases, saline hysterosonography can easily differentiate polyps from submucosal myomas. Polyps are hyperechoic, while fibroid submucosal myomas have tissue characteristics similar to those of the myometrium or other myomas in the uterus. Furthermore, hysterosonography facilitates surgical planning by providing the exact location and depth within the myometrium.

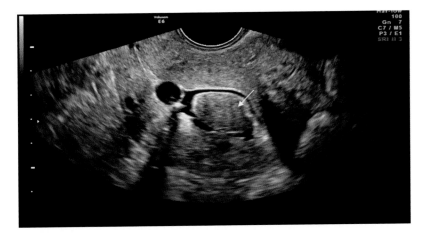

FIGURE 5.7 Submucous uterine myoma at ultrasound and saline hysterosonography. (Reproduced with permission from Seshadri et al. *Eur J Obstet Gynecol Reprod Biol.* 2015;185:66–73.)

VIDEO 5.2
Saline ultrasonography in a patient with multiple uterine polyps. (https://youtu.be/wPI0iWQrY48)

Saline hysterosonography for the detection of uterine polyps and submucosal myomas is usually compared to hysteroscopy, which is considered the gold standard in uterine cavity investigations. In a prospective evaluation of 65 women [29], hysterosonography had the same diagnostic accuracy as hysteroscopy and was markedly superior for polypoid lesions as compared with transvaginal sonography or x-ray HSG.

Two-dimensional and 3D saline hysterosonography were compared in another meta-analysis [30], in which both investigations were compared to hysteroscopy. Two-dimensional saline hysterosonography had high accuracy in detecting endometrial polyps and submucosal uterine myomas, with areas under the receiver-operated characteristic curve of 0.97 ± 0.02 and 0.97 ± 0.03, respectively.

Endometrial Hyperplasia

Endometrial hyperplasia is characterized by irregular, thickened, glandular, or heterogeneous endometrium with or without abnormal uterine bleeding. The ultrasonographic diagnosis is confirmed by histologic examination of an endometrial tissue sample. Saline hysterosonography has a diagnostic accuracy of 100%, as observed by Soares and colleagues [29].

Uterine Niche (Isthmocele)

The presence of a uterine scar defect following cesarean section is also known as a "niche" or "isthmocele." It is believed to originate in suboptimal surgical technique such as single-layer closing of the uterus, low cervical site of incision, and inadequate hemostasis [30] (Figures 5.8 and 5.9). An incompletely healed scar is a long-term complication of cesarean section and is associated with spotting at 6–12 months after the operation, dysmenorrhoea, chronic pelvic pain, dyspareunia, infertility, cesarean scar pregnancy, and

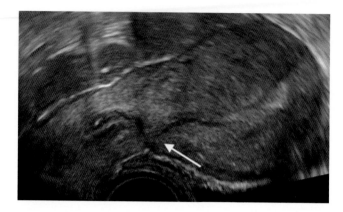

FIGURE 5.8   Suspected uterine niche in a woman who had a cesarean section several years before evaluation (arrow). Suspected defect is empty, endometrium is very thin, and sonohysterography is necessary for full assessment.

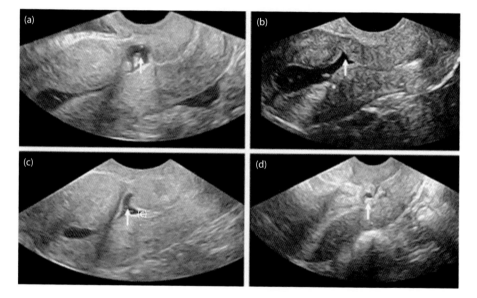

FIGURE 5.9   Visibility of uterine niche is greatly enhanced if liquid in the uterine cavity is present. Ultrasound scans showing the most common niche shapes: the semicircular niche (a), triangular niche (b), droplet-shaped niche (c), and inclusion cysts (d). (Reproduced with permission from Bij de Vaate AJ et al. *Ultrasound Obstet Gynecol.* 2011;37:93–9.)

uterine rupture [31]. Because of globally rising rates of cesarean deliveries, which have been reported to be 29%–30% in the United Kingdom and United States [32,33], up to 80% in China [34,35], and 80% in the private sector in Brazil [36], accurate detection of uterine niche ensures timely management of symptoms (Table 5.2).

TABLE 5.2

Etiology of Uterine Niche

- Low (cervical) location of the uterine incision during a cesarean section
- Incomplete closure of the uterine wall, due to single-layer, endometrial saving closure technique or use of locking sutures
- Surgical activities that may induce adhesion formation (i.e., nonclosure of peritoneum together with single-layer closure of uterine wall, inadequate hemostasis, applied sutures, use of adhesion barriers)
- Factors that possibly hamper normal wound healing and related angiogenesis

Note: For further information, see Vervoort AJ et al., *Hum Reprod.* 2015;30:2695–702.

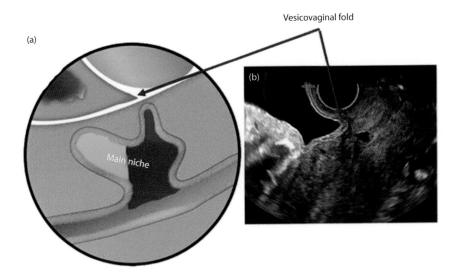

FIGURE 5.10 Main niche and vesicovaginal fold. (a) Red and green areas represent main niche, and blue area represents branch. (b) Green line indicates plica vesicouterina or uterovesical fold, while red line indicates vesicovaginal fold. (Reproduced with permission from Vervoort AJ et al. *Hum Reprod*. 2015;30:2695–702.)

Uterine niche can be diagnosed by ultrasound or hysteroscopy. Its ultrasound definition is the presence of a hypoechoic area within the myometrium of the lower uterine segment, reflecting a discontinuation of the myometrium at the site of a previous cesarean section, with myometrium indentations greater than or equal to 2 mm [31,37–39]. Criteria for evaluation of uterine niche were clarified in a Delphi consensus [40] (Figure 5.10). Niche length and depth, as well as residual and adjacent myometrial thickness, should be measured in the sagittal plane, while niche width should be measured in the transverse plane (Table 5.3).

Recently, the 3D technique and scoring classification system of uterine niche have been described [41]. This relies on the use of saline and standardized 3D imaging (Figure 5.11). It is worth noting that the authors prefer to perform this evaluation between the 17th and 25th days of the menstrual cycle, i.e., in the luteal phase. This necessitates the use of effective contraception but allows superior image quality.

TABLE 5.3

Uterine Niche Consensus Evaluation Criteria

Methods of measurement
- Endometrium should be ignored; niche measurements are based only on myometrium.
- Correct sagittal plane to perform niche measurement depends on the niche or niche branch itself (length, depth, or residual myometrium thickness).
- Transverse plane is used for only measuring the width of the niche.
- To measure uterine niche, there should be good visualization of lower uterine segment only; this applies to all uterine positions (anteversion, retroversion, or stretched).
- Position of transvaginal probe (in anterior or posterior fornix) affects correct plane for niche measurement.

Additional tools
- It is useful to vary pressure with the transvaginal probe in order to achieve the best plane for niche measurement.
- Doppler imaging can be useful to differentiate between uterine niche and other findings (hematomas, adenomyomas, adenomyosis, fibrotic tissue).

Gel/saline contrast sonography
- Useful in patients with uterine niche unless there is intrauterine fluid accumulation.
- No preference for either gel or saline or type of catheter.
- Best location of catheter is just in front of niche (caudal to its most distal part) or cranial to its most proximal part, at start of gel/saline contrast infusion, then pulling catheter slowly backward toward base of niche.

Source: Modified from Jordans IPM et al. *Ultrasound Obstet Gynecol*. 2019;53:107–15.

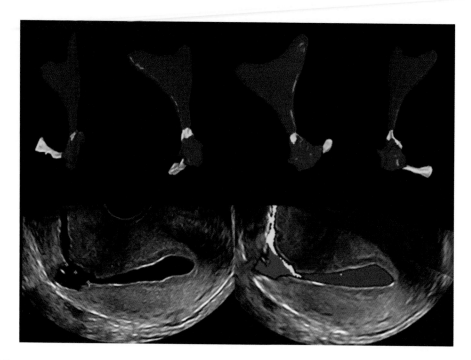

FIGURE 5.11 Volume estimation of uterine cavity (red), uterine niche (blue), and isthmus cavity with cervical canal (yellow) using three-dimensional saline contrast sonohysterography. The morphology of the niche may be clinically relevant, and potential future pregnancies should be monitored closely. (Modified with permission from Ludwin A et al. *Ultrasound Obstet Gynecol.* 2019;53[1]:139–43.)

Intrauterine Adhesions

Intrauterine adhesions are a complication of endometritis or pelvic inflammatory disease, and of repeated curettages of the uterine cavity. Other causes can include endometrial ablation and repeated uterine wall surgery, as well as incomplete surgical termination of pregnancy. The appearance of intrauterine adhesions at saline hysterosonography varies. They can be visualized as hyperechoic bands that stretch across the uterine cavity (Figure 5.12) or as liquid-filled pockets within the uterine cavity. In severe cases, they can even obliterate the whole uterine cavity.

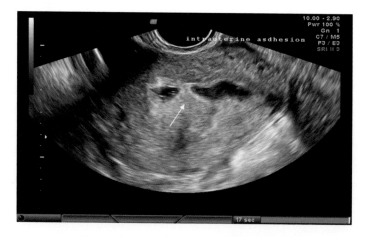

FIGURE 5.12 Intrauterine adhesions. (Reproduced with permission from Seshadri et al. *Eur J Obstet Gynecol Reprod Biol.* 2015;185:66–73.)

These lesions cannot be detected by transvaginal ultrasound [29]. Because the adhesions interfere with the normal elasticity of the uterine wall, hysterosonography can be painful for patients with intrauterine adhesions. Compared to the gold standard hysteroscopy, hysterosonography is less sensitive [29], with sensitivity of 75%, specificity of 93.4%, and positive predictive value of 43%. Three-dimensional ultrasonography might be more helpful in the evaluation of intrauterine adhesions as reported in a small study [42].

Uterine Malformations

Müllerian duct anomalies are found in up to 7% of infertile women [43,44]. In 2013, the three simultaneously used classifications of uterine malformations were merged into a new classification based on anatomy and embryological origin [45]. The joint work by the European Society of Human Reproduction and Embryology (ESHRE) and the European Society for Gynaecological Endoscopy (ESGE) recognizes the following main classes (Figure 5.13):

- U0, normal uterus
- U1, dysmorphic uterus: T-shaped and infantile-type uterus
- U2, septate uterus: the length of internal indentation (septum) is more than half (greater than 50%) of the uterine wall thickness; external contour (wall of fundus) is straight or with indentation less than half (less than 50%) of the thickness of the uterine wall
- U3, bicorporeal uterus: the indentation of fundus (external indentation) is more than half (greater than 50%) of the uterine wall thickness
- U4, hemi-uterus
- U5, aplastic uterus
- U6, for still unclassified cases

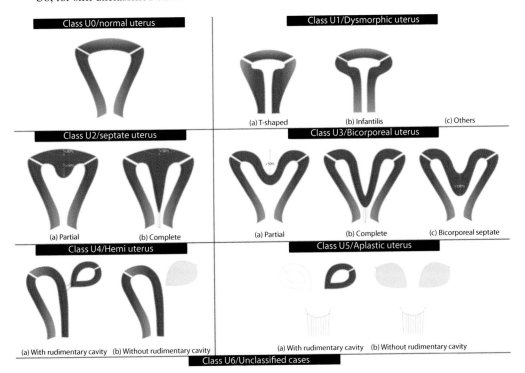

FIGURE 5.13 ESHRE/ESGE classification of uterine anomalies: schematic representation. (Reproduced from Grimbizis GF et al. *Hum Reprod.* 2013;28[8]:2032–44, under Open Access.)

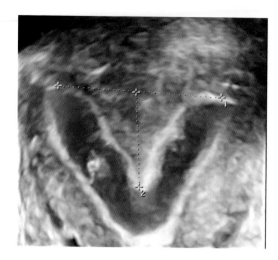

FIGURE 5.14 Septate uterus. (Reproduced with permission from Seshadri et al. *Eur J Obstet Gynecol Reprod Biol.* 2015;185:66–73.)

Arcuate uterus, a condition that is sometimes associated with subfertility [46,47], can be classified as either a normal or a dysmorphic uterus with minor deformity. The most common uterine anomalies of infertile women are those with septa of differing lengths. These are also the most common anomalies in patients with miscarriage (up to 18%) [48] (Figure 5.14).

For uterine malformations, saline hysterosonography has a high pooled sensitivity (0.85%, 95% confidence interval [CI]: 0.79–0.90) and specificity (1.00%, 95% CI 0.99–1.00), [49] and it is significantly more accurate than transvaginal ultrasonography or HSG [29].

The overall accuracy of saline hysterosonography is good (summary receiver operated characteristic curve $0.97+0.01$) [49]. A Cochrane analysis evaluated the use of 3D hysterosonography. The meta-analysis revealed no statistically significant differences between 2D and 3D saline hysterosonography. The authors concluded that margins of improvement for 3D are limited because 2D hysterosonography is already accurate.

Conclusion

In conclusion, it is relatively easy to master the technique of saline hysterosonography in an office setting. The method is accurate for detecting and properly diagnosing a wide range of uterine abnormalities and uterine cavity defects. Because 2D hysterosonography has high overall accuracy, 3D offers little advantage over 2D.

REFERENCES

1. Armstrong SC, Showell M, Stewart EA, Rebar RW, Vanderpoel S, and Farquhar CM. Baseline anatomical assessment of the uterus and ovaries in infertile women: A systematic review of the evidence on which assessment methods are the safest and most effective in terms of improving fertility outcomes. *Hum Reprod Update.* 2017;23(5):533–47.
2. Saunders RD, Shwayder JM, and Nakajima ST. Current methods of tubal patency assessment. *Fertil Steril.* 2011;95(7):2171–9.
3. Donald I, MacVicar J, and Brown TG. Investigation of abdominal masses by pulsed ultrasound. *Lancet.* 1958;1:1188–95.
4. Campbell S. A short history of sonography in obstetrics and gynaecology. *Facts Views Vis Obgyn.* 2013;5(3):213–29.
5. Nannini R, Chelo E, Branconi F, Tantini C, and Scarselli GF. Dynamic echohysteroscopy: A new diagnostic technique in the study of female infertility. *Acta Eur Fertil.* 1981;12(2):165–71.

6. Richman TS, Viscomi GN, deCherney A, Polan ML, and Alcebo LO. Fallopian tubal patency assessed by ultrasound following fluid injection. Work in progress. *Radiology.* 1984;152:507–10.

7. Deichert U, Schleif R, van de Sandt M, and Juhnke I. Transvaginal hysterosalpingo-contrast-sonography (Hy-Co-Sy) compared with conventional tubal diagnostics. *Hum Reprod.* 1989;4:418–24.

8. Papaioannou S, Afnan M, and Jafettas J. Tubal assessment tests: Still have not found what we are looking for. *Reprod Biomed Online.* 2007;15(4):376–82.

9. Savelli L, Pollastri P, Guerrini M et al. Tolerability, side effects, and complications of hysterosalpingocontrast sonography (HyCoSy). *Fertil Steril.* 2009;92(4):1481–6.

10. Koskas M, Mergui JL, Yazbeck C, Uzan S, and Nizard J. Office hysteroscopy for infertility: A series of 557 consecutive cases. *Obstet Gynecol Int.* 2010;2010:168096.

11. Sahu L, Tempe A, and Gupta S. Hysteroscopic evaluation in infertile patients: A prospective study. *Int J Reprod Contracept Obstet Gynecol.* 2012;1:37–41.

12. Dessole S, Farina M, Capobianco G, Nardelli GB, Ambrosini G, and Meloni GB. Determining the best catheter for sonohysterography. *Fertil Steril.* 2001;76(3):605–9.

13. Spieldoch RL, Winter TC, Schouweiler C, Ansay S, Evans MD, and Lindheim SR. Optimal catheter placement during sonohysterography: A randomized controlled trial comparing cervical to uterine placement. *Obstet Gynecol.* 2008;111(1):15–21.

14. Ahmadi F, Rashidy Z, Haghighi H, Hemat M, and ShamsiPour M. Uterine cavity assessment in infertile women: Sensitivity and specificity of three-dimensional HyCoSy versus hysteroscopy. *Iran J Reprod Med.* 2013;11:977–82.

15. Saunders RD, Nakajima ST, and Myers J. Experience improves performance of hysterosalpingo-contrast sonography (HyCoSy): A comprehensive and well-tolerated screening modality for the subfertile patient. *Clin Exp Obstet Gynecol.* 2013;40(2):203–9.

16. Gange SN, and Baum N. Verbal anesthesia: How and when to use it in urological procedures. *JOJ Urol Nephrol.* 2018;4(5). doi:10.19080/JOJUN.2018.04.555647

17. Opolskiene G, Radzvilaite S, Bartkeviciene D, Ramasauskaite D, Zakareviciene J, and Drasutiene G. Pain experience during saline-contrast sonohysterography differs between premenopausal and postmenopausal women. *J Clin Ultrasound.* 2016;44(5):267–71.

18. Marci R, Marcucci I, Marcucci AA et al. Hysterosalpingocontrast sonography (HyCoSy): Evaluation of the pain perception, side effects and complications. *BMC Med Imaging.* 2013;13:28.

19. Sladkevicius P, Ojha K, Campbell S, and Nargund G. Three-dimensional power Doppler imaging in the assessment of fallopian tube patency. *Ultrasound Obstet Gynecol.* 2000;16:644–7.

20. Socolov D, Boian I, Boiculese L, Tamba B, Anghelache-Lupascu I, and Socolov R. Comparison of the pain experienced by infertile women undergoing hysterosalpingo contrast sonography or radiographic hysterosalpingography. *Int J Gynaecol Obstet.* 2010;111(3):256–9.

21. Rodgers R, Ludlow J, Gee A, Ramsay P, and Benness C. Clinical case presentation: Life threatening group A sepsis secondary to HyCoSy. *Australas J Ultrasound Med.* 2014;17(3):131–3.

22. Jareethum R, Suksompong S, Petyim S, Prechapanich J, Laokirkkiat P, and Choavaratana R. Efficacy of mefenamic acid and hyoscine for pain relief during saline infusion sonohysterography in infertile women: A double blind randomized controlled trial. *Eur J Obstet Gynecol Reprod Biol.* 2011;155(2):193–8.

23. Moro F, Selvaggi L, Sagnella F et al. Could antispasmodic drug reduce pain during hysterosalpingo-contrast sonography (HyCoSy) in infertile patients? A randomized double-blind clinical trial *Ultrasound Obstet Gynecol* 2012;39(3):260–5.

24. Ludwin I, Ludwin A, Wiechec M et al. Accuracy of hysterosalpingo-foam sonography in comparison to hysterosalpingo-contrast sonography with air/saline and to laparoscopy with dye. *Hum Reprod.* 2017;32:758–69.

25. Yung SS, Lai SF, Lam MT et al. Randomized, controlled, double-blind trial of topical lidocaine gel and intrauterine lidocaine infusion for pain relief during saline contrast sonohysterography. *Ultrasound Obstet Gynecol.* 2016;47(1):17–21.

26. Guney M, Oral B, Bayhan G, and Mungan T. Intrauterine lidocaine infusion for pain relief during saline solution infusion sonohysterography: A randomized, controlled trial. *J Minim Invasive Gynecol.* 2007;14(3):304–10.

27. American College of Obstetricians and Gynecologists' Committee on Gynecologic Practice. Technology Assessment No. 12: Sonohysterography. *Obstet Gynecol.* 2016;128(2):e38–42.

28. Seshadri S, Khalil M, Osman A, Clough A, Jayaprakasan K, and Khalaf Y. The evolving role of saline infusion sonography (SIS) in infertility. *Eur J Obstet Gynecol Reprod Biol.* 2015;185:66–73.

29. Soares SR, Barbosa dos Reis MM, and Camargos AF. Diagnostic accuracy of sonohysterography, transvaginal sonography, and hysterosalpingography in patients with uterine cavity diseases. *Fertil Steril.* 2000;73(2):406–11.
30. Vervoort AJ, Uittenbogaard LB, Hehenkamp WJ, Brolmann HA, Mol BW, and Huirne JA. Why do niches develop in Caesarean uterine scars? Hypotheses on the aetiology of niche development. *Hum Reprod.* 2015;30:2695–702.
31. Bij de Vaate AJ, Brolmann HA, van der Voet LF, van der Slikke JW, Veersema S, and Huirne JA. Ultrasound evaluation of the Cesarean scar: Relation between a niche and postmenstrual spotting. *Ultrasound Obstet Gynecol.* 2011;37:93–9.
32. Betrán AP, Merialdi M, Lauer JA et al. Rates of caesarean section: Analysis of global, regional and national estimates. *Paediatr Perinat Epidemiol.* 2007;21:98–113.
33. Osterman MJ, and Martin JA. Primary cesarean delivery rates, by state: Results from the revised birth certificate, 2006–2012. *Natl Vital Stat Rep.* 2014;63:1–11.
34. Deng W, Klemetti R, Long Q et al. Cesarean section in Shanghai: Women's or healthcare provider's preferences? *BMC Pregnancy Childbirth.* 2014;14:285.
35. Feng XL, Wang Y, An L, and Ronsmans C. Cesarean section in the People's Republic of China: Current perspectives. *Int J Womens Health.* 2014;6:59–74.
36. Barros AJ, Santos IS, Matijasevich A et al. Patterns of deliveries in a Brazilian birth cohort: Almost universal cesarean sections for the better-off. *Rev Saude Publica.* 2011;45:635–43.
37. Naji O, Abdallah Y, Bij De Vaate AJ et al. Standardized approach for imaging and measuring Cesarean section scars using ultrasonography. *Ultrasound Obstet Gynecol.* 2012;39:252–9.
38. van der Voet LF, Vervoort AJ, Veersema S, BijdeVaate AJ, Brolmann HA, and Huirne JA. Minimally invasive therapy for gynaecological symptoms related to a niche in the caesarean scar: A systematic review. *BJOG* 2014;121:145–56.
39. Bij de Vaate AJ, van der Voet LF, Naji O et al. Prevalence, potential risk factors for development and symptoms related to the presence of uterine niches following Cesarean section: Systematic review. *Ultrasound Obstet Gynecol.* 2014;43:372–82.
40. Jordans IPM, de Leeuw R, Stegwee SI et al. Sonographic examination of uterine niche in non-pregnant women: A modified Delphi procedure. *Ultrasound Obstet Gynecol.* 2019;53:107–15.
41. Ludwin A, Martins WP, and Ludwin I. Evaluation of uterine niche by three-dimensional sonohysterography and volumetric quantification: Techniques and scoring classification system. *Ultrasound Obstet Gynecol.* 2019;53(1):139–43.
42. Sylvestre C, Child T, Tulandi T, and Tan S. A prospective study to evaluate the efficacy of two and three dimensional sonohysterography in women with intrauterine adhesions. *Fertil Steril.* 2003;79:1222–5.
43. Acién P. Incidence of Müllerian defects in fertile and infertile women. *Hum Reprod.* 1997;12(7):1372–6.
44. Saravelos SH, Cocksedge KA, and Li TC. Prevalence and diagnosis of congenital uterine anomalies in women with reproductive failure: A critical appraisal. *Hum Reprod Update.* 2008;14(5):415–29.
45. Grimbizis GF, Gordts S, Di Spiezio Sardo A et al. The ESHRE/ESGE consensus on the classification of female genital tract congenital anomalies. *Hum Reprod.* 2013;28(8):2032–44.
46. Tomazevic T, Ban-Frangez H, Ribic-Pucelj M, Premru-Srsen T, and Verderik I. Small uterine septum is an important risk variable for preterm birth. *Eur J Obstet Gynecol Reprod Biol.* 2007;135:154–7.
47. Gergolet M, Campo R, Verdenik I, Kenda Suster N, Gordts S, and Gianaroli L. No clinical relevance of the height of fundal indentation in subseptate or arcuate uterus: A prospective study. *RBM Online.* 2012;24:576–82.
48. Chan YY, Jayaprakasan K, Tan A, Thornton JG, Coomarasamy A, and Raine-Fenning N. Reproductive outcomes in women with congenital uterine anomalies: A systematic review. *Ultrasound Obstet Gynecol.* 2011;38:371–82.
49. Seshadri S, El-Toukhy T, Douiri A, Jayaprakasan K, and Khalaf Y. Diagnostic accuracy of saline infusion sonography in the evaluation of uterine cavity abnormalities prior to assisted reproductive techniques: A systematic review and meta-analyses. *Hum Reprod Update.* 2015;21(2):262–74.

6

Tubal Patency Assessment (Focusing on Hysterosalpingo-Contrast Sonography)

Zdravka Veleva

Introduction

The first recording of tubal patency test dates from 1849, when W.T. Smith treated intratubal adhesions using transcervical whalebone tubal catheterization [1]. Nowadays, clearly less invasive procedures are in place for tubal patency investigation.

Practical Advice

Tubal patency investigation constitutes a part of the investigation during saline hysterosonography. In order to indicate the assessment of the fallopian tubes by ultrasound, the term *hysterosalpingo-contrast sonography* (HyCoSy) is used. Chapter 5 detailed the typical way to perform the procedure as well as its contraindications (active infection, suspected malignancy, and conditions such as hydrosalpinx/pyosalpinx). This chapter focuses on the specific issues regarding the investigation of the fallopian tubes, which is carried out as part of fertility workup.

Through a catheter inserted in the cervical canal or in the uterine cavity, contrast media is injected into the uterus. From there, it flows into the fallopian tubes and ends in the pouch of Douglas, where it is reabsorbed by the peritoneum. For the purposes of HyCoSy, the use of a balloon catheter prevents the reflux of contrast medium back into the vagina, because it seals off the cervical canal during the procedure. Positioning is more effective and less painful if the balloon is placed in the upper part of the cervical canal or at the level of the internal os [2]. In this way, higher pressures can be attained within the uterus, and less contrast medium is needed.

During HyCoSy, the bright echoes generated by the contrast solution fill in the lumen of the fallopian tube and make it visible. The tube itself remains poorly identifiable. Fallopian tubes are evaluated one by one (Figure 6.1).

The sonographer should observe the following:

- The pressure needed to advance the contrast medium into the tube. When the patient has patent tubes and saline/air are used as contrast, it often seems that the contrast flows freely into the pouch of Douglas. However, in cases with fully blocked tubes, contrast solution cannot be further injected after filling the uterine cavity. This could be associated with strong pain. The sonographer should anticipate this outcome and proceed with care.
- Ideally, the whole length of the tube should be visualized, including its abdominal end, and the flow of contrast into the pouch of Douglas should also be seen. This will rule out malformations such as tubal diverticula or polyps or postinfectious dilated/blocked areas of the tube. However, due to the tortuous route of tubal lumen, this is not always easy, especially with two-dimensional (2D) ultrasound. Repositioning of the ultrasound probe is often necessary (Figure 6.2).

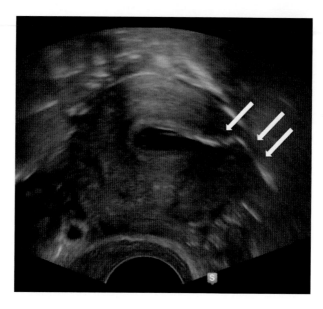

FIGURE 6.1 The interstitial and proximal parts of the fallopian tube during two-dimensional hysterosalpingo-contrast sonography with saline/air.

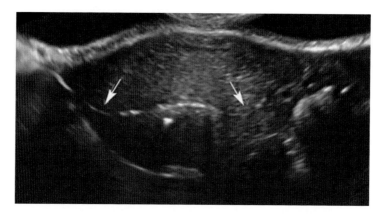

FIGURE 6.2 Hysterosalpingo-contrast sonography with saline/air. The narrow lumen of the fallopian tube is clearly seen.

- In case visualization of the entire tube is not possible, at least the flow of contrast into the pouch of Douglas should be noted. Care should be taken not to confuse flow from the right and from the left side, which might be challenging in patients with adhesions.

- Tubal spasm should be excluded in cases with suspected partial or complete tubal blockage. Tubal spasm is the temporary, reflectory occlusion of tubal lumen upon contact with the contrast liquid. It usually resolves after a couple of minutes and can be prevented by administration of an NSAID or spasmolytic medication before the procedure. Whenever the contrast solution does not seem to advance into the fallopian tubes, the operator should wait for 2–3 minutes and then resume the test. Alternatively, the test can be rescheduled to another day, and warmed contrast solution should be used. Little is known about tubal peristalsis in the absence of active investigation. However, a review on tubal evaluation in subfertility [3] revealed that pregnancy rates of women with tubal spasms undergoing expectant management are lower than those observed in fertile women. Laparoscopy is no longer considered the golden standard for tubal patency investigation because of its invasiveness. Its use as alternative to HyCoSy is limited to cases with another laparoscopy indication because the patient cannot provide feedback during general anesthesia.

Pain and Verbal Anesthesia

Direct correlation exists between pain during HyCoSy and tubal patency [4]. Performing the procedure in a calm, warm environment and having an assistant conduct verbal anesthesia can reduce significantly any discomfort experienced by the patient.

Contrast

The most widely used contrast is saline, which for the purposes of tubal evaluation should contain air. This is the cheapest and most globally accessible positive contrast agent used for ultrasound-based examination of tubal patency [5,6]. Air can be mixed with saline either by vigorously shaking the syringe or by injecting saline followed by air and then saline again. Other contrast media are clearly more expensive, but the benefit of using them is their higher viscosity and the longer time that they remain in the tubes—up to 5 minutes, compared with a few seconds with saline/air [7]. Results can be further improved by using color Doppler imaging or 3D/four-dimensional (4D) technology. However, use of Doppler is not recommended in cases where saline/air are used. Air bubbles create a lot of ultrasonographic noise, which makes tubal structures unidentifiable. For maximal comfort for the patient, the contrast solution can be warmed up to body temperature before investigation. Currently, there are no conclusive data showing that a warm solution prevents tubal spasm.

Contrast Solutions Other Than Saline Used in Hysterosalpingo-Contrast Sonography

Echovist and Levovist (Bayer Schering Pharma, Berlin, Germany) consist of galactose microparticles suspended either in galactose solution (Echovist) or in sterile water (Levovist). Just before use, these solutions are made by mixing and vigorously shaking the microparticles with the solvent. These solutions can remain in the reproductive tract for about 5–10 minutes and within 30 minutes completely dissolve in the body. They are contraindicated in patients with galactosemia.

ExEm gel and foam (GynaecologIQ, Delft, the Netherlands) were developed specifically for imaging the fallopian tubes [7]. The preparations consist of hydroxyethylcellulose, glycerol, and purified water and remain in the fallopian tubes for about 5 minutes. ExEm gel and foam have no known side effects.

Gelofusine (B. Braun Melsungen AG, Germany) is a solution of succinylated gelatin, which has been traditionally used as a volume expander in blood plasma replacement.

SonoVue (Bracco International BV, Amsterdam, the Netherlands) is based on stabilized sulfur hexafluoride microbubbles surrounded by a phospholipid shell with a mean size of 2.5 μm. Their saline suspension is also prepared just before examination.

Albunex (manufacturing discontinued) was a solution of air-filled albumin microspheres prepared from sonicated 5% human serum albumin.

Optison (GE Healthcare, Chicago, Illinois) is another human albumin–based contrast solution. It contains microspheres of heat-treated human albumin containing perflutren gas as the active substance. Because it is albumin-based, the solution is potentially allergenic.

Definity (Lantheus Medical Imaging Inc., Billerica, Massachusetts) is perflutren gas-filled lipid-coated microspheres.

See Videos 6.1 and 6.2.

VIDEO 6.1
HyCoSy with patent Fallopian tubes, example 1. (https://youtu.be/ECEAhwYrc0U)

VIDEO 6.2
HyCoSy with patent Fallopian tubes, example 2. (https://youtu.be/A_SOAPmgZ5I)

Expected Findings

The majority of patients will have patent tubes since the frequency of tubal occlusion has diminished due to the more aggressive treatment of nonspecific or chlamydial salpingitis. Reports from 1970 have indicated that as many as 60% of women with unexplained infertility had tubal occlusion as diagnosed by laparoscopy [8]. In 1977, 38.7% of women attending an infertility clinic were diagnosed with blocked tubes [9]. This trend continues to date. In Finland, the proportion of *in vitro fertilization/intracytoplasmic sperm injection* (IVF/ICSI) cycles performed for tubal factor infertility decreased from 21.4% in the year 2000 to only 5.1% in 2017 (Figure 6.3). Therefore, care should be taken when noting the patient's history regarding any pelvic inflammatory disease (PID) episodes and their medical care. Some guidelines on HyCoSy recommend the prophylactic administration of antibiotics in patients with history of PID/salpingitis [10]. An alternative approach is the active treatment of any genital infection before HyCoSy is performed. Tubal occlusion or altered position can also be suspected in patients with severe endometriosis, or in women with considerable pelvic adhesion of other origin.

Rare Fallopian Tube Findings

Most of these conditions can be diagnosed only by laparoscopy. It is worth remembering, however, that not all tubal blockages observed during saline HyCoSy are inflammatory in origin.

- *Unilateral absence of the fallopian tube and ovary*: This condition can be caused by adnexal torsion with subsequent reabsorption of necrotic tissue, or by a developmental complication such as a vascular incident causing regional ischemia, or Müllerian and mesonephric system development arrest [11]. A thorough investigation for urinary malformations should take place in these cases.

- *Unilateral partial absence of the fallopian tube*: A literature search by Nawroth et al. in 2006 [12] identified 18 patients with partial atresia of the fallopian tube. In 78% of cases, atresia was unilateral, with the rest of patients having partial atresia in both tubes. Unilateral absence of part of the tube was associated with uterine abnormalities (uni- or bicornuate uterus) in 22% of patients. The suspected mechanism of partial absence is either a congenital condition or a consequence of tubal torsion followed by necrosis and reabsorption of tubal tissue.

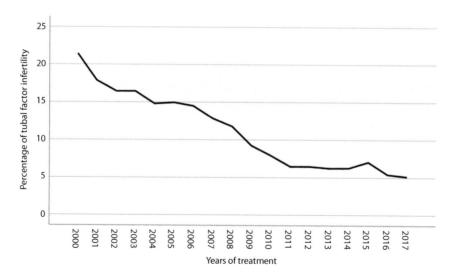

FIGURE 6.3   Percentage of tubal factor infertility in Finland as main indication in *in vitro* fertilization/intracytoplasmic sperm injection procedures. (Data from the LUMI database [Finnish IVF research database].)

- *Accessory tubal fimbrial ostium*: In a series of 1113 patients who underwent laparoscopic investigation for infertility, 21 (1.9%) had fallopian tube accessory ostium. Most of these women (90.5%, 19/21) were also diagnosed with pelvic endometriosis. An accessory ostium was identified in 19 (4.7%) of 403 women with endometriosis versus 2 (0.3%) of 710 women without endometriosis ($P = 0.001$) [13]. Surgery can be considered in such cases for good fertility outcome. In a study of 21 infertile women with accessory ostia, Cohen reported a live birth rate of 47% with natural conception after tubal microsurgery [14]. Using a laparoscopic approach in 18 patients with accessory ostium, Zheng et al. reported a clinical pregnancy rate of 66.7% with natural conception and intrauterine insemination [13].
- *Accessory fallopian tube*: Although the true prevalence of accessory fallopian tubes in the general population is unknown, a recent study found that its prevalence was as high as 1.9% in 1113 patients who underwent diagnostic laparoscopy for infertility workup [15]. It is believed that the lumen of most accessory fallopian tubes is obliterated at least partially.
- *Tubal polyps*: Seen on approximately 2% to 3% of radiologic hysterosalpingograms [16], interstitial fallopian tubal polyps might be related to infertility. Histologic studies of interstitial polyps reveal endometrial glands and stroma proliferating from endometrial foci in the fallopian tube [17].
- *Salpingitis isthmica nodosa*: This is a nodular thickening of the proximal (isthmic) part of the fallopian tube and is usually unilateral. A characteristic finding is multiple nodular diverticular spaces representing irregular benign extensions of tubal epithelium into the myosalpinx, mainly at the isthmic/proximal portion of the fallopian tube, though up to the proximal two-thirds may be affected. This condition has been associated with infertility and increased risk of tubal pregnancy. However, it cannot be evaluated reliably with 2D HyCoSy because of the naturally tortuous course of the fallopian tube [18].

Intraobserver Agreement on Findings

A literature search revealed that intraobserver agreement of HyCoSy findings has been investigated in only one study [19]. Twenty-nine patients underwent saline HyCoSy twice with a 3-month interval between examinations, and there was a good overall intraobserver agreement. Substantial agreement was found for bilateral ($\kappa = 0.66$) and right tubal patency and occlusion ($\kappa = 0.70$), but interestingly, for left tubal patency and occlusion, intraobserver agreement was found to be only fair ($\kappa = 0.37$). Possible explanations included a true difference in the prevalence in tubal occlusion between right and left in the population examined and the fact that investigation begins on the right side, which leaves limited time available for the left-side examination. The investigator's right-handedness was also included in the list of explanations.

Interobserver Agreement

A survey of MEDLINE did not return any evaluation of interobserver agreement on results from HyCoSy. A possible explanation may be the fact that the value of the method to clinical practice is clear, and there is no need to validate observations of different physicians.

Accuracy of HyCoSy

Findings of review articles are summarized in Table 6.1.

Hysterosalpingo-Contrast Sonography Compared to Laparoscopy

Laparoscopy with chromotubation (dye-laparoscopy) is considered the gold standard in tubal patency assessment. There is evidence that HyCoSy is as reliable as laparoscopy [22,24]. In a review article [20], HyCoSy was directly compared with laparoscopy and chromotubation in nine studies, representing 582

TABLE 6.1

Accuracy of Hysterosalpingo-Contrast Sonography (HyCoSy)

Study	Sensitivity (95% CI)	Specificity (95% CI)
Maheux-Lacroix et al., 2014 [20]		
HyCoSy versus HSG	0.92 (0.82–0.96)	0.95 (0.90–0.97)
HyCoSy versus LC	0.95 (0.78–0.99)	0.93 (0.89–0.96)
HyCoSy with Doppler versus LC	0.93 (0.84–0.98)	0.95 (0.92–0.98)
HyCoSy without Doppler versus LC	0.86 (0.74–0.93)	0.89 (0.83–0.93)
3D-HyCoSy versus LC	0.89 (0.77–0.95)	0.94 (0.86–0.98)
2D-HyCoSy versus LC	0.88 (0.80–0.94)	0.92 (0.87–0.95)
Saline versus LC	0.91 (0.92–0.96)	0.93 (0.88–0.96)
Other contrast media versus LC	0.87 (0.76–0.94)	0.92 (0.86–0.96)
Wang et al., 2016 [21]		
3D- and 4D-HyCoSy versus LC	0.92 (0.90–0.94)	0.92 (0.89–0.93)
Alcázar et al., 2016 [22]		
3D-HyCoSy versus LC or HSG	0.98 (0.91–1.00)	0.90 (0.93–0.95)
Ludwin et al., 2017 [23]		
2D HyCoSy with saline/air versus LC	0.93 (0.68–0.99)	0.86 (0.81–0.91)
2D/3D-HyFoSy versus LC	0.87 (0.60–0.98)	0.94 (0.90–0.97)
2D/3D-HDF HyFoSy versus LC	0.94 (0.73–1.00)	0.97 (0.94–0.99)

Abbreviations: CI, confidence interval; HDF, high-definition flow Doppler; HSG, x-ray hysterosalpingography; HyFoSy, hysterosalpingo-foam sonography; LC, laparoscopy with chromotubation.

women and 1055 tubes. Sensitivity was 0.95 (confidence interval [CI] 0.87–0.99) and specificity 0.93 (CI 0.89–0.96). In nearly all studies, HyCoSy was evaluated against laparoscopy and chromotubation.

Agreement between Different Modalities of HyCoSy

In Maheux-Lacroix's review of tubal patency assessment [20], diagnostic accuracy of HyCoSy was evaluated in 30 articles, of which 13 used saline as contrast, 15 used galactose particles (Echovist, Bayer Schering Pharma), and one used sulfur hexafluoride solution (SonoVue, Bracco International BV, Amsterdam, the Netherlands). In addition, 13 studies used Doppler flow as part of investigation, while in 5 articles, 3D probes were also used. Overall, the study investigated HyCoSy in 1551 women and 2740 tubes. Use of Doppler sonography compared with its nonuse had higher sensitivity and specificity, but the difference barely reached statistical significance ($P = 0.0497$). Estimates were also not statistically different when comparing 3D with 2D ($P = 0.7$) and saline/air with other contrasts ($P = 0.7$).

Choice of 3D or 4D ultrasound investigation was evaluated in another review article [21] that included 23 studies, including 1153 women with 2259 detected fallopian tubes. There were no differences in sensitivity and specificity between 3D and 4D ultrasound HyCoSy, or between contrast agents. Three-dimensional HyCoSy might offer improvement in image quality, because it allows visualization of the entire tube. By contrast, with 2D HyCoSy, the tortuous tubal structure often cannot be observed entirely in any scanning window [25]. Three-dimensional evaluation is faster [26], avoids difficult probe movements, and is less dependent on operator skill while allowing automation of the scanning process [25,27,28] (Figure 6.4). Four-dimensional evaluation also provides an evaluation of the dynamics of contrast flow and is particularly useful in identifying the morphology of the fallopian tubes among patients with myometrial venous reflux [29,30].

In a meticulous series of evaluations of 132 women/259 fallopian tubes, 2D/3D hysterosalpingo-foam sonography (HyFoSy) and 2D/3D-high-definition flow Doppler (HDF)-HyFoSy were compared with laparoscopy and chromotubation and with 2D saline/air HyCoSy [23]. The contrast agent used in HyFoSy was ExemFoam (GynaecologIQ, Delft, the Netherlands) that has been reported to have very high accuracy in comparison to laparoscopy and chromotubation [31]. Ludwin and colleagues observed the highest

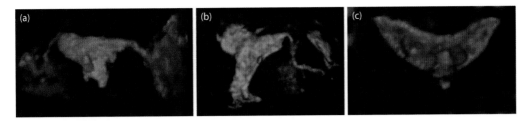

FIGURE 6.4 Automated three-dimensional coded contrast imaging hysterosalpingo-contrast sonography: reconstructed volumes of contrast medium in uterus and tubes in a case of bilateral tubal patency (a), and unilateral (b) and bilateral (c) tubal occlusion. (Reproduced with permission from Exacoustos C et al. *Ultrasound Obstet Gynecol.* 2013;41:328–35.)

diagnostic accuracy with 2D/3D-HDF-HyFoSy (96.9%), which was equal to the accuracy of laparoscopy with chromotubation [23]. Saline/air 2D-HyCoSy had an accuracy of 86.8%.

Since there is a multitude of hysterosonographic evaluation modalities, a simple guide was proposed by Ludwin and colleagues [23]. They recommend saline/air HyCoSy as a first-line examination because it is not expensive but at the same time has an excellent negative predictive value of 98%–99.5%. This means that if tubal patency is seen with saline/air HyCoSy, the method is accurate enough for diagnosing patent fallopian tubes. If, on the other hand, tubal occlusion is visible during saline/air injection, the authors concluded that another diagnostic method (HDF-foam HyCoSy or laparoscopy) might be necessary for the definitive diagnosis.

Saline HyCoSy Compared to Hysterosalpingography

The review of Maheux-Lacroix and colleagues observed similar diagnostic accuracy of HyCoSy and hysterosalpingography, with sensitivity of 0.92 (CI 0.82–0.96) and specificity of 0.95 (CI 0.90–0.97) [20]. Reported pain scores have shown either similarities in patient experiences and no difference in pain [30] or better tolerability in HyCoSy [33]. However, the advantages of ultrasound assessment are clear, as it allows simultaneous evaluation of the ovaries, myometrium, and pouch of Douglas, which can reveal important pathologic findings such as polycystic ovaries, ovarian cysts, myomas, or uterine anomalies [34]. Saline HyCoSy was associated with greater sensitivity and specificity for the detection of intrauterine pathologies, as mentioned in Chapter 5. Furthermore, by performing ultrasound examinations, one can avoid the use of ionizing radiation and the potentially allergenic iodinate contrast.

The costs of saline HyCoSy and hysterosalpingography can vary but are nonetheless considered similar [35]. The cost of HyCoSy can be further reduced by using air/saline as a medium rather than sonographic contrast media [36]. However, regardless of the contrast used, HyCoSy is the most cost-effective intervention because of the associated other benefits of ultrasound examination.

Benefit of HyCoSy

Although HyCoSy is considered a diagnostic and not a therapeutic procedure [37], there have been reports of pregnancies within a short time after the procedure. The possible beneficial effect of tubal flushing was first described in 1951 in a study of salpingograms [38], but the same possible mechanism of action applies to HyCoSy: contrast material passing through the fallopian tubes breaks and carries away small internal adhesions or stimulates in another way the function of the tube. Typically, pregnancies are reported in couples with otherwise unexplained infertility, and it is difficult to provide a good estimation of what their pregnancy rate would be without the procedure.

This issue was studied in a series of 180 couples with unexplained infertility of at least 1 year [39]. Of these, 40 patients (22.2%) became spontaneously pregnant within 6 months after HyCoSy. The mean time to conception was 75 days, but about half (45%) of pregnancies occurred within the first 30 days. In another follow-up of Australian patients, 50% of women who had no prior pregnancies at the time of HyCoSy became pregnant within 6 months after the procedure [40].

The latest Cochrane analysis on the effect of tubal flushing for subfertility analyzed treatments in 2494 women [41]. Patients who had tubal flushing with an oil-soluble contrast media had a higher rate of live birth and ongoing pregnancy than women who had no intervention, but in both cases, the evidence was of very low quality. However, it was estimated that this patient population would have a 17% chance of an ongoing pregnancy with expectant management but that the rate would increase to between 29% and 55% if they have tubal flushing with oil-soluble contrast media. Such an effect was not observed in patients who were treated with water-soluble contrast media, but again, the evidence was of very low quality. Until new evidence from larger studies emerges, we can conclude that HyCoSy for tubal patency is a diagnostic and not a therapeutic procedure [37].

Conclusion

In conclusion, HyCoSy is a powerful method for evaluating tubal patency, and it has already replaced laparoscopy with chromotubation as the method of choice. HyCoSy can be performed in the office together with an ultrasound examination of the uterus, ovaries, and other pelvic structures. Using 3D/4D technology, the method can be automated, and images can be stored for further reference.

REFERENCES

1. Smith W. The new uterine operation. On a new method of treating sterility by the removal of obstruction of the fallopian tubes. *Lancet.* 1849;53(1342):603–5.
2. Dessole S, Farina M, Capobianco G, Nardelli GB, Ambrosini G, and Meloni GB. Determining the best catheter for sonohysterography. *Fertil Steril.* 2001;76(3):605–9.
3. Papaioannou S, Afnan M, and Jafettas J. Tubal assessment tests: Still have not found what we are looking for. *Reprod Biomed Online.* 2007;15(4):376–82.
4. Moro F, Selvaggi L, Sagnella F et al. Could antispasmodic drug reduce pain during hysterosalpingo-contrast sonography (HyCoSy) in infertile patients? A randomized double-blind clinical trial. *Ultrasound Obstet Gynecol.* 2012;39(3):260–5.
5. Jeanty P, Besnard S, Arnold A, Turner C, and Crum P. Air-contrast sonohysterography as a first step assessment of tubal patency. *J Ultrasound Med.* 2000;19:519–27.
6. Sladkevičius P, Zannoni L, and Valentin L. B-flow ultrasound facilitates visualization of contrast medium during hysterosalpingo-contrast sonography. *Ultrasound Obstet Gynecol.* 2014;44:221–7.
7. Exalto N, Stappers C, van Raamsdonk LAM, and Emanuel MH. Gel instillation sonohysterography: First experience with a new technique. *Fertil Steril.* 2007;87:152–5.
8. Peterson EP, and Behrman SJ. Laparoscopy of the infertile patient. *Obstet Gynecol.* 1970;36, 363–7.
9. Templeton AA, and Kerr MG. An assessment of laparoscopy as the primary investigation in the subfertile female. *Br J Obstet Gynaecol.* 1977;84:760–2.
10. American College of Obstetricians and Gynecologists' Committee on Gynecologic Practice. Technology Assessment No. 12: Sonohysterography. *Obstet Gynecol.* 2016;128(2):e38–42.
11. Pabuccu E, Kahraman K, Taskın S, and Atabekoglu C. Unilateral absence of fallopian tube and ovary in an infertile patient. *Fertil Steril.* 2011;96(1):e55–7.
12. Nawroth F, Nugent W, and Ludwig M. Congenital partial atresia of the Fallopian tube. *Reprod Biomed Online.* 2006;12(2):205–8.
13. Zheng X, Han H, and Guan J. Clinical features of fallopian tube accessory ostium and outcomes after laparoscopic treatment. *Int J Gynaecol Obstet.* 2015;129(3):260–3.
14. Cohen BM. Microsurgical reconstruction of congenital tubal anomalies. *Microsurgery.* 1987;8(2):68–77.
15. Rottenstreich M, Smorgick N, Pansky M, and Vaknin Z. Isolated torsion of accessory fallopian tube in a young adolescent. *J Pediatr Adolesc Gynecol.* 2016;29:e57–58.
16. Brubaker LM, and Clark RL. Effects of interstitial fallopian tube polyps on isthmic tubal diameter. *Fertil Steril.* 2005;83(5):1500–3.
17. Gillett WR. The surgical treatment of tubal polyps. *Aust N Z J Obstet Gynaecol.* 1989;29:79–81.
18. Gardner D, Weissman A, Howles CM, and Shoham Z. *Textbook of Assisted Reproductive Techniques,* 4th ed. Vol. 2: clinical perspectives. Boca Raton, FL: CRC Press, Taylor & Francis Group; 2012. p. 234.
19. Tekay A, Spalding H, Martikainen H, and Jouppila P. Agreement between two successive transvaginal salpingosonography assessments of tubal patency. *Acta Obstet Gynecol Scand.* 1997;76:572–5.

20. Maheux-Lacroix S, Boutin A, Moore L et al. Hysterosalpingosonography for diagnosing tubal occlusion in subfertile women: A systematic review with meta-analysis. *Hum Reprod.* 2014;29(5):953–63.

21. Wang Y, and Qian L. Three- or four-dimensional hysterosalpingo contrast sonography for diagnosing tubal patency in infertile females: A systematic review with meta-analysis. *Br J Radiol.* 2016;89:20151013.

22. Alcázar JL, Martinez-Astorquiza Corral T, Orozco R, Dominguez-Piriz J, Juez L, and Errasti T. Three-dimensional hysterosalpingo-contrast-sonography for the assessment of tubal patency in women with infertility: A systematic review with meta-analysis. *Gynecol Obstet Invest.* 2016;81(4):289–95.

23. Ludwin I, Ludwin A, Wiechec M et al. Accuracy of hysterosalpingo-foam sonography in comparison to hysterosalpingo-contrast sonography with air/saline and to laparoscopy with dye. *Hum Reprod.* 2017;32:758–69.

24. Lo Monte G, Capobianco G, Piva I, Caserta D, Dessole S, and Marci R. Hysterosalpingo contrast sonography (HyCoSy): Let's make the point! *Arch Gynecol Obstet.* 2015;291(1):19–30.

25. Exacoustos C, Di Giovanni A, Szabolcs B, Binder-Reisinger H, Gabardi C, and Arduini D. Automated sonographic tubal patency evaluation with three-dimensional coded contrast imaging (CCI) during hysterosalpingocontrast sonography (HyCoSy). *Ultrasound Obstet Gynecol.* 2009;34:609–12.

26. Sladkevicius P, Ojha K, Campbell S, and Nargund G. Three-dimensional power Doppler imaging in the assessment of fallopian tube patency. *Ultrasound Obstet Gynecol.* 2000;16:644–7.

27. Watrelot A, Hamilton J, and Grudzinskas JG. Advances in the assessment of the uterus and fallopian tube function. *Best Pract Res Clin Obstet Gynaecol.* 2003;17:187–209.

28. Exacoustos C, Di Giovanni A, Szabolcs B et al. Automated three-dimensional coded contrast imaging hysterosalpingo-contrast sonography: Feasibility in office tubal patency testing. *Ultrasound Obstet Gynecol.* 2013;41:328–35.

29. Zhang Y, Li R, Tian HY, Lv LH, and Zhou YJ. Evaluation of tubal patency with transvaginal four-dimensional hysterosalpingo-contrast sonography. *Hebei Med J.* 2014;36:2654–56.

30. Zhang XX, Chen JY, Zhang J et al. Assessment of transvaginal four-dimensional hysterosalpingo-contrast sonography in evaluation of fallopian tube patency. *J Pract Obstetrics Gynecol.* 2015;31:198–201.

31. Van Schoubroeck D, Van den Bosch T, Meuleman C, Tomassetti C, D'Hooghe T, and Timmerman D. The use of a new gel foam for the evaluation of tubal patency. *Gynecol Obstet Invest.* 2013;75:152–6.

32. Ayida G, Kennedy S, Barlow D, and Chamberlain P. A comparison of patient tolerance of hysterosalpingo-contrast sonography (HyCoSy) with Echovist-200 and X-ray hysterosalpingography for outpatient investigation of infertile women. *Ultrasound Obstet Gynecol.* 1996;7:201–4.

33. Ahinko-Hakamaa K, Huhtala H, and Tinkanen H. The validity of air and saline hysterosalpingo-contrast sonography in tubal patency investigation before insemination treatment. *Eur J Obstet Gynecol Reprod Biol.* 2007;132:83–7.

34. Saunders RD, Shwayder JM, and Nakajima ST. Current methods of tubal patency assessment. *Fertil Steril.* 2011;95:2171–9.

35. Lim CP, Hasafa Z, Bhattacharya S, and Maheshwari A. Should a hysterosalpingogram be a first-line investigation to diagnose female tubal subfertility in the modern subfertility workup? *Hum Reprod.* 2011;26(5):967–71.

36. Spalding H, Martikainen H, Tekay A, and Jouppila P. A randomized study comparing air to Echovist as a contrast medium in the assessment of tubal patency in infertile women using transvaginal salpingosonography. *Hum Reprod.* 1997;12:2461–4.

37. Armstrong SC, Showell M, Stewart EA, Rebar RW, Vanderpoel S, and Farquhar CM. Baseline anatomical assessment of the uterus and ovaries in infertile women: A systematic review of the evidence on which assessment methods are the safest and most effective in terms of improving fertility outcomes. *Hum Reprod Update.* 2017;23(5):533–47.

38. Weir WC, and Weir DR. Therapeutic value of salpingograms in infertility. *Fertil Steril.* 1951;2(6):514–22.

39. Giugliano E, Cagnazzo E, Bazzan E, Patella A, and Marci R. Hysterosalpingo-contrast sonography: Is possible to quantify the therapeutic effect of a diagnostic test? *Clin Exp Reprod Med.* 2012;39(4):161–5.

40. Tanaka K, Chua J, Cincotta R, Ballard EL, and Duncombe G. Hysterosalpingo-foam sonography (HyFoSy): Tolerability, safety and the occurrence of pregnancy post-procedure. *Aust N Z J Obstet Gynaecol.* 2018;58(1):114–8.

41. Mohiyiddeen L, Hardiman A, Fitzgerald C et al. Tubal flushing for subfertility. *Cochrane Database Syst Rev.* 2015;(5):CD003718.

7

The Infertile Male

Thoraya Ammar, C. Jason Wilkins, Dean C.Y. Huang, and Paul S. Sidhu

Introduction

A multicenter study by the World Health Organization concluded that in 20% of infertile couples, a cause was predominantly male and in 27%, abnormalities were found in both partners. A male factor is likely to be present in approximately 50% of infertile couples [1]. A physical cause for male infertility can only be identified in a third of patients, with testicular failure (primary hypogonadism) being the most common identifiable cause [2]. In the remainder, idiopathic male infertility is the umbrella term to describe the condition. Ultrasound is the initial and often only imaging modality for the investigation of the infertile male and plays a vital role in identifying potentially correctable causes of infertility, especially congenital anomalies and disorders that obstruct sperm transport.

Initial Evaluation

The first step in screening for male infertility involves a simple semen analysis that is compared against the World Health Organization (WHO) 2010 reference values [1]. If this is abnormal, the process is repeated. Unless azoospermia or severe oligospermia is identified, when an earlier repeat test is indicated, the test should be repeated after 3 months, when a full spermatozoa cycle is completed. If male subfertility is established from the semen analysis, urological referral is commenced. Thereafter, evaluation of the infertile male starts with a detailed history and physical examination, followed by laboratory tests and imaging in order to identify any correctable causes. Laboratory tests routinely include follicle-stimulating hormone (FSH) and testosterone levels with further tests carried out when needed. Male infertility may be divided into pretesticular, testicular, and post-testicular in origin. There are many causes of male infertility—congenital or acquired urogenital abnormalities, genetic and immunological factors, endocrine disturbances, genital tract infections, and erectile dysfunction—and they are summarized in Table 7.1 [3].

Imaging Evaluation

Imaging in male infertility is essential in establishing the cause and may also be used in determining and guiding the best method for treating the female partner, such as image-guided sperm aspiration from the epididymis or seminiferous tubules, allowing *in vitro* fertilization or intracytoplasmic sperm injection [3].

Ultrasound holds its place as the primary imaging modality in investigating the causes of male infertility. Essentially it remains noninvasive, safe, widely available, and effective in detecting and identifying causes relevant to male infertility. Magnetic resonance imaging (MRI) is useful in problem-solving. Imaging-guided interventions, such as fluoroscopic-guided testicular vein embolization in the management of testicular varicoceles, offer additional therapeutic options.

TABLE 7.1

Causes of Male Infertility

Pretesticular causes	Acquired endocrinopathies
	Genetic endocrinopathies
	Disorders of production or secretion of gonadotrophin-releasing hormone
	Disorders of luteinizing hormone, follicle-stimulating hormone, and androgen function
Testicular causes	Varicocele
	Genetics
	Cryptorchidism
	Exposure to gonadotoxins
Post-testicular causes	Obstruction
	Immunologic infertility
	Disorders of ejaculation
	Erectile dysfunction

Ultrasound Techniques

Ultrasound is almost always the initial imaging investigation in male infertility, with superb resolution aiding accurate assessment. Testicular morphology, patency of the efferent ducts, and prostatic anomalies are readily identified, and erectile dysfunction may be ascertained with a dynamic investigation. Ultrasound techniques used are as follows:

1. Scrotal ultrasound B-mode, color and spectral Doppler ultrasound, and contrast-enhanced ultrasound (termed *multiparametric ultrasound*) [4]
2. Transrectal ultrasound
3. B-Mode and dynamic color and spectral Doppler ultrasound of the penis

Scrotal Ultrasound

The European Association of Urology deem scrotal ultrasound a mandatory examination in the investigation of the infertile male. Scrotal ultrasound is excellent for the initial evaluation of the scrotum and can directly demonstrate abnormalities within the testis and the peritesticular structures.

B-Mode Ultrasound

This is performed with a high-frequency (7–12 MHz) linear-array transducer with adequate length for longitudinal measurement of the testes. The patient is examined in a supine position. The testes should be examined in orthogonal transverse and longitudinal planes and with color flow Doppler evaluation and volume measurements performed routinely (Figure 7.1) [3].

On ultrasound examination of the normal testis, the testis has a homogeneous echotexture with the head of the epididymis related to the upper pole of the testis measuring 5–12 mm and the body of the epididymis running along the posterior aspect of the testis measuring 2–4 mm in depth. The epididymis is slightly hyperechoic in relation to the testis. The rete testis when seen runs in the mediastinum testis and is hypoechoic compared to the rest of the testis.

During ultrasound examination of the scrotum, the following should be evaluated:

- Testicular volume

  Volume measurement is usually calculated as length × height × width × 0.523. A total volume (both testes) of greater than 30 mL and a single testicular volume of 12–30 mL is generally considered normal [5] (Figure 7.1).

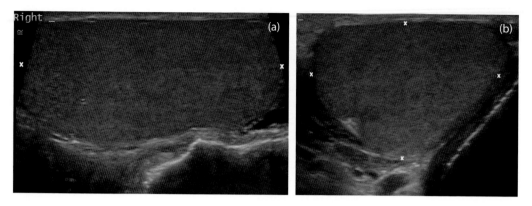

FIGURE 7.1 Normal ultrasound images of the testis in longitudinal (a) and transverse (b), with measurement cursors in position (x-x). Volume measurement is calculated as length × height × width × 0.523 giving a volume of approximately 18mL for a single testis.

- The rete testis and epididymis for dilatation and enlargement due to obstruction
- The presence and morphology of the vas deferens
- The presence of varicoceles, and grading of reflux
- Intra- or extratesticular lesions
- The presence of microlithiasis

Doppler and Contrast-Enhanced Ultrasound

Some studies have suggested a correlation between testicular perfusion and spermatogenesis. Doppler ultrasound has been used for guiding testicular sperm extraction and improves the success of this procedure [6]. There is growing evidence that contrast-enhanced ultrasound (CEUS) improves testicular sperm extraction by targeting vascularized areas and highlighting the microvasculature within the testicle. Areas of hyperperfusion most likely contain spermatozoa residuals [7]. In this technique, 4.8 mL SonoVue (Bracco SpA, Milan) contrast agent is administered as an intravenous bolus, which will last up to 3 minutes, allowing time for extraction. This dose can be repeated if required after 5 minutes.

CEUS and elastography are now established techniques in the characterization of scrotal lesions, initially detected on B-mode ultrasound [8,9]. This is generally thought not part of the routine ultrasound examination but mainly used as a problem-solving technique once a lesion is identified on B-mode ultrasound.

Transrectal Ultrasound

Transrectal ultrasound (TRUS) enables high-resolution imaging of the prostate, seminal vesicles, and vas deferens and is the modality of choice in identifying features of obstructive azoospermia.

Features visualized on TRUS suggestive of obstruction are

- Seminal vesicle enlargement
- Midline prostatic cysts
- Ejaculatory duct calcification associated with obstruction

The patient is positioned in a left lateral decubitus position. A high-frequency endorectal transducer covered with a condom should be used. Systematic evaluation of the terminal vas deferens, seminal vesicles, ejaculatory duct, and prostate are carried out in the axial and sagittal planes (Figure 7.2). TRUS is also used to guide prostatic cyst aspiration.

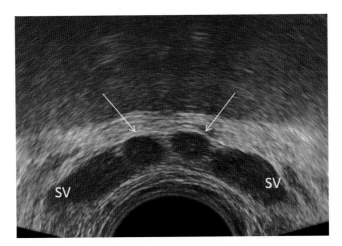

FIGURE 7.2   Normal ultrasonographic anatomy of the seminal vesicles (SV) and vasa deferens (VD). Transverse image from transrectal ultrasound, obtained superior to the prostate, shows symmetric seminal vesicles and more medially located vas deferens (arrows).

B-Mode and Dynamic Color Doppler Ultrasound of the Penis

Penile ultrasound is performed for the evaluation of erectile dysfunction [10,11]. Ultrasound of the penis should include

1. Assessment for structural penile abnormalities of the paired corpora cavernosa and the corpora spongiosum
2. Arterial assessment to identify problems with arterial inflow on the spectral Doppler waveform trace
3. Venous leakage inferred by assessing the arterial Doppler signal, to identify any malfunction of the venous occlusive mechanism [12]

In order to reduce any anxiety associated with this examination, the procedure should be conducted in a quiet and private room. Of note, there is a small risk of priapism following intracavernosal injection of the stimulant used, commonly prostaglandin E1 (PGE1), which is injected to elicit an erectile response. This should be included in the consent process, and patients should be advised to return to the emergency department if the erection persists for longer than 4 hours.

B-mode ultrasound is initially performed to exclude structural abnormalities such as fibrotic plaque disease, focal cavernosal fibrosis or calcification, and tunica albuginea disruption [13]. Intracavernosal injection of PGE1 is then undertaken. In our practice, the transducer is placed on the ventral surface of the base of the penis and a color and spectral Doppler ultrasound of the cavernosal artery is undertaken. Some authors prefer to image the penis from the dorsal aspect [7].

It is important to undertake angle correction to allow for accurate velocity measurements. The peak systolic and end diastolic velocities are assessed every 5 minutes after the administration of PGE1 for up to 30 minutes [2]. In normal erections, the peak systolic velocity is more than 35 cm s^{-1}, and the end diastolic velocity (EDV) is negative or close to 0 cm s^{-1} [7]. Although complete reversal of EDV is not always observed, in our experience with young patients, EDV reversal is the rule if an adequate grade of erection is achieved (Figure 7.3).

Magnetic Resonance Imaging Techniques

MRI is useful for both detection and characterization of prostatic cysts if seen on a TRUS as well as evaluation of the vas, seminal vesicles, and ejaculatory ducts (Figure 7.4).

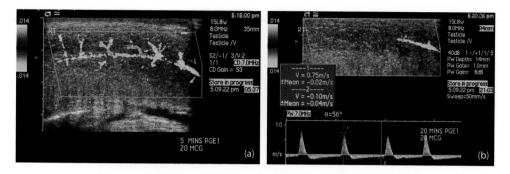

FIGURE 7.3 Ultrasound evaluation of a normal cavernosal artery response after intracavernosal injection of prostaglandin E1 (a). Reversal of end diastolic velocity is demonstrated (b).

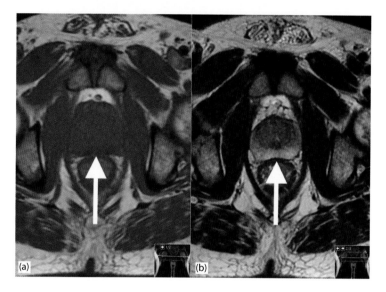

FIGURE 7.4 Normal T1 (a) and T2 (b) axial magnetic resonance images through the prostate (arrow).

Causes of Male Infertility and Their Ultrasound Imaging Findings

Normal spermatogenesis is a crucial prerequisite for achieving male fertility. In order to achieve normal spermatogenesis, successful storage and maturation of the sperm within the epididymis, normal sperm transport, and normal accessory gland function are essential.

Urogenital tract abnormalities causing infertility can be subdivided into obstructive azoospermia (OA) and nonobstructive azoospermia (NOA). Obstructive azoospermia is less frequent than NOA and represents only 15%–20% of cases of azoospermia. OA manifests due to blockage of sperm transport or due to abnormalities of the epididymis, vas deferens, or ejaculatory duct. NOA results from defective sperm production by the testicles.

The importance in differentiating these entities and correctly identifying the cause is that OA may be amenable to surgical correction.

Obstructive Azoospermia

Imaging is directed at a mechanical reason for the obstruction, and evaluation of the entire tract from the testis to the distal ductal system is essential. In patients with OA, testicular ultrasound is often abnormal. Almost

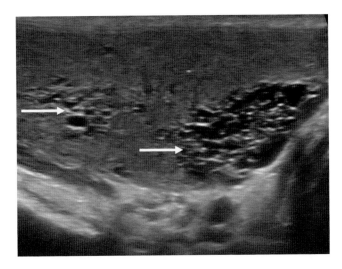

FIGURE 7.5 Heterogeneous testis with ectasia of the rete testis (arrows) in keeping with long-standing obstruction.

all patients with OA have an abnormal epididymis on B-mode ultrasound. The epididymal abnormalities include tubular ectasia of the epididymal head, tapering of the epididymal tail, absence of the epididymis, and presence of heterogeneous mass along the epididymal course, possibly a tumor such as a benign adenomatoid lesion, or a focal area of chronic infection (Figure 7.5). Testicular volume tends to be preserved in OA [14].

Although B-mode ultrasound is a useful preliminary test in diagnosing OA and differentiating it from NOA, TRUS is the modality of choice for assessing the actual cause of OA. A scrotal ultrasound finding suggesting OA is usually followed by a TRUS with the aim of differentiating proximal from distal obstruction. Vasoepididymostomy may be offered to patients with proximal obstruction. In those with distal obstruction, TRUS and/or MRI will define whether urogenital cysts are present, and if so, they can be aspirated under ultrasound guidance, though the results are often short lived. Ultrasound-guided aspiration for sperm harvesting is also possible. If no cysts are identified, then transurethral resection of the ejaculatory ducts can be performed on the assumption there is distal duct abnormality causing obstruction.

Using TRUS, a systematic evaluation of the terminal vas deferens, seminal vesicles, ejaculatory ducts, and prostate can be carried out in both axial and sagittal planes (Figure 7.6).

Obstruction may occur at any level in the reproductive tract from the epididymis proximally to the ejaculatory duct distally. At each of these levels, obstructive causes can be categorized into congenital and acquired (Table 7.2). The level of obstruction has direct relevance to the possible treatment of correctable causes, with proximal obstruction being amenable to vasoepididymostomy, while distal obstruction is often treated by transurethral resection of the ejaculatory ducts (TURED).

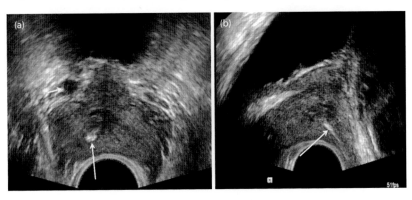

FIGURE 7.6 Transrectal ultrasound axial (a) and sagittal (b), demonstrating calcification within the ejaculatory duct (long arrows) with dilatation of the vas deferens proximally (short arrow).

TABLE 7.2

Classification of Obstructive Azoospermia

Classification	Conditions
Epididymal Obstruction	
Congenital	Idiopathic epididymal obstruction
Acquired	Postinfective (epididymitis)
	Postsurgical (epididymal cysts)
Vas Deferens Obstruction	
Congenital	Congenital absence of the vas deferens
Acquired	Postvasectomy
	Postsurgical (hernia, scrotal surgery)
Ejaculatory Duct Obstruction	
Congenital	Prostatic cysts (Müllerian cysts)
Acquired	Postsurgical (bladder neck surgery)
	Postinfective

Epididymal Obstruction

Infection is a common cause of obstruction anywhere along the course of the male reproductive tract, especially the epididymis (Figure 7.7). Acute gonococcal or subacute chlamydial infections can lead to scarring and subsequent obstruction (Figure 7.8). Iatrogenic epididymal obstruction may be sustained after surgical removal of an epididymal cyst.

Epididymal obstruction is treated surgically. Vasoepididymostomy is a microsurgical technique where the epididymis is anastomosed to the vas bypassing the level of obstruction. Pregnancy can be achieved by 20%–40% of patients after vasoepididymostomy without using assisted reproductive techniques [9].

Vas Deferens Obstruction

Vasectomy is the most common cause of vasal obstruction. The postvasectomy epididymis has a characteristic dilated inhomogeneous appearance on ultrasound described as ectasia of the epididymis (Figure 7.9). About 2%–8% of patients request reversal of vasectomy. Although vasectomy reversal is technically possible, prolonged obstruction secondary to vasectomy is associated with testicular fibrosis

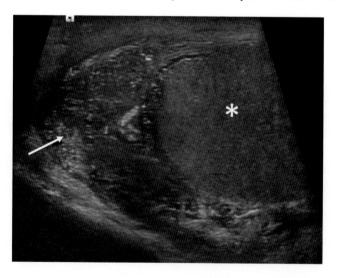

FIGURE 7.7   Scrotal ultrasound demonstrating thickening and enlargement of the epididymal head (arrow) in infective epididymitis; testis as shown (*).

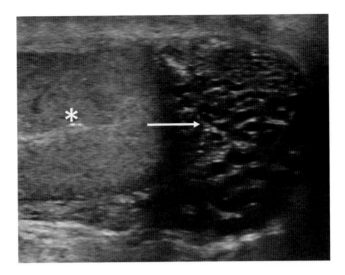

FIGURE 7.8 Longitudinal scan demonstrating a small testis (*) and focal dilatation of the epididymis (arrow) in keeping with chronic obstruction secondary to infection.

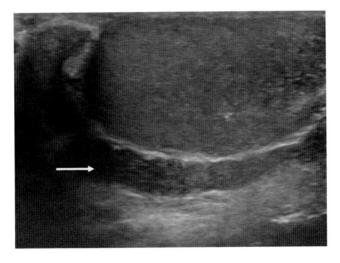

FIGURE 7.9 Longitudinal ultrasound demonstrating a dilated inhomogeneous epididymis (arrow) characteristic of the postvasectomy appearance.

and impairment of germ cell function. Therefore, reduced fertility may persist following reversal. Other acquired causes include inguinal hernia, scrotal sac surgery, and chronic infection (Figure 7.10).

The most common cause of congenital vas deferens obstruction is congenital bilateral absence of the vas deferens (CBAVD). CBAVD is seen in 2% of male patients being investigated for infertility. Up to 82% of patients with CBAVD have at least one mutation within the cystic fibrosis gene [15]; therefore, patients with CBAVD must be considered for cystic fibrosis screening and genetic counseling prior to sperm retrieval/intracytoplasmic sperm injection (ICSI) treatment given the possibility of conceiving offspring with cystic fibrosis [16].

In patients with CBAVD, scrotal ultrasound demonstrates dilatation of the efferent ducts with the epididymis stopping abruptly at the junction of the body and tail beyond which no vas deferens is seen. TRUS of the caudal junction of the vas deferens and the seminal vesicles shows absence of the ampulla of the vas deferens [17]. CBAVD is nearly always associated with abnormalities of the seminal vesicle and ejaculatory duct [18,19]. Vas deferens agenesis is known to be associated with renal anomalies

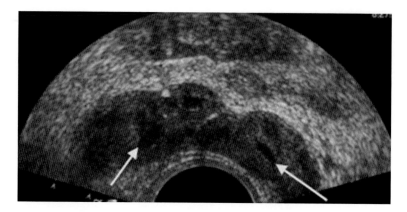

FIGURE 7.10   Bilateral thickening dilatation of the vas deferens (arrows) on transrectal ultrasound in keeping with vesiculitis.

including agenesis, cross-fused ectopia, and ectopic pelvic location. In view of this, renal ultrasound is recommended when agenesis of the vas deferens is diagnosed.

In a similar fashion to epididymal obstruction, vas deferens obstruction may also be amenable to microsurgical reconstruction [20].

Ejaculatory Duct Obstruction

Ejaculatory duct obstruction (EDO) is relatively uncommon, with the incidence of complete bilateral EDO reported as less than 1% in infertile men [21].

Congenital causes of ejaculatory duct obstruction include duct atresia or stenosis as well as compression by midline prostatic cystic lesions, for example, cysts of the prostatic utricle (previously named Müllerian duct cysts), cystic dilatation of the prostatic utricle (PU), and ejaculatory duct cysts [22]. Cystic obstruction of the ejaculatory tracts is usually congenital.

Cysts and Cystic Dilatation of the Prostatic Utricle

PU cysts and cystic dilatation of the PU are both midline anomalies. PU cysts and cystic dilatation of the PU may be difficult to distinguish on TRUS, as they both appear as spherical cystic structures within the midline of the prostate. However, PU cysts may grow above the prostate and are prone to hemorrhage; therefore, distinction from cystic dilatation of the PU can be made on the bases of the cyst size and contents. MRI is a useful technique for characterization of these cysts (Figure 7.11).

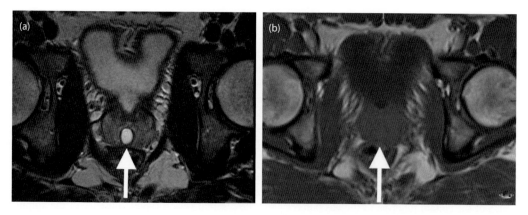

FIGURE 7.11   A midline cyst lying within the prostatic utricle (arrow). This returns high signal intensity on the T2-weighted images (a), and low signal on the T1-weighted images (b), in keeping with cystic dilatation of the prostatic utricle.

Ejaculatory Duct Cysts

Ejaculatory duct cysts are far less common than PU cysts or cystic dilatation of the PU [23]. Ejaculatory duct cysts are midline or paramedial prostatic cysts derived from the Wolffian duct and urogenital sinus, into which the ejaculatory ducts empty; therefore, these cysts will contain spermatozoa. Confirmation of the diagnosis of an ejaculatory duct cyst can be obtained by demonstrating spermatozoa from cyst fluid on TRUS aspiration. They can become large and may extend beyond the prostate [24]. Although large cysts can be aspirated transrectally under ultrasound guidance, the recurrence is high, and results are often short lived [24].

Acquired causes include calculi in the distal ejaculatory ducts at the level of the ampulla, which may be associated with dilatation of the proximal duct and evidence of obstruction [18]. Iatrogenic causes include surgery to the base of the bladder and infections acquired postcatheterization [2].

Despite the low overall incidence of ejaculatory duct obstruction, correct diagnosis is important, as it can be treated by transurethral resection of the ejaculatory duct. This is followed by the appearance of spermatozoa in the ejaculate in approximately 50%–73% of cases with a 25% pregnancy rate [20].

Nonobstructive Azoospermia

Nonobstructive azoospermia can be divided into

1. Testicular abnormalities
2. Varicoceles
3. Primary testicular tumors

Testicular Abnormalities

Cryptorchidism

The term *cryptorchidism* is derived from the Greek words *kryptos* meaning "hidden" and *orchis* meaning "testis." Cryptorchidism is the most common congenital abnormality of the male urogenital tract at birth. The failure of testicular descent into the cooler environment of the scrotal sac is thought to impair spermatogenesis and predispose to malignancy. In men with bilateral cryptorchidism, the rate of paternity is approximately 50%, but unilateral cryptorchidism results in little, if any, impairment of fertility [2].

Scrotal ultrasound confirms the clinical diagnosis of cryptorchidism by demonstrating the absence of the testis within the scrotal sac. As most undescended testes are located within the inguinal canal, ultrasound may also directly visualize the testis in this location (Figure 7.12). Either abdominal computed tomography (CT) or MRI evaluation is useful in cases where the undescended testis is not identified with ultrasound, as the testis may lie within the abdomen.

Testicular Atrophy

Testicular atrophy is associated with reduced spermatogenesis and a reduction in fertility. Atrophy may occur following previous inflammation, with liver cirrhosis, with estrogen treatment, with hypopituitary disorders, and normally with aging. On ultrasound, there is a global reduction in the volume of the testis (Figure 7.13). A decrease in both testicular reflectivity and vascularity are common findings. The epididymis usually appears normal [5].

Orchitis and Epididymo-Orchitis

Infection and inflammation of the genital tract are considered the most frequent causes of reduced male fertility, without conclusive epidemiology data [25]. Clinical and pathological evidence exists to support the concept that chronic testicular inflammatory conditions disrupt spermatogenesis and irreversibly alter the number and quality of spermatozoa [25]. Chronic epididymitis and epididymo-orchitis can also result

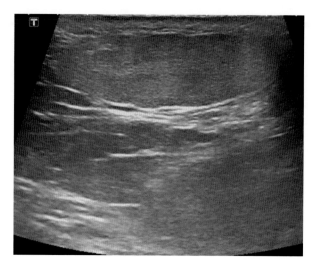

FIGURE 7.12   Ultrasound image of the groin in a patient with undescended testis demonstrates an isoechoic, small testis in keeping a normal undescended testis.

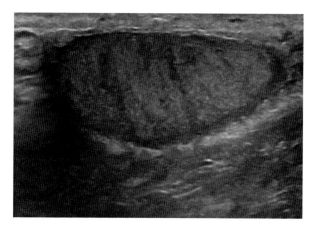

FIGURE 7.13   Scrotal ultrasound image demonstrating global reduction in volume with global heterogeneity of the testis.

in testicular atrophy, and epididymitis may result in post-inflammatory epididymal obstruction causing obstructive azoospermia.

A range of organisms including *Neiserria gonorrhoea* and *Chlamydia trachomatis* are implicated in acute epididymo-orchitis. Less frequent causes such as mumps and sarcoidosis tend to cause bilateral changes [26]. Early diagnosis and appropriate management of epididymo-orchitis are important, as early therapeutic intervention may prevent loss of fertility. B-mode ultrasound findings of epididymo-orchitis include testicular enlargement and heterogeneity of echo-texture associated with an enlarged hypoechoic or hyperechoic epididymis. Doppler ultrasound shows increased blood flow to both testis and epididymis (Figure 7.14).

Varicocele

A varicocele is an abnormal venous dilatation of the pampiniform venous plexus, which may lead to symptoms of pain and discomfort, failure of ipsilateral testicular growth and development, and possibly reduced fertility. A varicocele is a common finding in approximately 20% of adolescents and adult men, and in up to 40% of infertile patients [27]. The direct connection between varicocele and infertility is not clear. There is weak evidence to suggest that in men with a varicocele and unexplained subfertility, treatment may improve the chances of a spontaneous pregnancy, with some studies reporting an

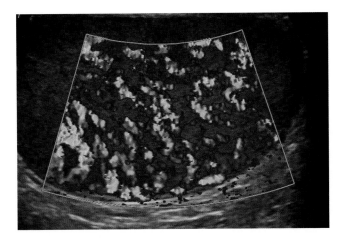

FIGURE 7.14 Longitudinal ultrasound image of orchitis demonstrating heterogeneous echotexture, testicular enlargement, and increased color Doppler flow.

improvement in spermatozoa quality post-treatment [27]. The American Urological Association and the American Society of Reproductive Medicine still recommend varicocele repair for patients with palpable varicoceles and an abnormal semen parameter.

Diagnosis of a varicocele is made on clinical examination and is usually confirmed by ultrasound. On B-mode ultrasound imaging, a varicocele is seen as serpiginous tubules posterior to the testis and may extend to the inferior pole of the testis with at least two or three veins of the pampiniform plexus measuring greater than 2–3 mm in diameter (Figure 7.15). Color Doppler ultrasound is a routine component of the examination as identification of flow reversal on Valsalva improves diagnostic accuracy. The degree of venous reflux during the Valsalva maneuver may be graded grades 1–5 by the Sarteschi classification, one of the most commonly used systems [28,29]:

Grade 1

- No evidence of scrotal varicosities
- Prolonged reflux in inguinal vessels only during Valsalva

Grade 2
- Small varicosities reaching superior pole of testis, increasing in diameter during Valsalva
- Positive venous reflux in supratesticular region only during Valsalva

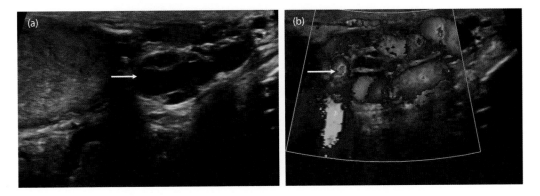

FIGURE 7.15 On B-mode ultrasound imaging, a varicocele is seen as serpiginous tubules posterior to the testis (arrow, a). Color Doppler ultrasound confirms flow within varicocele (arrow, b).

Grade 3

- Enlarged veins near inferior pole of testis in standing position
- Positive reflux only during Valsalva

Grade 4

- Enlarged vessels in supine position
- Dilatation increases in upright position and during Valsalva
- Enhancement of reflux during Valsalva
- Reduced testicular size may be present

Grade 5

- Venous dilatation in the supine position
- Basal venous reflux not altering substantially in standing position or during Valsalva

Treatment may be surgical or radiological with similar rates of success and of recurrence.

Primary Testicular Tumors

Men with infertility have an increased risk of testicular cancer, even after excluding the common risk factors for testicular cancer and infertility, such as a history of undescended testes and chromosomal aberrations.

Similarly, patients presenting with a primary testicular tumor often have decreased semen quality and reduced fertility that appear to be specific for germ cell tumors—that is, seminomas and teratomas [2]. Ultrasound is sensitive for the detection of testicular lesions. Ultrasound techniques such as color Doppler ultrasound (CDUS) (Figure 7.16), CEUS, and tissue elastography (TE), in conjunction with B-mode imaging, can be used for characterization of testicular lesions, and although they do not always provide a definitive diagnosis, they may help differentiate benign from malignant lesions. Features of testicular malignancy are varied. Most but not all tumors are homogeneous and of low reflectivity when compared with the surrounding testicular parenchyma, with increased vascularity on CDUS and enhancement on CEUS. Elastography is an ultrasound modality that maps the elastic properties and stiffness of soft tissue, the stiffer or harder a lesion, the more likely it is to be malignant.

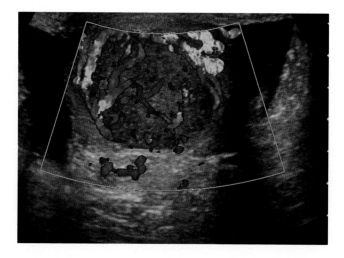

FIGURE 7.16   Longitudinal ultrasound image of a testicular mass demonstrating increased color Doppler flow within it. This was a histologically proven seminoma.

As testicular cancer usually affects young men, the preservation of semen prior to therapy (either surgery or radiotherapy) is an important consideration, and semen cryopreservation may be indicated.

Pretesticular Infertility

This is referred to as hypogonadotropic hypogonadism and is due to extragonadal endocrine disruption. This may be due to adrenal, pituitary, or hypothalamic disorders. Ultrasound's role in pretesticular infertility is limited to demonstrating a small testicular size, which can aid the diagnosis when combined with hormonal indices and abnormal semen parameters.

Conclusion

The investigation of infertile male patients is essential in order to identify potentially treatable causes of infertility and to guide therapy. A key element in the pathway is separation of nonobstructive from obstructive azoospermia. Scrotal ultrasound is sensitive in differentiating OA from NOA, with further modalities such as TRUS and MRI defining levels of obstruction and often the cause in cases of OA. Scrotal ultrasound findings may prompt treatment of varicocele, testicular maldescent, or tumor.

REFERENCES

1. *WHO Laboratory Manual for the Examination and Processing of Human Semen.* 5th ed. Geneva, Switzerland: World Health Organization; 2010.
2. Edey AJ, and Sidhu PS. Male infertility: Role of imaging in the diagnosis and management. *Imaging.* 2008;20:139–46.
3. Ammar T, Sidhu PS, and Wilkins CJ. Male infertility: The role of imaging in diagnosis and management. *Br J Radiol.* 2012;85:S59–68.
4. Sidhu PS. Multiparametric ultrasound (MPUS) imaging: Terminology describing the many aspects of ultrasonography. *Ultraschall in Med.* 2015;36:315–7.
5. Sidhu PS. Diseases of the testis and epididymis. In: Baxter GM, Sidhu PS, eds. *Ultrasound of the Urogenital System.* Stuttgart, Germany: Thieme; 2006, pp. 153–80.
6. Zhang S, Du J, Tian R, Xie S, Li F, and Li Z. Assessment of the use of contrast enhanced ultrasound in guiding microdissection testicular sperm extraction in nonobstructive azoospermia. *BMC Urol.* 2018;18:48.
7. Patel DV, Halls J, and Patel U. Investigation of erectile dysfunction. *Br J Radiol.* 2012;85(Spec Issue 1):S69–78.
8. Sidhu PS, Cantisani V, Dietrich CF et al. The EFSUMB Guidelines and Recommendations for the Clinical Practice of Contrast-Enhanced Ultrasound (CEUS) in Non-Hepatic Applications: Update 2017 (Long Version). *Ultraschall in Med.* 2018;39:e2–e44.
9. Sâftoiu A, Gilja OH, Sidhu PS et al. The EFSUMB Guidelines and Recommendations for the Clinical Practice of Elastography in Non-Hepatic Applications: Update 2018. *Ultraschall in Med.* 2019;40(4):425–53.
10. Wilkins CJ, Sriprasad S, and Sidhu PS. Colour Doppler ultrasound of the penis. *Clin Radiol.* 2003;58:514–23.
11. Wilkins CJ, and Sidhu PS. Diseases of the penis with functional evaluation. In: Baxter GM, Sidhu PS, eds. *Ultrasound of the Urogenital System.* Stuttgart, Germany: Thieme; 2006, pp. 181–92.
12. Halls J, Bydawell G, and Patel U. Erectile dysfunction: The role of penile Doppler ultrasound in diagnosis. *Abdom Imaging.* 2009;34:712–25.
13. Chavhan GB, Parra DA, Mann A, and Navarro OM. Normal Doppler spectral waveforms of major pediatric vessels: Specific patterns. *Radiographics.* 2008;28:691–706.
14. Liu J, Wang Z, Li M, Zhou M, and Zhan W. Differential diagnostic value of obstructive and nonobstructive azoospermia by scrotal ultrasound. *Ultrasound Q.* 2017;33(4).

15. Donat R, McNeill AS, Fitzpatrick DR, and Hargreave TB. The incidence of cystic fibrosis gene mutations with congenital bilateral absence of the vas deferens in Scotland. *Br J Urol.* 1997;79:74–7.

16. de Souza DAS, Faucz FR, Pereira-Ferrari L, Sotomaior VS, and Raskin S. Congenital bilateral absence of the vas deferens as an atypical form of cystic fibrosis: Reproductive implications and genetic counseling. *Andrology.* 2018;6(1):127–35.

17. Cornud F, Amar E, Hamida K, Thiounn N, Helenon O, and Moreau JF. Imaging in male hypofertility and impotence. *Br J Urol.* 2000;86:153–63.

18. Kuligowska E, and Fenlon HM. Transrectal US in male infertility: Spectrum of findings and role in patient care. *Radiology.* 1998;207:173–81.

19. Hendry WF. Disorders of ejaculation: Congenital, acquired and functional. *Br J Urol.* 1998;82:331–41.

20. Report on management of obstructive azoospermia. *Fertil Steril.* 2006;86(5 suppl):S259–63.

21. Jarow JP, Espeland MA, and Lipschultz LI. Evaluation of the azoospermic patient. *J Urol.* 1989;142:62–5.

22. Kurpisz M, Havryluk A, Nakonechnyj A, Chopyak V, and Kamieniczna M. Cryptorchidism and long-term consequences. *Reprod Biol.* 2010;10(1):19–35.

23. Stewart VR, and Sidhu PS. The testis: The unusual, the rare and the bizarre. *Clin Radiol.* 2007;62:289–302.

24. Weidner W, Pilatz A, and Altinkilic B. Andrologie: Varikozele. *Der Urologe.* 2010;49(1):163–5.

25. Dogra VS, Gottlieb RH, Oka M, and Rubens DJ. Sonography of the scrotum. *Radiology.* 2003;227(1):18–36.

26. Schuppe HC, Meinhardt A, Allam JP, Bergmann M, Weidner W, and Haidl G. Chronic orchitis: A neglected cause of male infertility? *Andrologia.* 2008;40(2):84–91.

27. Kohn TP, Kohn JR, and Pastuszak AW. Varicocelectomy before assisted reproductive technology: Are outcomes improved? *Fertil Steril.* 2017;108(3):385–91.

28. Sarteschi M, Paoli R, Bianchini M, and Menchini Fabris GF. Lo studio del varicocele con eco-color-Doppler. *Giornale Italiano di Ultrasonologia.* 1993;4:43–9.

29. Freeman SJ, Bertolotto M, Richenberg J et al. Ultrasound evaluation of varicoceles: Guidelines and Recommendations of the European Society of Urogenital Radiology Scrotal and Penile Imaging Working Group (ESUR-SPIWG) for detection, classification and grading. *European Radiology.* 2019;30:11–25.

8

Ultrasonographic Monitoring of Follicle Growth in Controlled Ovarian Hyperstimulation

Arianna D'Angelo

Introduction

Ovulation occurs in the menstrual cycle when a selected mature follicle breaks and releases a viable and competent oocyte from the ovary. It is commonly divided into three phases [1].

Follicular phase occurs at the beginning of each cycle, when a group of the most mature follicles (also known as "antral follicles") are recruited. This phase usually lasts 6–8 days. During this phase, the follicles most sensitive to follicle-stimulating hormone (FSH) undergo further development, producing estradiol (E2) and inhibin B while the remaining follicles become atretic. This phase is followed by the ovulatory phase that occurs in midcycle. The E2 produced by the dominant follicle triggers through a positive feedback mechanism the massive release of the luteinizing hormone (LH) by the pituitary gland. The LH surge triggers ovulation within 34–38 hours. The wall of the preovulatory follicle is broken, and the oocyte is rapidly released. In the last phase known as the luteal phase, the corpus luteum secretes both E2 and progesterone, resulting in a negative feedback mechanism that suppresses the FSH release until the next menstruation. The fall in the level of circulating progesterone causes menstruation in the absence of fertilization, embryo implantation, and human chorionic gonadotropin (hCG) secretion. This physiological process is described in Figure 8.1.

During assisted reproduction treatments (ARTs), more follicles are going to be needed; hence, different protocols for superovulation are used. The standard protocol involves the use of a gonadotropin-releasing hormone analog agonist (GnRH-a) to downregulate the pituitary gland to prevent premature ovulation followed by daily superovulation injections of gonadotropins (Gn). The antagonist protocol involves the use of the superovulation drugs (Gn) from the beginning of the menstrual cycle. When the leading follicle reaches 12–14 mm, the GnRH analog antagonist is started to avoid premature luteinization while all follicles reach maturation. The short protocol involves the use of superovulation drugs (Gn) and GnRH-a from the beginning of the menstrual cycle (days 1–3) until all follicles reach maturation. Ovulation is then triggered by using hCG (recombinant or urinary) simulating LH activity, 36 hours before the egg's retrieval. The different phases of the menstrual cycle and the superovulation cycle can be monitored by USS. It is very important for successful outcomes that the USS monitoring is performed accurately.

Follicular Ultrasound Monitoring

Controlled ovarian hyperstimulation (COH) is achieved by daily subcutaneous injections of recombinant or urinary gonadotropins (Gn). The dose is individualized, and the aim is to recruit 5–15 follicles. USS is used to assess the number and average diameter of the developing follicles for timing of egg retrieval. The estimated pregnancy rate per cycle using standard COH is approximately 30% [2], but when using minimal ovarian stimulation, the pregnancy rate per cycle is lower, approximately 10% [3]. This is why the accuracy of follicular ultrasound monitoring is very important for the ultimate outcome. In addition, ovaries might overrespond to the stimulation protocol, causing ovarian hyperstimulation syndrome

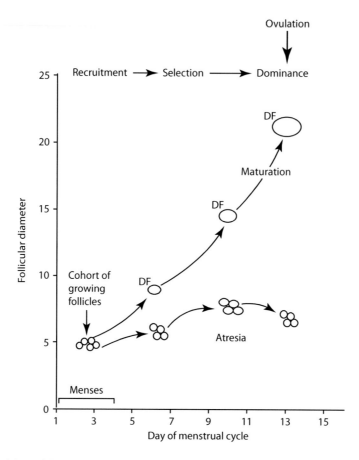

FIGURE 8.1 Physiology of the natural cycle.

(OHSS), which can be a life-threatening condition [4], and hence, the importance of having a reliable and secure tool to monitor superovulation. Martins et al. [5] performed a literature search up to April 2013 for randomized controlled trials (RCTs) on this topic. Studies that compared different methods for monitoring COH, including ultrasound assessment of follicles (alone or combined with hormonal assessment), in at least one group were included in the meta-analysis. The objective of the meta-analysis was to evaluate the efficacy and safety of monitoring COH using ultrasonography. Of the 1515 records found, only six studies fulfilled the inclusion criteria and were analyzed.

The authors concluded that monitoring COH only with ultrasonography is unlikely to make any difference in the chances of achieving a clinical pregnancy and in the number of oocytes retrieved compared to monitoring with ultrasonography and hormonal assessment. Moreover, they suggest the need for more studies on this topic.

This conclusion was reiterated by Vandekerckhove et al. [6] by showing in a nonrandomized, comparative prospective study (416 patients) that adding serum E2 measurements to ultrasound monitoring did not change the number of mature oocytes collected in *in vitro* fertilization (IVF)/intracytoplasmic sperm injection (ICSI) treatments. They compared the outcome of IVF/ICSI in two parallel control groups. Group one used combined monitoring (ultrasound plus serum E2 monitoring), and group two used only ultrasound monitoring. The average difference in the number of mature oocytes between the groups was −0.4 (95% confidence interval [CI]: −1.7 to 1). However, the conclusion was that still larger studies are required to confirm these findings.

A Cochrane review published in 2008 [7] concluded that there is no evidence from randomized trials to support cycle monitoring by ultrasound plus serum estradiol as more efficacious than cycle monitoring by ultrasound only on outcomes of live birth and pregnancy rates. However, these conclusions were drawn based on two studies out of 1119 potential reports. This highlights the difficulties in designing and performing a large well-designed RCT that reports on live birth rates and pregnancy, with economic evaluation of the COHts involved and the views of the women undergoing cycle monitoring.

In the opinion of the author, until such a trial is performed, cycle monitoring by transvaginal ultrasound plus serum E2 may need to be retained as a precautionary good practice point and for prevention of OHSS.

Different Measurement Techniques

The mean rate of follicular growth is linear at approximately 1.5 mm per day [8]. The diameter of a follicle can be measured in one, two, or three directions. Several studies have shown that measuring a follicle in three directions correlates well with follicular volume [9,10]. However, it can be very time consuming to perform three measurements in a busy fertility clinic, so it is common practice to perform only two perpendicular measurements of the largest diameter.

Duijkersa et al. [11] investigated the differences in the mean follicular diameter when the follicle was measured in one, two, or three directions, respectively. They explored whether measurements in two or three directions gave additional information compared to measurements in one or two directions. They enrolled 36 volunteers (mean age 28 years old). Assessments were carried out in a pretreatment cycle. Transvaginal ultrasonography was performed every other day from the first day of the cycle onward until ovulation was observed. Two experienced investigators performed all measurements. At first, the follicle was visualized in the sagittal plane, and the two perpendicular diameters were measured in the largest plane. Then, the probe was turned approximately 90° to visualize the follicle in the coronal plane. Again, the largest diameter and the diameter perpendicular to the first were measured. The mean diameter in three directions was calculated as the mean of two diameters in the sagittal plane and the largest diameter in the coronal plane. The differences in follicular diameter between measurement in one and two directions and between one and three directions were statistically significant ($P < 0.0001$); the difference between two and three directions was not statistically significant. The mean difference and the standard deviation of the difference increased with the follicular diameter when measurements in one and two or three directions were compared.

So, the conclusion was that even though three-directional measurement of a follicle is most accurate, measuring in three directions is more time consuming and may be rather difficult if a large number of follicles is present in the ovary. The margin of error when comparing measurement in one and two directions and one and three directions was 1.2 mm, which is rather small. However, the mean difference increased with the size of the follicle, which could result in planning an inappropriate time for the egg retrieval procedure.

Two pitfalls of the study was that it was performed on unstimulated cycles, and their conclusion cannot be applied with confidence to multifollicular ovaries, as images of the follicles are distorted by the large number of follicles. In addition, the standard way to measure follicles to get a mean diameter should be the measurements in three orthogonal planes: caudocephalic, anteroposterior, and right to left. Measuring the largest diameter in the coronal plane could simply be replicating one of the other diameters.

A more recent article proposed to study follicular measurement and number in two-dimensional (2D)/three-dimensional (3D) sonography [12]. The main difference between 3D and 2D sonography is that skilled and experienced sonographers create their own 3D impressions of the organ of interest when they scan in 2D. In contrast, 3D sonography uses special computer software to render a 3D image of the examined organ and to project a multiplanar view on the screen. Using conventional 2D sonography, the operator rotates the transvaginal probe gradually to scan each ovary, identifies each follicle, and then measures its dimensions. This sonographic method is time consuming and could be uncomfortable for the patient. In contrast, a 3D study requires only a single clear view of each ovary while the probe captures the sonographic data, and the ovarian follicles are counted offline at a later time.

In this study, the same patient group was examined to assess the correlation of ovarian follicle counts from conventional real-time 2D sonography and stored 3D volume data sets by the same observer. The digital technology essential to the development of 3D sonography also means that 3D imaging permits storage of large data sets without loss of information to allow a subsequent offline analysis. The authors' data showed that with an increasing number of ovarian follicles, possible follicle-counting mistakes increase.

The results show that most of the differences in ovarian follicle counts occurred when the total follicle counts increased to approximately 10 total follicles. It would help to decide what cut-off difference in the number of follicles is considered clinically acceptable without interfering with patient treatment. A review of the literature does not give a definite number. With a cut-off difference of five follicles, 2D and 3D counts differed by 10% when performed by the same experienced operator.

As such, it is up to the individual practitioner to decide what difference in follicle counts between the various methods compared in this study would be acceptable. It is clear that training an inexperienced operator to correctly interpret and count ovarian follicles using stored 3D data sets offline would by far be less time consuming than training somebody in real-time 2D ovarian follicle counting.

This study's conclusions were that offline ovarian follicle counts from stored 3D volume data are similar to those obtained by 2D real-time sonography. In addition, 3D offline ovarian follicle counts are correctly interpreted by an operator with basic sonographic skills. Very limited time is needed to acquire the expertise to correctly interpret 3D volumes for performing ovarian follicle counts.

Software for Automated Follicular Measurements

A novel method of automatic ovarian follicle counting and follicular volume calculation has been introduced by some ultrasound machine manufacturers [13,14]. Sono-AVC (automated volume count) follicle (GE) helps provide semiautomated measurements and calculates follicles in a simulated ovary volume (Figure 8.2).

Because the follicles in the ovaries are filled with fluid, Sono-AVC identifies the hypoechogenic follicles within the selected ovarian volume, automatically analyzes the volume data, identifies the boundaries between follicles, and provides an estimate of their measurements and volume [15,16].

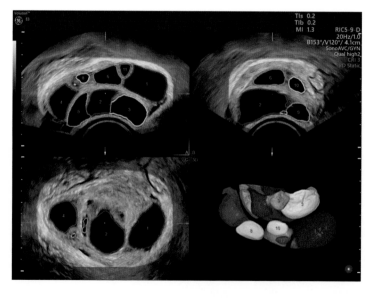

FIGURE 8.2   Sono AVC follicle. (Used with permission of GE Healthcare. Voluson is a trademark of GE Healthcare.)

The volume measurement is based on the amount of voxels within the identified follicle. Therefore, the measurement represents the actual volume of the follicle, regardless of its shape [15]. In addition, it is possible to add or remove follicles manually. Once the region of interest (ROI) is selected, the software is applied to the data set. The automatic analysis lasts approximately 6 seconds; afterward, the individual follicles are represented. After the software has made automatic calculations of the entire ovary, the operator can remove all extraovarian artifacts from the data set. Each volume has its own color [17], making Sono-AVC an ideal tool for studying follicular development within the ovary [18].

Frank Vandekerckhove et al. [19] performed a systematic review of the latest evidence investigating the role of automatic follicular measurements within ART. They mainly investigated the accuracy of Sono-AVC and how it compares, with the gold standard being the 2D sonography follicular measurement.

The electronic database PubMed was searched between 1966 and 2014; 74 articles were fully studied, and 32 articles were included in the data analysis.

They concluded that Sono-AVC software showed excellent accuracy. Comparing the technology with the 2D USS follicle measurements, Sono-AVC showed significantly lower intra- and interobserver variability. There was a significant advantage in the time gained, both for doctor and patient. In addition, by storing the images, Sono-AVC offered the possibility of including a quality control and continuous training for standardization of follicular monitoring.

However, as shown by Raine-Fenning et al. [16], there is no significant difference in clinical outcome (pregnancy rate). He showed that the number of mature oocytes collected, the number of fertilized oocytes, and the clinical pregnancy rates were similar with both 2D ultrasound and Sono-AVC methods.

Automated follicle tracking using Sono-AVC identifies a comparable number of follicles to real-time 2D ultrasound. However, timing final follicle maturation and egg retrieval on the basis of these automated measures does not appear to improve the clinical outcome of ART.

Finally, Rodríguez-Fuentes et al. [20] concluded that when image quality is good, measurements obtained by the automated mode are comparable to those obtained manually in 62% of cases. Automated monitoring is significantly quicker than conventional manual monitoring. Follicles with a measured volume greater than or equal to 0.6 cc (cubic centimeters) on the day of hCG administration are associated with the finding of mature oocytes at the time of egg retrieval.

Sono-AVC allows reliable evaluation of stimulated ovaries and may help establish new criteria for timing hCG administration based on follicular volume estimation rather than follicular diameter. They concluded that some software improvements are needed to improve universal patient use.

Reproducibility of Results

Undoubtedly, inter- and intraobserver variability will be encountered, but its extent needs to be calculated to assess its significance. Given the extent to which ultrasound is employed during fertility treatment, precision of ultrasound is important in order to accurately assess management of patients. Furthermore, measurements and images retrieved by ultrasonography are used to conclude the optimal timing of procedures such as egg retrieval; accurate measurement of the endometrium is difficult if the image quality is not optimal. Inaccuracy can be detrimental to IVF success and therefore patient well-being, affecting patient mental health or even physical health if a repeat cycle is required.

It should also be taken into consideration that scans, which need to be repeated due to inadequacy, result in excess patient exposure, not to mention additional waste of resources. Bates et al. [21] writes about the safety considerations that should be employed; these include ensuring that ultrasound scans are only performed by adequately trained personnel who must keep the scanning time to a minimum. Although the sonographer has a great deal of responsibility, there is currently no ultrasonographer-based quality assurance (QA) program available in this area of infertility treatment. This might be because ultrasound is considered a safe modality of imaging; unlike most imaging modalities, it does not deliver radiation and does not require nephrotoxic chemicals for visual enhancement. It has been claimed that in diagnostic ultrasound, the greater hazard to the patient is that presented by an untrained or poorly trained operator. Furthermore, it has been recognized that a successful sonographer-based ultrasound service should incorporate: (1) recognized training; (2) continuing education; (3) regular, frequent ultrasound practice; (4) use of protocols or schemes of work; and (5) good audit and quality control procedures.

Arredondo et al. [22] carried out a study to determine the intra- and interobserver reproducibility of ovarian follicle diameter measurements in natural menstrual cycles. Two blinded observers each calculated follicle diameter measurements on 70 patients. The results showed that there was excellent correlation: intraobserver correlation coefficient for both observers was 0.99, and the interobserver correlation coefficient was 0.98. It was concluded that the reproducibility of ovarian follicle diameter measurements was clinically acceptable. Farrell et al. [23] investigated the reliability and validity of 2D ultrasound volumetric measurements using balloon models. Thirty different sets of ultrasound images were obtained from 15 water-filled balloons with volumes ranging from 19 to 697 mL. Two observers who were blinded to the true volumes of the balloons performed the measurements independently. The intraclass correlation coefficient was used to assess the intra- and interobserver reliability. Results showed the intraclass correlation coefficient ranged from 0.992 to 0.998 for reliability and validity, whereas the Pearson correlation coefficient for validity was 0.996. In conclusion, high levels of reliability and validity were obtained for ultrasound balloon volume measurements.

Driscoll et al. [24] carried out a study about the variation in the determination of follicular diameter using an ultrasonic phantom. The ultrasonic phantom is a solid, ultrasound-permeable block of rubberized material with embedded wires and cylinders. Twenty-four operators with varying training completed the measurements; five were trained ultrasonographers, ten were experienced clinical nurse specialists, seven were experienced medical practitioners, and two were scientists with no experience in ultrasound methods. The results demonstrated a large variation ranging between 10% and 25% coefficient of variation on distances between 10 and 32 mm, suggesting the need for an external QA program for ultrasound in assisted reproductive technology programs.

The contribution of image magnification to the repeatability of caliper placement was assessed by Herman et al. [25]. Fetal nuchal translucency thickness was measured on 27 women undergoing first-trimester ultrasound scans by two qualified examiners. Measurements were taken twice by each examiner: first on a regular-sized image and subsequently on the same still image magnified. There were significantly smaller mean values obtained from the magnified images compared to the regular-sized images. Therefore, magnification gives a more accurate and more repeatable measurement.

Herman et al. [25] recommended blind repeated measurements on still images as a tool for self-assessment, quality control, and training.

Bredella et al. [26] stated that common technical errors can exacerbate the potential for inaccuracy in measurement: inadequate depth setting and consequent imprecise calipers placement. It was concluded that correct calipers placement can be achieved at repeat examination with use of an appropriate depth setting.

In 2008, Levine et al. [27] carried out a study to assess factors affecting the quality of performance of sonography. Images obtained from 31 sonographers were analyzed to assess the impact of multiple factors on quality, location of examination, type of training, practice experience, and speciality. Results concluded that no significant differences were found on the basis of training type, years in practice, or number of examinations read; however, it was found that sonographers who specialized in women's imaging performed best.

A small study was carried out at the University Hospital of Wales in the Obstetrics and Gynaecology department in 2008 to investigate inter- and intraobserver variation between different categories of health-care professionals performing ultrasound. The 11 participants included in this project ranged from consultants in gynecology to trainees in gynecological ultrasound; all participants had differing levels of experience measured in years practicing ultrasound and frequency at which scans were carried out per week. This was to ensure the results obtained for the dependability of ultrasound were more reliable. Furthermore, it meant the correlation between image quality/measurement accuracy and experience could be analyzed and assessed.

Subjects were asked to be involved in one experiment involving two components to assess the different areas of interest: inter-/intraobserver variability, image optimization, and measurement accuracy. The experiment required subjects to carry out an ultrasound scan on a pelvic ultrasound mannequin (Blue

Phantom transvaginal mannequin CAE, Sarasota, Florida). The ultrasound mannequin is a contraption that provides a realistic medical training device for use by medical staff to gain experience in the skills and techniques required when performing gynecological ultrasound examinations. The mannequin comprises a full-scale model of the female pelvis containing organs such as ovaries with follicles, uterus, and so on, in their normal occurring relative positions. Organs are constructed with a variable density substance to simulate the true sonic density of these organs. It is a valuable training and learning tool, which accurately imitates the imaging properties of an actual transvaginal ultrasound examination. Using the mannequin will enable intra- and interobserver variability, image quality, and measurement to be calculated accurately as the parameters remain constant. It allows analysis without the ethical implications and inconvenience of performing in patients.

Participants carried out an ultrasound scan on the mannequin recording follicular diameter of the largest follicle (based on two measurements). This was performed on two occasions with an interval of 5–7 days. This interval was present in order to accurately assess intraobserver variability. The information gathered from individual subjects was combined and analyzed to calculate intraobserver variability. The data collected between participants were compared to evaluate interobserver variability.

Bates et al. [21] writes how the sonographer should be able to optimize the image by using focal zones and other image processing options and the importance of placing the focal zone at the depth of interest. Narrowing the width of the beam at a certain depth has a focusing effect similar to that obtained using a lens, which improves the resolution in the plane of interest [28]. Gain settings are used to compensate for the loss of sonic energy experienced at deeper levels, as the beam has to travel further and through an increasing amount of tissue; it allows structures to be visualized with the meaningful gray levels. Too much gain causes hyperechoic areas to form, which can give the appearance of filled-in regions, whereas too little gain causes hypoechoic regions, making solid regions appear clear. Artifacts are misleading or incorrect information on the image and can cause a reduction in image quality. Ultrasound is particularly susceptible to artifacts, and many are operator induced [28]. As a result, the factors that needed to be taken into consideration when assessing the image quality and were therefore included in the scoring criteria are shown in Figures 8.3 and 8.4. This study showed that there is a significant positive correlation between image quality and measurement accuracy ($R = 0.730, N = 12, P < 0.01$, two-tailed) (Figure 8.5). Further analysis was performed on the above variables comparing them against years of ultrasound practice to find whether an association could be found. A nonsignificant correlation was demonstrated when comparing image quality with years of performing clinical ultrasound (Figure 8.6).

A nonsignificant correlation was found between image quality and scan frequency ($R = 0.133, P = 0.680$, $N = 12$), as shown in Figure 8.7. Similarly, no significant correlation was evident when comparing frequency of scans with measurement accuracy ($R = 0.233, P = 0.465, N = 12$), as illustrated in Figure 8.8. Figure 8.9 shows no correlation between measurement accuracy and years of ultrasound experience.

This is comparative to the studies performed by Hertzberg et al. [29] and Levine et al. [27], who both concluded that performance did not correlate with experience (<5, 5–10, and >10 years). This suggests that performance may have associated factors other than experience. Hertzberg et al. [29] discerns that sonographer competency needs to be calculated specifically rather than basing it on experience alone.

Using the information collected from the study conducted at the University Hospital of Wales on the qualification of each participant, bar charts were plotted to observe whether a relationship could be seen when compared with image quality and measurement accuracy. From the bar charts (Figures 8.10 and 8.11), a relationship can be depicted that as the level of qualification increases, so does image quality and measurement accuracy. However, this correlation is just an observation with no calculation of significance. Breitkopf et al. [30] also found a correlation between year of residency and measurement accuracy, with lower-level residents committing more errors, such as incorrect image plane and caliper placement.

Servaes et al. [31] investigated the hypothesis that follicular tracking by well-trained nurses/midwifes was reliable for clinical decisions in assisted conception and examined the reproducibility of 2D follicle measurements using a new 3D tool imitating real-life ovarian scanning (ultrasound recordings). This was a prospective observational study where for each of the four patients enrolled, the number and average diameter of the follicles greater than or equal to 10 mm were assessed by 2D measurements by the same observer, and subsequently, 3D ultrasound images were stored by an expert sonographer. The volumes were calculated and stored anonymously. The 3D tool enabled the midwives to scan the whole ovary offline and to decide which image was used for 2D measurements. Imitating real-life ovarian scanning, the midwives determined the number of follicles and the average size of the follicles greater than or equal to 10 mm in a setup that was very close to clinical practice. No significant differences were found in the evaluation of the number and mean diameter of all follicles or the diameter of the largest follicle measured. Junior and senior midwives were compared, and no differences were found in both groups

Adequate magnification of area of interest	Poor = 0 (Area of interest too small ~1/4 screen) 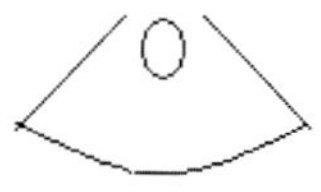	Suboptimal = 1 (Region of interest ~1/2 screen) 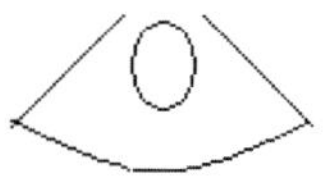	Good = 2 (Region of interest filling ~3/4screen) 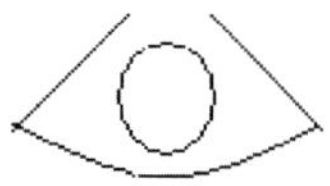
Region of interest in center of field	Poor = 0 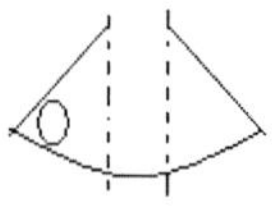	Suboptimal = 1 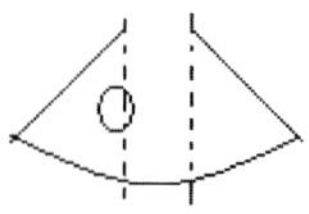	Good = 2 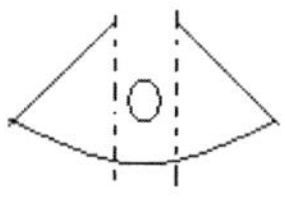
Image detail-defined as the clarity of organ outlines and ease with which boundaries of structures are seen and defined	Poor = 0	Suboptimal = 1	Good = 2
Artifacts	Extensive = 0	Few = 1	None = 2
Focus settings	Poor = 0 (not over area of interest) 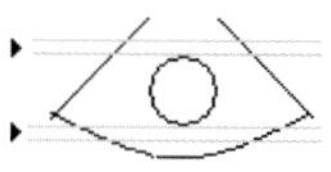	Satisfactory = 1 (at level of area of interest) 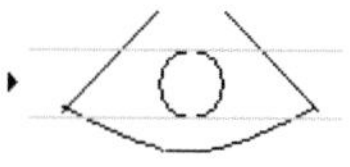	
Gain compensation settings	Poor = 0 (too bright or too dark)	Satisfactory=1	
Annotation	Not present = 0 Incorrect = 0	Present and correct = 1	

FIGURE 8.3   Image quality scoring sheet.

(a)

Caliper placement	Both calipers not to the edge = 0	One caliper placed on edge = 1	Both calipers on edges = 2 (outer to outer in the case of ovaries and inner to inner in the case of follicle/cyst)
For ovarian measurements, is the image in correct plane e.g., transverse × 1 measurements and sagittal × 2 measurement	No = 0	Yes = 1	
Or			
For endometrial thickness measurement, is the correct measurement technique applied? (perpendicular to lining)			
Largest possible diameter measured	No = 0	Yes = 1	
Sufficient zoom applied	No = 0	Yes = 1 (region of interest ½ of the screen or more)	

(b)

Caliper placement	Both calipers not to the edge = 0	One caliper placed on edge = 1	Both calipers on edges = 2 (outer to outer in the case of ovaries and inner to inner in the case of follicle/cyst)
Largest possible diameter measured	No = 0	Yes = 1	
Is second measurement perpendicular to first measurement?	No = 0	Yes = 1	

FIGURE 8.4 Measurement accuracy scoring sheet: (a) first measurement and (b) second measurement (if applicable).

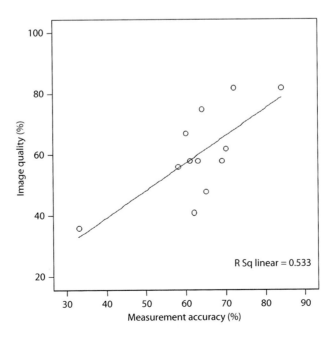

FIGURE 8.5 Correlation between image quality and measurement accuracy.

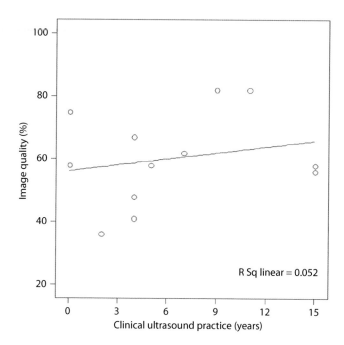

FIGURE 8.6   Correlation between image quality and years of ultrasound experience.

(interobserved variability). No significant differences were found between the two measurement moments (intraobserver variability). The study concluded that follicle measurements provided reliable information for the gynecologists to consider when making decisions during assisted conception treatments. One limitation of this study was that the measurements were taken on prerecorded 3D images, but it would have been unfeasible to have performed the same examination by seven different sonographers with the

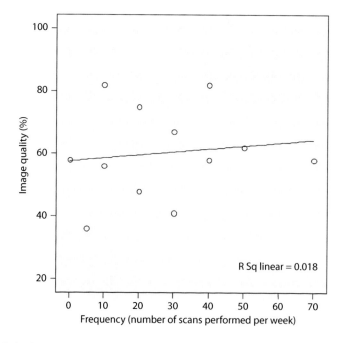

FIGURE 8.7   Correlation between image quality and number of scans performed weekly.

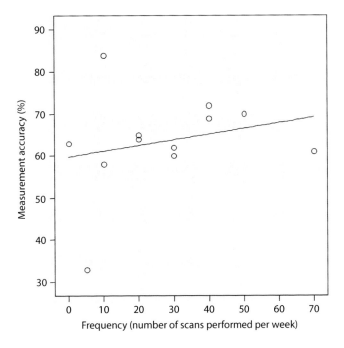

FIGURE 8.8   Correlation between measurement accuracy and number of scans performed weekly.

same patient at the same time. These data support the view that appropriately trained nurses/midwives can perform 2D follicle measurements for superovulation monitoring in a reproducible way and that the 3D tool can be used for quality control.

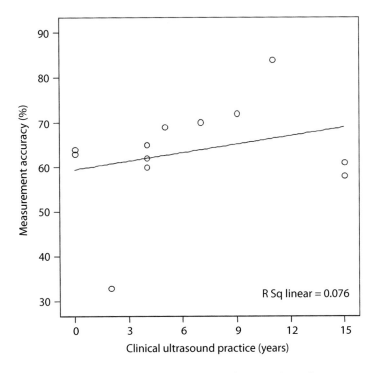

FIGURE 8.9   Correlation between measurement accuracy and years of ultrasound experience.

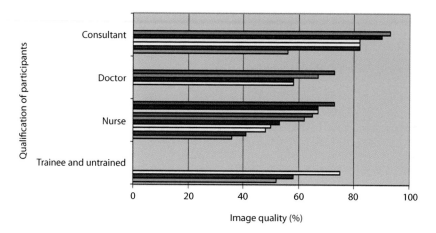

FIGURE 8.10   Comparison between image quality and qualification of participants.

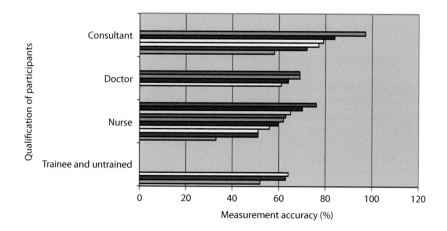

FIGURE 8.11   Comparison between measurement accuracy and qualification of participants.

Future Developments: Self-Operating Endovaginal Telemonitoring

The possibility of monitoring ovarian response remotely by training and teaching the patient to perform her own individual ultrasound scan was speculated for the first time by Gerris et al. [32].

More recently, the same authors [33] published the first randomized controlled study comparing self-operated endovaginal telemonitoring (SOET) at home with traditional sonographic (non-SOET) follow-up. Patients were considered eligible to take part in the study if they were less than 41 years of age, had two ovaries, and were undergoing ICSI treatment. They also needed wireless internet connection at home and basic computer skills. Previous OHSS and polycystic ovarian syndrome (PCOS) were not excluded from the study.

The authors described that enrolled patients were given a diary to fill in the data for calculating direct and indirect costs. Patients were shown how to make video images and how to upload and send them back. They were given a laptop, a vaginal sonography probe with USB connection, condoms, and gel. Patients scanned first their right ovary, then the uterus, then the left ovary. Midwives and nurses taught the patients how to introduce and handle the probe, and they were available for any queries. Most patients learned quickly once they knew how to handle the probe within the vagina. Patients entering the SOET arm were monitored using the homemade recordings only until the day of egg recovery. Videos were downloaded and opened in order for the principal investigators to perform the 2D measurements of the follicles.

One hundred and twenty-one patients were analyzed (59 SOET, 62 non-SOET). The most common reason for not taking part in the SOET group was the uncertainty of being able to produce good-quality images; some patients were at their first attempts or at their last attempts. The two groups had similar general characteristics. The authors reported that two patients did not succeed in the SOET group, having to make some extra visits: the first was a poor responder, and the second had follicles that were almost mature but failed to identify them.

In the SOET group, there was a 25% ongoing pregnancy rate versus 26% in the non-SOET group. Clinical outcome measures did not statistically differ between the two groups. Patients were assessed also for satisfaction, feeling of empowerment, active participation of the partner, stress, and discretion. Feedback was positive for everything except for the stress. The stress was due to logistics and to a new technique; however, the stress levels decreased when the follicles became more visible.

The authors looked also at the economic aspect of this novel technique. They found that taking into consideration the cost of care providers, transportation/gas, and time taken from work, the average total cost per SOET attempt was approximately half that of a non-SOET attempt. They concluded that despite the results being very encouraging, technological improvements are still needed, and external validation needs to be undertaken. Another interesting conclusion was to apply the automated follicular size measurements, based on 3D rather than on 2D measurements as discussed earlier in this chapter.

Simulation for Training

As highlighted in this chapter, education and training are paramount for successfully monitoring ovarian response during superovulation in ART, and indeed for reaching the ultimate target of a live birth. The ScanTrainer simulator (Intelligent Ultrasound plc, Cardiff, United Kingdom) was introduced in 2010 as a novel development for ultrasound training. The simulator teaches health-care professionals the complex, hard-to-learn ultrasound scanning skills, without the need for a patient and with minimal expert supervision. It dramatically speeds up the skills learning process, saving hospitals time and resources in producing better-trained sonographers prior to patient contact. It uses a replica ultrasound probe attached to a force-feedback (haptic) device, together with ultrasound images that have been generated during real-time scanning. The simulator replicates the real-time physical feedback of probe manipulation and contact with a patient, allowing trainees to develop the necessary hand-eye coordination and manual dexterity. The ultrasound software provides a real patient ultrasound scan with virtual anatomy images for each learning module.

Another important feature of the simulator is the integrated feedback that allows the trainees to review their performance through detailed feedback on each task within an assignment. At the end of each assignment, the trainee's performance is assessed against a gold standard, and detailed feedback is provided. Trainees can review their performance and then retake the assignment, if unsuccessful. Tutors can tailor the training experience to their trainees' specific requirements by creating customized tutor groups and customized training modules for different levels of trainees.

ScanTrainer modules are available for all skill levels—from core skills and advanced skills to differential diagnosis. Core and advanced modules are broken down into easy-to-follow tutorials, assignments, and tasks, designed to teach the trainee in an interactive way, where the trainee is given the freedom to learn a task by experiencing different attempts and by making mistakes.

Summary of Findings

- Cycle monitoring by transvaginal ultrasound plus serum estradiol may need to be retained as a precautionary good practice point for prevention of OHSS.
- Although three-directional measurement of a follicle is the most accurate, the margin of error when comparing measurement in one and two directions and one and three directions is small.
- With an increasing number of ovarian follicles, possible follicle-counting mistakes increase.

- Automated follicle tracking using Sono-AVC identifies a comparable number of follicles to real-time 2D ultrasound. However, timing final follicle maturation and egg retrieval on the basis of these automated measures does not appear to improve the clinical outcome of ART.

- Ultrasound performance does not seem to correlate with operator experience only, but a relationship can be depicted that as the level of qualification increases, so does image quality and measurement accuracy.

- Appropriately trained nurses/midwives can perform 2D follicle measurements for superovulation monitoring in a reproducible way. The 3D tool can be used for quality control.

- SEOL has the potential widely employed in the future to reduce cost in ART.

- The simulator teaches doctors and sonographers the complex, hard-to-learn ultrasound scanning skills, without the need for a patient and with minimal expert supervision.

REFERENCES

1. Bull JR, Rowland SP, Scherwitzl EB, Scherwitzl R, Danielsson KG, Harper J. Real-world menstrual cycle characteristics of more than 600,000 menstrual cycles. NPJ Digit Med. 2019;2:83.
2. Gnoth C, Maxrath B, Skonieczny T et al. Final ART success rates a 10 years survey. *Hum Reprod.* 2011;26:2239–46.
3. Pelinck MJ, Vogel NE, Hoek A et al. Cumulative pregnancy rates after three cycles of minimal stimulation IVF and results according to subfertility diagnosis a multicentre cohort study. *Hum Reprod.* 2006; 21:2375–83.
4. D'Angelo A. OHSS prevention strategies: Cryopreservation of all embryos. *Semin Reprod Med.* 2010;28(6):513–8.
5. Martins WP, Vieira CVR, Teixeira DM et al. Ultrasound for monitoring controlled ovarian stimulation: A systematic review and meta-analysis of randomized controlled trials. *Ultrasound Obstet Gynecol.* 2014;43:25–33.
6. Vandekerckhove F, Gerris J, Vansteelandt S, and De Sutter P. Adding serum estradiol measurements to ultrasound monitoring does not change the yield of mature oocytes in IVF/ICSI. *Gynecol Endocrinol.* 2014;30(9):649–52.
7. Kwan I, Bhattacharya S, McNeil A, and van Rumste MM. Monitoring of stimulated cycles in assisted reproduction (IVF and ICSI). *Cochrane Database Syst Rev.* 2008;(2):CD005289. doi:10.1002/14651858. CD005289.pub2
8. Meldrum DR, Chetkowski RJ, Steinold KA, and Randle D. Transvaginal ultrasound scanning of ovarian follicles. *Fertil Steril.* 1984;42:803–5.
9. O'Herlihy C, de Crespigny LC, Lopata A et al. Preovulatory follicular size: A comparison of ultrasound and laparoscopic measurements. *Fertil Steril.* 1980;34:24–6.
10. Kyei-Mensah A, Zaidi J, Pittrof R et al. Transvaginal three-dimensional ultrasound: Accuracy of follicular volume measurements. *Fertil Steril.* 1996;65:371–6.
11. Duijkersa IJM, Louwe LA, Braatc DDM, and Klipping C. One, two or three: How many directions are useful in transvaginal ultrasound measurement of ovarian follicles? *Eur J Obstet Gynecol Reprod Biol.* 2004;117:60–3.
12. Moawad NS, Gibbons H, Liu J, and Lazebnik N. Comparison of 3- and 2-dimensional sonographic techniques for counting ovarian follicles. *J Ultrasound Med.* 2009;28:1281–8.
13. Raine-Fenning N, Jayaprakasan K, Clewes J et al. Sono-AVC: A novel method of automatic volume calculation. *Ultrasound Obstet Gynecol.* 2008; 31:691–6.
14. Deutch TD, Joergner I, Matson DO et al. Automated assessment of ovarian follicles using a novel three-dimensional ultrasound software. *Fertil Steril.* 2009;92:1562–8.
15. Ata B, and Tulandi T. Ultrasound automated volume calculation in reproduction and in pregnancy. *Fertil Steril.* 2011;95:2163–70.
16. Raine-Fenning N, Jayaprakasan K, Campbell BK et al. Timing of oocyte maturation and egg collection during controlled ovarian stimulation: A randomized controlled trial evaluating manual and automated measurements of follicle diameter. *Fertil Steril.* 2010;94(1):184–8.

17. Deb S, Jayaprakasan K, Campbell BK et al. Intraobserver and interobserver reliability of automated antral follicle counts made using three-dimensional ultrasound and Sono-AVC. *Ultrasound Obstet Gynecol.* 2009;33:477–83.

18. Raine-Fenning N, Jayaprakasan K, Chamberlain S et al. Automated measurements of follicle diameter: A chance to standardize? *Fertil Steril.* 2009;91:1469–72.

19. Vandekerckhove F, Bracke V, and De Sutter P. The value of automated follicle volume measurements in IVF/ICSI. *Front Surg Gynecol Obstet.* 2014;1:18. doi:10.3389/fsurg.2014.00018

20. Rodríguez-Fuentes A, Hernández J, Gracia-Guzman R et al. Prospective evaluation of automated follicle monitoring in 58 in vitro fertilization cycles: Follicular volume as a new indicator of oocyte maturity. *Fertil Steril.* 2010;93:616–20.

21. Bates J., Deane C, and Lindsell D. *Extending the provision of ultrasound services in the UK.* London, UK: British Medical Ultrasound Society; 2003.

22. Arredondo F, Loret de Mola JR, Frasure H, and Liu J.H. Intra-observer and inter-observer reproducibility of ultrasound measurements of ovarian follicle diameter. *Fertil Steril.* 2004;82(Suppl 2):S169.

23. Farrell T, Leslie JR, Chien PFW, and Agustsson P. The reliability and validity of three dimensional volumetric measurements using an *in vitro* balloon and *in vivo* uterine model. *Br J Obstet Gynaecol.* 2001;108:573–82.

24. Driscoll GL, Tyler JPP, and Carpenter D. Variation in the determination of follicular diameter: An inter-unit pilot study using an ultrasonic phantom. *Hum Reprod.* 1997;12(11):2465–8.

25. Herman A, Maymon R, Dreazen E et al. Image magnification does not contribute to the repeatability of caliper placement in measuring nuchal translucency thickness. *Ultrasound Obstet Gynecol.* 1998;11:266–70.

26. Bredella MA, Feldstein VA, Filly RA et al. Measurement of endometrial thickness at US in multicenter drug trials: Value of central quality assurance reading. *Radiology..* 2000;217:516–20.

27. Levine D, Asch E, Mehta TS et al. Assessment of factors that affect the quality of performance and interpretation of sonography of adnexal masses. *J Ultrasound Med.* 2008;27:721–8.

28. Chudleigh T, and Thilaganathan B. *Obstetrics Ultrasound How, Why and When.* 3rd ed. Edinburgh, Scotland: Elsevier; 2004.

29. Hertzberg BS, Kliewer MA, Bowie JD et al. Physician training requirements in sonography: How many cases are needed for competence? *Am J Radiol.* 2000;174:1221–7.

30. Breitkopf DM, Smith ER, and Herbert WNP. Measurement of endometrial stripe thickness by obstetrics and gynecology residents. *Am J Obstet Gynaecol.* 2005;193(5):1866–9.

31. Servaes K, Van Schoubroeck D, Welkenhuysen M et al. How reproducible are 2-dimensional ultrasonographic follicular diameter measurements from stored 3-dimensional files of ovarian scanning? *Gynecol Obstet Invest.* 2014;77(3):163–8.

32. Gerris J, Geril A, and De Sutter P. Patient acceptance of self-operated endovaginal telemonitoring (SOET): Proof of concept. *Facts Views Vis Obstet Gynecol.* 2009;1:161–70.

33. Gerris J, Delvigne A, Dhont N et al.. Self-operated endovaginal telemonitoring versus traditional monitoring of ovarian stimulation in assisted reproduction: An RCT. *Hum Reprod.* 2014;29(9):1941–8.

9

Oocyte Pick-Up Technique

Costas Panayotidis

Definition

Oocyte retrieval (OR) is an ultrasound-guided technique in which oocytes are aspirated using a needle connected to a suction pump.

Many different abbreviations exist in published papers to describe OR, including transvaginal oocyte retrieval (TVOR), egg collection, egg aspiration, and oocyte pick-up (OPU). By consensus in 2019 the European Society of Human Reproduction and Embryology (ESHRE) working group [1] adopted OPU as one common terminology to describe this procedure.

History and Background of the Technique

The first ultrasound retrieval method used a needle designed for OPU under the guidance of a transabdominal ultrasound study. This technique was called transabdominal oocyte retrieval (TA-OR) [2,3]. Then in 1983, OPU was first performed transvaginally for *in vitro fertilization* (IVF) cycles under transvaginal ultrasound guidance [4–6]. Since then, technological advances in ultrasound machines and IVF therapy protocols have made significant progress [7–11].

Because of good OR yield, the need for only light sedation [12–14], and the fact that it is less invasive than laparoscopic OR, transvaginal ultrasound-guided oocyte retrieval has now become the technique of choice for obtaining oocytes for IVF.

However, TA-OR is still an alternative method for patients with certain risk factors, such as an increased body mass index and displacement of the ovaries [15] or Müllerian malformations [16,17].

Introduction

Despite its prominence as the first-choice retrieval method, OPU has only recently been evaluated in terms of standardization of practice or what should be considered the best technique [1]. Recent literature research [18] showed that published papers were heterogeneous in their content and structure, not allowing any meta-analysis. No paper described from the ultrasound point of view the OPU technique, and the majority of research focused on the IVF success rates [19–21]. Moreover, no information was given about the specifics of the ultrasound technique (e.g., frequency, type of probe, focal zone area, plane, position of the patient, or description of the reasons for complications) and how to achieve the optimum quality image for effective retrieval. In addition, ultrasound proficiency and acquired gynecological ultrasound competencies vary throughout European countries, making it more difficult to identify ultrasound standards relative to OPU.

IVF centers are expected to have high standards for their ultrasound practice (although differences in practice may be detected between university hospitals, public- or private-sector hospitals, and/or between European countries). Ultrasound practice should follow the recommendations and relevant guidelines of the national ultrasound organizations for the specific location.

The author of this chapter undertook a systematic review of the literature and conducted a Delphi method survey [22–26] with a group of 15 expert specialists on OPU, using a 53-item questionnaire completed in three rounds. The results sourced the proposal of 32 recommendations on standards of practice. These were formulated based on the literature review and the expert opinions [18]. In 2018, these recommendations of OPU practice were considered and discussed by a learned body, the European Society of Human Reproduction and Embryology (ESHRE), and formed the basis of its clinical guideline publication [1].

This chapter follows a structured approach aiming at describing OPU from an ultrasound point of view, focusing on the most acceptable practice and describing the most common complications and how to avoid them.

Patient Setup

From the literature search, it has been noted that a thorough ultrasound study pretreatment should be performed in order to assess the appropriate IVF ovarian stimulation protocol, to determine whether there is anatomical malformation or malposition of the ovaries, and to assess ovarian placement after previous fertility surgery [27]. Three-dimensional ultrasound could be applied to assess the overall anatomy and help the operator preoperatively. The time to perform this should be under the discretion of the IVF subspecialist, ranging between 4 and 6 months prior to IVF [28].

The patient's position during OPU needs to be comfortable for both patient and operator. Gynecological positioning in the semilithotomy or lithotomy position can facilitate the OPU maneuvers and ensure cable positioning is out of the way. However, little is known about the quality of vaginal examination and patient position, as demonstrated by Panayotidis [29].

It seems more appropriate for a specialized examination or interventional vaginal ultrasound techniques to bring the patient's buttocks to the edge of the examination table. A suitably designed gynecological table should be used. OPU can be done by the operator in a sit-down or stand-up position. However, the majority of reproductive specialists prefer to sit down.

Although some postures could be an operator's preference, the basic rules of ergonomics and back care protection should be applied. This should be investigated in the future with respect to OPU complications, inability to perform all the maneuvers during OPU, timing of OPU, and work-related injury (back or shoulder) for those operators who perform many OPU procedures on a weekly basis.

Practically, it is easier to manipulate the ultrasound probe with the hands in projection toward the probe (parallel) versus bending the wrist using the probe at a lateral angle. Figure 9.1 shows how the transducer is held for OPU and Figure 9.2 shows different views of the ultrasound fields are created. Figures 9.3 and

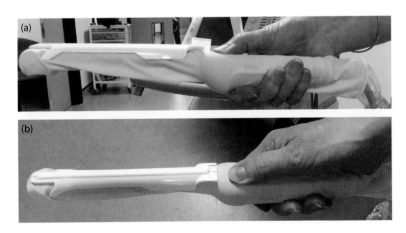

FIGURE 9.1 Holding the transvaginal probe. (a) The proximity of the different tissues and organs is seen better on the monitor holding the probe as shown. (b) In addition to having better tactile perception if the operator is placing the transducer parallel with his or her hand, the transducer then becomes an extension of the operator's fingers.

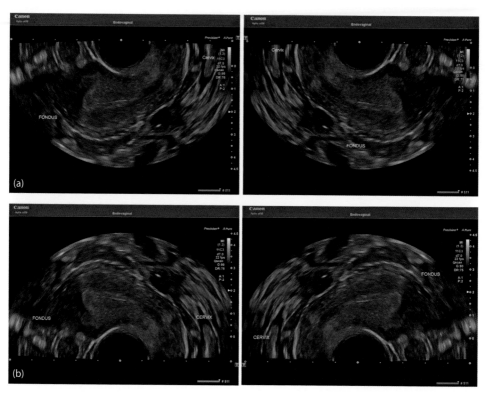

FIGURE 9.2   Variations of the ultrasound field representation with transducer represented on the top and from bottom with mirror image on right or left.

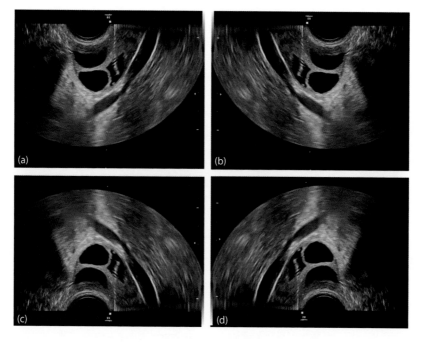

FIGURE 9.3   (a–d) Oocyte pick-up and probe orientation.

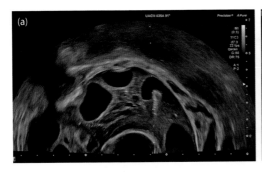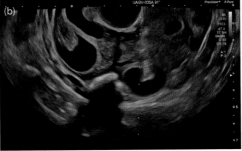

FIGURE 9.4 OPU with ultrasound field seen from (a) the bottom and (b) the top of the monitor in a left ovarian oocyte puncture.

9.4 show the different views of orientation with the ultrasound field at the bottom or at the top of the screen while performing the OPU.

An empty bladder improves the image quality during transvaginal examination, as it decreases the posterior enhancement (ultrasound artifact), which occurs on a partially emptied bladder at its posterior wall. The patient needs to empty her bladder prior to OPU also to reduce the risk of bladder injuries; if OPU is done under general anesthesia, a urine catheter can be used to empty the bladder (in and out). Vaginal cleansing can be done with normal saline prior to OPU. Further evaluation should be focused on the usage of antiseptic methods and how this may influence the rate of post-OPU complications [18,30–34].

OPU is mostly performed under sedation [33,35,36] and seldom (patient request or clinically indicated) under general anesthesia. Ambulatory procedures are preferable for the patients, as their recovery is shorter in comparison with general anesthesia. Advances in anesthesiology regarding drug preparations for sedation should be followed by IVF centers in order to provide a drug combination that results in minimal side effects to the patient, such as drowsiness, nausea, or pain. In order to avoid the risk of allergic reaction, nonlatex gloves and probe covers should be used.

Ultrasound Machine

The ultrasound machine should be adequate for the purpose of OPU with high imaging accuracy. Most of the reproductive specialists work with a standard machine (meaning nonportable), because the computer processing power is superior, and the generated images are of better quality. Different manufacturers provide powerful ultrasound machines, with some having perfected recent advances in ultrasound technology to the level that excellent images are generated even from portable devices. No specific ultrasound model (company) is considered better than others at the present time. Many factors determine the choice of an ultrasound machine, as it is a significant investment. In particular, budgetary restrictions, clear image quality, and safety parameters are major considerations in determining the final decision.

During OPU, the ultrasound field of view and anatomical orientation are set from the top or bottom part of the monitor depending on the preference of the operator (Figures 9.5 through 9.7).

Some of the reproductive specialists use an ultrasound field seen from the bottom part of the monitor, where the deepest structures of the pelvis are represented at the top part of the monitor (Figure 9.7). However, in most of the basic gynecological ultrasound studies, the ultrasound field is represented at the top of the monitor.

The representation of the probe from the bottom part of the monitor may help the controlled manipulation of the probe. The initial structures are seen exactly at the beginning of the probe as seen on the monitor and the tactile sensation during the scanning and needle manipulation is more realistically represented.

The orientation (lateralization left to right side) is another parameter that can be set depending on the operator's preference. According to Panayotidis [18], the patient's right side is represented on the left-hand side of the monitor most of the time. It is important not to confuse the image representation when the operator changes and aspirates the contralateral ovary. The needle is preferably introduced from the median part of the ovary in order to avoid any accidental trauma of the lateral iliac vessels. Therefore, the transvaginal probe has to be rotated accordingly.

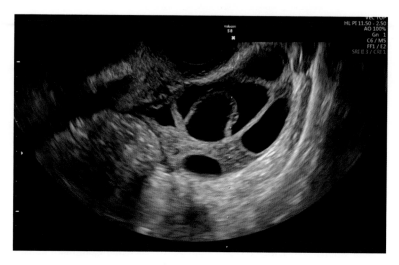

FIGURE 9.5 The left ovary is seen clearly with multiple stimulated follicles. The needle guide is visible prior the introduction of the needle. (Note that the left side of the probe is represented on the right side of the monitor.)

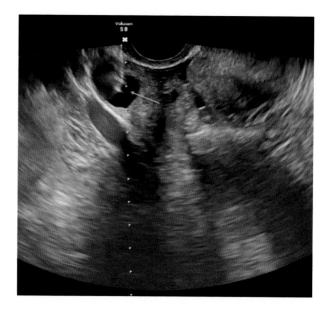

FIGURE 9.6 Right oocyte pick-up: The orange arrow depicts the needle edge within the follicle; the tip of the probe (black half circle) is shown at the top of the ultrasound field. The right iliac vessel is visible at the proximity, and the edge of the needle is clearly seen. The anterior edge of the transvaginal probe is represented at the left part of the monitor.

The ultrasound frequency used for OPU varies between 5 and 7 MHz in order to obtain sufficient resolution and depth penetration. Additional filters and image adjustment settings can be activated in order to improve the image. Most operators use high rather than low frequency [18].

The ability to adjust the image is operator dependent. Ultrasound machines with automatic settings to improve and enhance the image in real time during scanning are not yet available. Some operators enhance the image to the maximum before starting the egg collection; others may need a larger field of view and therefore initially use low frequency for deeper penetration. The selection should depend on how the operator approaches the ovaries, and adjustment should be done before or during OPU in order to facilitate the accurate visualization of the OPU needle. The ability to constantly improve the image is recommended by the British Medical Ultrasound Society [37], and it is an obvious requirement

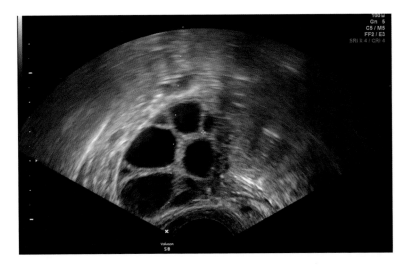

FIGURE 9.7   The right ovary is seen with the probe represented from the low part of the ultrasound field. Note that the proximity to the probe is less than 2 cm, and the needle guide is already in place (yellow x).

for good-quality ultrasound imaging. The harmonic setup frequency in many machines is activated automatically and overall improves the smoothness of the image. Harmonic filters can improve the image with different frequencies; nonetheless, very experienced operators do not always consider it. Some may feel that the tip of the needle is not well seen or that the surface of the follicle is less clearly seen, as the contrast and image are less bright.

Another setting for image improvement is adjustment of the ultrasound beam focus. Most operators use one focal area during their OPU practice [18]. Focus can be adjusted on the lowest expectant level of the needle positioning, making it possible to see the edge of the ovary and the lowest follicle more clearly. It seems that double focus does not improve the OPU image in real time.

A large ultrasound field of view (more in depth as possible) is preferable to identify all parts of the ovarian surface and peripheral organs (tubes, uterus, iliac vessels, and bladder). If in doubt, Doppler study before starting the OPU will identify vascular structures near the ovary, which look remarkably similar to superficial follicles [38,39]. In cases of polycystic ovaries, the color Doppler can be of value in helping to avoid penetration within the central vascular areas between the follicles, as seen in Figure 9.8.

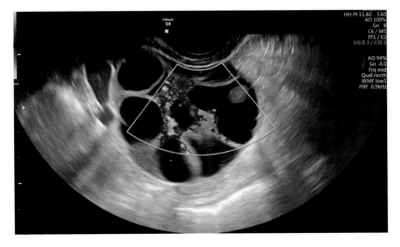

FIGURE 9.8   Color Doppler helps to identify the vascular areas within the ovary in between the follicles. The OPU is conducted avoiding these vessels to decrease the risk of internal bleeding and pain to the patient.

The need to record the OPU procedure and store images or video clips (cine loop setup) was not considered important in the past. However, with the technological advances in ultrasound machines, a video recording is easy to capture. In case of complications, the image or video review can be used for training and future recognition of similar unfortunate situations, can explain the failure of the OPU technique, and can be used for audit in respect to quality assessment of the ultrasound image. The use of recorded images and videos in gynecological practice and interventional ultrasound techniques should no longer be controversial [40]. The recording of the procedure could distinguish between unavoidable accidents and real mistakes; despite the fear of medicolegal actions, if the recorded video shows errors, the video recording can also give valuable information on how to prevent complications and how to learn to improve the technique [41–46]. Some may be of the opinion that the operator tends to prefer automatic movements minimizing the use of additional buttons (cine or other setup image adjustments); however, recording and auditing an individual OPU technique and image quality are an invaluable practice and need further exploration.

The Transducer

The transvaginal transducer should be designed with ergonomics in mind, enabling easy manipulation during the scanning and ovarian puncture, secure attachment of a needle guide, and unrestricted application of a fit-for-purpose, sterile, preferably nonlatex cover that incorporates inside it sonographic gel on the transducer tip.

An older but readily available method for a probe cover was to use a finger of a sterile surgical glove. This practice should be avoided because of the risk that it creates air bubbles in the gel (between the probe and glove part), which compromises the ultrasound view. Specialized probe covers should be preferred. The transducer needle guide should be simple to attach after a sterile cover has been applied. The transducer should be cleaned and disinfected between procedures following the local protocols. Chapter 19 elaborates on infection control methods, which all health-care professionals working in IVF units must be familiar with.

Aspiration Needles

The operator should be familiar with the different aspiration needle designs. Translucent tubing should be attached to the needle so the operator can see the content and color of the fluid being aspirated. The single-lumen needle is the most common type in use for OPU [12,18,30,31,33]. Different sizes with different flexibility characteristics are available on the market, most commonly a 17- or 18-gauge needle is used [47].

Double-lumen needles or variations of them use a constant infusion of culture media into the follicle at the same time as the follicular fluid is being aspirated. This technique increases the turbulence within the follicle with a potential benefit of dislodging the oocyte-cumulus complex from the follicle wall. The technological advances in needle design made it possible to incorporate Teflon tubing between the needle and the sampling tube with less mechanical trauma to the oocyte during aspiration. Operators who perform a flushing technique generally prefer to use culture medium during flushing most of the time. The flushing media is aspirated out to retrieve the egg, and if it was not identified in the initial aspirate.

Aspiration needles have near the tip a small band of highly reflective surface (the echo tip sign) that makes the visualization of the distal end easier to see as the needle enters the ovary and once it is in the follicles (Figure 9.9).

Aspiration needles have differences in diameter 17–20 gauge (gg). As long as the inner diameter of the needle is 0.8–1 mm, the oocyte cumulus complex should be unaffected, provided that the aspiration pressure is less than 120 mm Hg with 20 gg/35 mm (thin in) or 17 gg/35 mm (standard outer) if a different needle diameter was trialed [48]. Potential disadvantages of the flushing technique include longer procedure time with additional anesthesia or sedation medication and more tissue handling [49–51]. A longer procedure time potentially results in increased operator tiredness and/or span of attention, especially in units where there are many procedures in any one day.

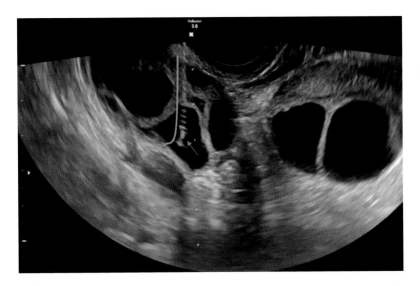

FIGURE 9.9 The needle tip is visible (orange curve line is parallel to the needle). The aspiration of the fluid is done from the opposite side of the hyperechogenic curve tip (see blue arrow). It is important to know from where the aspiration happens in order to have appropriate control of the needle rotation. This observation helps to minimize the risk of incomplete suction of the follicle.

It was thought that flushing during the oocyte aspiration technique increases the likelihood of oocyte collection. However, several studies have shown no significant differences in the number of oocytes retrieved, fertilization rate, or pregnancy rates between those where flushing had been used as compared to no flushing [20,32,52–54]. Meta-analysis showed no significant difference in oocyte gain if flushing was used in poor responders [55] or in minimal stimulation IVF [56]. Most operators do not use the flushing technique [18], and a recent meta-analysis [51] did not show significant benefit from performing follicular flushing.

The operator must be familiar with the tactile resistance when the ovary/follicle is penetrated with the needle, be able to manipulate the transducer to generate the relevant ultrasound image, and have a steady hand for the aspiration/flushing process. A fingertip handle on the distal end of the needle can facilitate the puncture with good clinical touch.

Suction Pump and Vacuum Pressure

The suction pump creates a negative pressure to facilitate aspiration of follicles. Usually, this pressure can be modulated, but most commonly, a setting of −90 to −120 mm Hg is enough [32] for good recovery with no harm on the oocyte-cumulus complex. Most operators use a digital pump with a variety of pressure settings, the predominant being toward −140 mm Hg. There is no consensus as to what specific aspiration pressure or needle gauge is optimal during OPU. Audit or records of this correlated with total oocyte yield should be subject for future research [57].

During suction, the follicle collapses and its volume decreases, and then conversely increases during flushing. The relationships between suction pressure, needle diameter, and oocyte yield were explored by Rose [57], concluding that the highest oocyte recovery rate occurs using higher pressures and larger needles, but this comes at the cost of damaging the cumulus-oocyte complex. It is likely that this damage is caused by the sheer stress forces exerted on the cumulus-oocyte complex due to parabolic forces associated with laminar flow within the needle, and is likely worsened by irregular forces during intervals of turbulent flow occurring with entry into the needle. Most reproductive medicine specialists maintain stable suction pressure. In case of low ovarian response or smaller follicles, some may increase the suction pressure hoping to achieve a better oocyte yield.

The Technique

The transvaginal transducer must have an appropriate cover and needle guide already in place (Figure 9.1). OPU cannot be done by a single operator, and a trained assistant should be available to help. The transducer tip should be in good contact with the cervix and vaginal fornixes giving access to the ovaries. Having the transvaginal probe contact with the fornix and paracervical space helps to stabilize the ovary prior to the OPU. The need for abdominal pressure may be required if the ovary is mobile and not fixed on the lateral pelvis. A quick but thorough ultrasound study before starting OPU is important to confirm numbers of large/small follicles and to allow the operator to choose the best access point for needle penetration. The operator should be familiar with needle characteristics prior to OPU, and the needle path guide on the monitor should be visible. The highly reflective end of the needle tip should be visible during needle progression toward the ovarian cortex. Aspiration should start, preferably with the automatic aspiration pump when the needle tip is within the first follicle. The follicle wall collapses during this process, and the operator can identify the color of the fluid through the aspiration tube. After suction of the first follicle, the egg is positively identified by the embryologist, mostly located nearby, and the needle progresses to the next follicle avoiding a reentry through the ovarian cortex and avoiding lateral movements that could slice the ovarian stroma. Repositioning of the transducer is needed in order to penetrate as central as possible within the next follicle space. The probe should be kept steady and not advancing with the needle exposed outside the needle guide. Manipulation of the OPU needle should be gentle and steady, avoiding abrupt movements, and its tip should always be visible. All follicles should be aspirated except those that are difficult to reach or if small, under 10 mm. The needle should be flushed when moving from one ovary to the other to clear any potential blockage caused by blood clots.

The Aspiration Technique

The operator needs to be familiar with the change of the follicle volume during aspiration and be able to control this as much as necessary to move the needle tip to the next follicle, repeating the same maneuver again. Identification of the distal needle part during the aspiration is essential for preventing uncomplete follicular aspirations and mainly avoiding wall remains/membranes that can obstruct the tip. In cases of polycystic ovaries where there are many adjacent follicles, twisting only the tip of the needle does not seem to be sufficient as some fluid can be trapped in between follicles. The ultrasonographic artifact created by the needle tip varies when the needle is rotated 90° to 180° and depends on which angle the tip is interacting with the ultrasound field. At 180°, the view is clear as in Figure 9.9, but when it is on a 90° angle, the real end of the needle is lower than what is seen on the screen. The tip of the needle may have a cone shape as demonstrated in Figures 9.10 and 9.11. See Videos 9.1 and 9.2 as well.

VIDEO 9.1

OPU demonstration of needle artifact and aspiration. (https://youtu.be/H-DsqCBQvtI)

VIDEO 9.2

Demonstration of OPU aspiration technique. (https://youtu.be/7mo4_P1rkoQ)

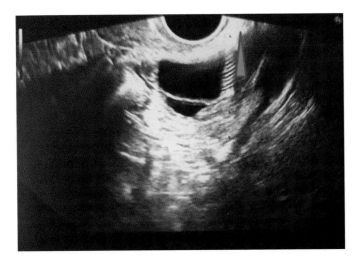

FIGURE 9.10 Here the end of the needle is seen as a cone (see blue arrow and cone) with an enlarged base on the distal end; however, the real tip of the needle is a couple of millimeters lower.

Most operators prefer to start OPU from the ovary nearest to the vaginal vault rather than the one with the largest follicles or complex appearances. There is no specific preference of right or left ovary, which is operator rather than anatomical choice. Most experts in the reproductive field use both planes, longitudinal and coronal, while performing OPU in order to confirm the anatomy and ovarian cortex boundaries and thus undertake the procedure safely. The application of vacuum pressure should start just before entering a follicle [20,57], which minimizes fluid loss in the pelvis [57].

Additional ultrasound-guided aspiration procedures in adjacent structures may be undertaken just before OPU with hysteroscopy [58] or after OPU, such as aspiration of hydrosalpinx under experienced hands, or ovarian cyst. In some rare cases, endometrioma may be aspirated only to facilitate aspiration of follicles under the endometrioma (Figure 9.12). The combination of these investigations and treatments may enhance the chances of pregnancy after embryo transfer.

Aspiration of hydrosalpingeal fluid in case of hydrosalpinx during ovarian stimulation and at the time of oocyte retrieval has been attempted and shown to improve pregnancy rates [59,60].

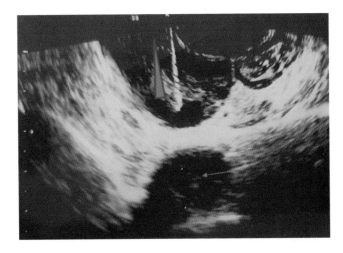

FIGURE 9.11 There is a mirror image of the ovary on the low part of the ultrasound field (blue arrow). The edge of the needle is showing a cone shape. Although the needle is maintained in the middle of the follicle, there is the potential risk of trauma on adjacent structures during the last moments of the oocyte pick-up, as the follicles are collapsing around the needle.

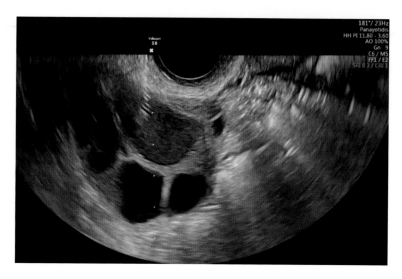

FIGURE 9.12   The endometrioma was on the top part of this ovary, and the access to the follicles would be compromised with the fluid aspirated through the endometrioma. In this case, a separated needle was used for aspiration of the endometrioma content, then with a new clean needle access to the healthy follicles was achieved. The patient had additional IV antibiotic cover for infection prophylaxis.

Complications

OPU complications had been reported [31,36,61], whether intraoperative and/or postoperative injuries such as vascular [62], hemoperitoneum [63,64], vaginal bleeding [65], or pelvic abscess [66,67].

Under experienced hands, the complication rate is very low, ranging from 0.06% to 0.2% for intraperitoneal bleeding and 0.03% to 0.6% for pelvic infections [1]. The frequency of complications, most frequent to least frequent, include hemoperitoneum or pelvic bleeding, infection such as ovarian or pelvic abscesses, and to a lesser extent, bladder perforation with some rare cases of retroperitoneal hematomas or bowel perforation. Patients at higher risk of complications include those with endometriomas, history of laparoscopic surgery for endometriosis and salpingitis, Müllerian malformations, and uterine fibroids, and those who are obese.

Few retrospective studies looked into the incidence of post-OPU complications, such as hemoperitoneum [31,33,36,63,65,68], and some recommended the use of ultrasound postoperative OPU to detect potential intra-abdominal bleeding. An article on potential health hazards of assisted reproduction [69] reported on the long-term effects of repeated oocyte collections on pelvic structures. It was possible to assess the pelvis at laparoscopic embryo transfer following IVF. In 54 women, four peritoneal fluid samples showed growth of coagulase-negative *Staphylococcus* and β-hemolytic streptococci. One further sample tested positive for *Chlamydia trachomatis*. All women remained asymptomatic, and three conceived and delivered healthy babies. Eight spontaneous pregnancies were reported up to 18 months after an unsuccessful attempt.

Endometriomas during OPU modify the mobility and kinetics of the ovary (Figure 9.12) and pose an additional risk of infection. History of past laparoscopic surgery may modify the location and anatomical relations of the organs (adhesions, scar tissues, less mobility of the ovary, or additional neovascularization), making it potentially more difficult to complete the OPU. An unusual location of fibroids modifying the anatomical relations with adnexa or creating ultrasound artifacts in the image, such as shadowing or increased attenuation, may be an additional difficulty for safe OPU. Obesity can modify the clarity of the image (higher fat deposits, omentum, and peritoneal fat), decreasing the resolution.

In these situations, patients should be counseled about the extra risks while carrying the OPU as well as consented about the need for external abdominal pressure to facilitate access to the ovaries (bring them closer to the probe or stabilize them) or the option to undertake the OPU under general anesthesia.

The Role of Doppler Study and/or Three-Dimensional Ultrasound Imaging

Routine color Doppler ultrasound can help to detect vascular areas and visualize major vessels in proximity of the ovaries. In a small study [39], Doppler use with OPU did not predict (45%) patients with moderate peritoneal bleeding, as this may not appear from vessels but from ovarian surface puncture. Approximately 15% of vaginal bleeding was detected and correctly predicted during oocyte aspiration when color Doppler OPU guidance was accessible technology [39]. Transvaginal color Doppler was introduced in gynecological imaging more than 10 years ago [70–72] and was initially used to evaluate follicular vascular perfusion [73], uterine artery flow, and the association of blood flow with IVF outcomes [74]. However, few operators used it as routine practice during OPU. Some operators perform a Doppler study to observe the follicles of each ovary immediately postaspiration and attempt to detect active bleeding; however, color Doppler remained largely an investigational tool with limited clinical added value, as some believe that it can be time consuming.

A Doppler-equipped ultrasound machine has become readily available to many IVF centers. Selecting a safe trajectory for the OPU needle devoid of large vessels is essential. The idea that Doppler ultrasound might reduce the risk of blood vessel injury during follicular aspiration seemed promising [38], but the authors did not measure peritoneal blood loss, and the validity of their proposal was never appropriately tested.

Other authors reflected on the value of three-dimensional (3D) or color Doppler study to determine if these imaging techniques have value in preventing complications associated with OPU [38,39,75]. Interestingly, 90% of experts did not agree that 3D ultrasound could prevent OPU complications [18]. Only a few practitioners used 3D prior to OPU in the course of fertility assessment, mainly to detect uterine abnormalities and endometrial polyps.

With new innovations in imaging technology, color Doppler and 3D ultrasound will have the potential to enhance the evaluation of IVF ovarian stimulation protocols and safer performance of OPU [32,76,77].

After Care

After the OPU procedure, the patient is usually observed for a couple of hours in the IVF center [30]. A follow-up scan after about 3–4 hours could depict hematoma formation or help to estimate the volume of fluid or bleeding in the pouch of Douglas [31,33,36,78]. Some authors have suggested that Doppler study or 3D ultrasound may be of value in estimating blood loss volume from 2 hours post-OPU and up to 3 days [75,79] for early detection of hematoma.

Late postaspiration ultrasound scan may offer an estimate of bleeding and free fluid in the abdominal cavity. Estimation of pelvic fluid volume after OPU may warn of potential bleeding complications and alert further surveillance. Patients with fluid pockets measuring less than 2 cm may be classified as having mild bleeding, patients with at least one pocket of maximal depth of 2–4 cm (circle or ellipsoid pocket) may be defined as having moderate abdominal bleeding, while a maximal depth of 5 cm or more may indicate severe bleeding [33,39,75,79,80].

Conclusion

The literature review revealed that there was a scarcity of information on standards relating to OPU techniques. Recommendations on standards performing OPU were necessary, and recent guidelines were produced by the ESHRE group [1]. The most common complications are reported as being vascular, internal pelvic bleeding followed by pelvic infections and pelvic abscesses. A systematic approach in performing OPU will ensure a low incidence of complications.

REFERENCES

1. ESHRE Working Group on Ultrasound in ART; D'Angelo A, Panayotidis C, Amso N et al. Recommendations for good practice in ultrasound: Oocyte pick up. *Hum Reprod Open*. 2019;2019(4):hoz025. doi:10.1093/hropen/hoz025

2. Lenz S, Lauritsen JG, and Kjellow M. Collection of human oocytes for *in vitro* fertilisation by ultrasonically guided follicular puncture. *Lancet*. 1981;1(8230):1163–4.

3. Dellenbach P, Nisand I, Moreau L et al. Transvaginal, sonographically controlled ovarian follicle puncture for egg retrieval. *Lancet*. 1984;1:1467.

4. Gleicher N, Friberg J, Fullan N et al. EGG retrieval for *in vitro* fertilisation by sonographically controlled vaginal culdocentesis. *Lancet*. 1983;2(8348):508–9.

5. Wikland M, Enk L, and Hamberger L. Transvesical and transvaginal approaches for the aspiration of follicles by use of ultrasound. *Ann N Y Acad Sci*. 1985;442:82–94.

6. Dellenbach P, Nisand I, Moreau L, Feger B, Plumere C, and Gerlinger P. Transvaginal sonographically controlled follicle puncture for oocyte retrieval. *Fertil. Steril* 1985;5:656–62.

7. Lewin A, Laufer N, Rabinowitz R, Margalioth EJ, Bar I, and Schenker JG. Ultrasonically guided oocyte collection under local anesthesia: The first choice method for *in vitro* fertilization—A comparative study with laparoscopy. *EBM Reviews—Cochrane Central Register of Controlled Trials. Fertil Steril*. 1986;46(2): 257–61.

8. Sterzik K, Jonatha W, Keckstein G, Rossmanith W, Traub E, and Wolf A. Ultrasonically guided follicle aspiration for oocyte retrieval in an *in vitro* fertilization program: Further simplification. *Int J Gynaecol Obstet*. 1987;25(4):309–14.

9. Deutinger J, Reinthaller A, Csaicsich P et al. Follicular aspiration for *in vitro* fertilization: Sonographically guided transvaginal versus laparoscopic approach. *Eur J Obstet Gynecol Reprod Biol*. 1987;26:127–33.

10. Seifer DB, Collins RL, Paushter DM, George CR, and Quigley MM. Follicular aspiration: A comparison of an ultrasonic endovaginal transducer with fixed needle guide and other retrieval methods. *Fertil Steril*. 1988;49:462–7.

11. Chang MY, Chang SY, and Soong YK. Transvaginal ultrasound-directed oocyte retrieval for *in vitro* fertilization. *Taiwan Yi Xue Hui Za Zhi*. 1989;88(7):689–93.

12. Barber R, Porter R, Picker R, Robertson R, Dawson E, and Saunders D. Transvaginal ultrasound directed oocyte collection for *in vitro* fertilization: Successes and complications. *J Ultrasound Med*. 1998;7:377–9.

13. Cerne A, Bergh C, Borg K et al. Pre-ovarian block versus paracervical block for oocyte retrieval. *Hum Reprod*. 2006;21(11):2916–21.

14. Vlahos NF, Giannakikou I, Vlachos A, and Vitoratos N. Analgesia and anaesthesia for assisted reproductive technologies. *Int J Gynecol Obstet*. 2009;105:201–5.

15. Barton SE, Politch JA, Benson CB, Ginsburg ES, and Gargiulo AR. Transabdominal follicular aspiration for oocyte retrieval in patients with ovaries inaccessible by transvaginal ultrasound. *Fertil Steril*. 2011;95(5):1773–6.

16. Roman-Rodriguez C-F, Weissbrot E, Hsu C-D, Wong A, Siefert C, and Sung L. Comparing transabdominal and transvaginal ultrasound-guided follicular aspiration: A risk assessment formula. *Taiwan J Obstet Gynecol*. 2015;54:693–9.

17. Edris F, Holiva N, Baghdadi S et al. Single operator ultrasound guided transabdominal oocyte retrieval in patients with ovaries inaccessible transvaginally: A modified technique. *Gynecol Obstet (Sunnyvale)*. 2014;4(214):1–5.

18. Panayotidis C. Interventional Ultrasound: Standardisation of Oocyte Retrieval in Assisted Reproduction Treatments. *MSc Dissertation*. Cardiff University; 2017. doi:10.13140/RG.2.2.28861.31205. Accessed September 15, 2018. https://www.researchgate.net/publication/327142563_Interventional_Ultrasound_Standardisation_of_Oocyte_Retrieval_in_Assisted_Reproduction_Treatments

19. European Society of Human Reproduction and Embryology (ESHRE). Guideline Group on good practice in IVF labs. 2015, Chapter 7, page 14. Accessed September 15, 2018. https://www.eshre.eu/Guidelines-and-Legal/Guidelines/Revised-guidelines-for-good-practice-in-IVF-laboratories-(2015).aspx

20. Georgiou EX, Melo P, Brown J, and Granne IE. Follicular flushing during oocyte retrieval in assisted reproductive techniques. *Cochrane Database Syst Rev*. 2018;4(4):CD004634.

21. Robson SJ, Barry M, and Norman RJ. Power Doppler assessment of follicle vascularity at the time of oocyte retrieval in *in vitro* fertilization cycles. *Fertil Steril.* 2008;90(6):2179–82.
22. Dalkey NC, and Helmer O. An experimental application of the Delphi method to the use of experts. *Manage Sci.* 1963;9(3):458–67.
23. Brown BB. *Delphi Process: A Methodology Used for the Elicitation of Opinions of Experts.* An earlier paper published by RAND (Document No: P-3925, 1968, 15 pages); 1968. Accessed September 4, 2018. http://www.rand.org/pubs/papers/P3925.html
24. Sackman H. Delphi Assessment: Expert Opinion, Forecasting and Group Process. R-1283–PR; 1974. Accessed September 5, 2018. http://www.rand.org/content/dam/rand/pubs/reports/2006/R1283.pdf
25. Linstone HA, and Turoff M. *The Delphi Method: Techniques and Applications. Reading, MA*: Addison-Wesley; 1975. Accessed June 7, 2017. https://web.njit.edu/~turoff/pubs/delphibook/index.html
26. Jones J, and Hunter D. Consensus methods for medical and health services research. *BMJ.* 1995;5(311):376–80.
27. Branigan EF, Estes A, Walker K, and Rothgeb R. Thorough sonographic oocyte retrieval during *in vitro* fertilization produces results similar to ovarian wedge resection in patients with clomiphene citrate–resistant polycystic ovarian syndrome. *Am J Obstet Gynecol.* 2006;194:1696–701.
28. American Institute of Ultrasound in Medicine (AIUM) 2008. Guideline AIUM Practice Parameter for Ultrasonography in Reproductive Medicine. Accessed September 4, 2018. http://www.aium.org/resources/guidelines/reproductivemed.pdf
29. Panayotidis C. Vaginal examination, have we forgotten the basics? *Eur Clin Obstet Gynaecol.* 2007;3(2):103–10.
30. Tobler KJ, Zhao Y, Weissman A, Majumdar A, Leong M, and Shoham Z. Worldwide survey of IVF practices: Trigger retrieval and embryo transfer techniques. *Arch Gynecol Obstet.* 2014;290:561–8.
31. Ludwig AK, Glawatz M, Griesinger G, Diedrich K, and Ludwig M. Perioperative and post-operative complications of transvaginal ultrasound-guided oocyte retrieval: Prospective study of >1000 oocyte retrievals. *Hum Reprod.* 2006;21:3235–40.
32. Healy MW, Hill MJ, and Levens ED. Optimal oocyte retrieval and embryo transfer techniques: Where we are and how we got here. *Semin Reprod Med.* 2015;33(2):83–91.
33. Bodri D, Guillén JJ, Polo A, Trullenque M, Esteve C, and Coll O. Complications related to ovarian stimulation and oocyte retrieval in 4052 oocyte donor cycles. *Reprod Biomed Online.* 2008;2(17):237–43.
34. Weinreb EB, Cholst IN, Ledger WJ, Danis RB, and Rosenwaks Z. Should all oocyte donors receive prophylactic antibiotics for retrieval? *Fertil Steril.* 2010;94(7):2935–7.
35. Govaerts I, Devreker F, Delbaere A, Revelard Ph, and Englert Y. Short-term medical complications of 1500 oocyte retrievals for *in vitro* fertilization and embryo transfer. *EJOGR.* 1998;77(2):239–43.
36. Aragona C, Mohamed MH, Espinola MSB et al. Clinical complications after transvaginal oocyte retrieval in 7,098 IVF cycles. *Fertil Steril.* 2011;95(1):293–4.
37. British Medical Ultrasound Society (BMUS). Guidelines for Professional Ultrasound Practice (revised version December 2016). Accessed September 4, 2018. https://www.bmus.org/policies-statements-guidelines/professional-guidance
38. Shalev J, Orvieto R, and Meizner I. Use of color Doppler sonography during follicular aspiration in patients undergoing *in vitro* fertilization may reduce the risk of blood vessel injury. *Fertil Steril.* 2004;81(5)::1408–10.
39. Risquez F, and Confino E. Can Doppler ultrasound-guided oocyte retrieval improve IVF safety? *Reprod Biomed Online.* 2010;21:444–5.
40. Panayotidis C. Illustrations in gynaecology: Still controversial? *Gynaecol Surg.* 2005;2(3):165–8.
41. Koninckx PR. Video registration of surgery should be used as a quality control. *J Minim Invasive Gynecol.* 2008;15:248–53.
42. Makary MA. The power of video recording: Taking quality to the next level. *JAMA.* 2013;309(15):1591–2.
43. Kondo W, and Zomer MT. Video recording the laparoscopic surgery for the treatment of endometriosis should be systematic! *Gynecol Obstet (Sunnyvale).* 2014;4:220. doi:10.4172/2161-0932.1000220
44. Grantcharov T. 2015. Surgical Black Box Improves Performance and Safety? TEDxFortMcMurray. Accessed September 6, 2018. https://www.youtube.com/watch?v=O4gP6JkJ2YI
45. Vincent C, Moorthy K, Sarker SK, Chang A, and Darzi AW. Systems approaches to surgical quality and safety: From concept to measurement. *Ann Surg.* 2004;239:475–82.

46. Makary MA. Can video recording revolutionize medical quality. *BMJ.* 2015;351:h5169.
47. Awonuga A, Waterstone J, Oyesanya O, Curson R, Nargund G, and Parsons J. A prospective randomized study comparing needles of different diameters for transvaginal ultrasound-directed follicle aspiration. EBM Reviews—Cochrane Central Register of Controlled Trials. *Fertil Steril.* 1996;65(1):109–13.
48. Kushnir VA, Kim A, Gleicher N, and Barad DH. A pilot trial of large versus small diameter needles for oocyte retrieval. *Reprod Biol Endocrinol.* 2013;11:22.
49. Leung ASO, Daham MH, and Tan SL. Techniques and technology for human oocyte collection. *Expert Rev Med Devices.* 2016;13(8):701–3.
50. Levens ED, Whitcomb BW, Payson MD, and Larsen FW. Ovarian follicular flushing among low-responding patients undergoing assisted reproductive technology. *Fertil Steril.* 2009;91:1381–4.
51. Georgiou EX, Melo P, Brown J, Granne IE. Follicular flushing during oocyte retrieval in assisted reproductive techniques. *Cochrane Database Syst Rev.* 2018;4:CD004634.
52. Levy G, Hill MJ, Ramirez C et al. The use of follicle flushing during oocyte retrieval in assisted reproductive technologies: A systematic review and meta-analysis. *Hum Reprod.* 2012;27(8):2373–9.
53. Tan SL, Waterstone J, Wren M, and Parsons J. A prospective randomized study comparing aspiration only with aspiration and flushing for transvaginal ultrasound-directed oocyte recovery. *Fertil Steril.* 1992;58:356–60.
54. Haydardedeoglu B, Cok T, Kilicdag EB, Parlakgumus AH, Simsek E, and Bagis T. *In vitro* fertilization-intracytoplasmic sperm injection outcomes in single versus double-lumen oocyte retrieval needles in normally responding patients: A randomized trial. *Fertil Steril.* 2011;95:812–4.
55. Neumann K, and Griesinger G. Follicular flushing in patients with poor ovarian response: A systematic review and meta-analysis. *Reprod Biomed Online.* 2018;36(4):408–15.
56. Mendez Lozano DH, Brum Scheffer J, Frydman N, Fay S, Fanchin R, and Frydman R. Optimal reproductive competence of oocytes retrieved through follicular flushing in minimal stimulation IVF. *Reprod Biomed Online.* 2018;16(1):119–23.
57. Rose BI. Approaches to oocyte retrieval for advanced reproductive technology cycles planning to utilize *in vitro* maturation: A review of the many choices to be made. *J Assist Reprod Genet.* 2014;31:1409–19.
58. Ozgur K, Bulut H, Berkkanoglu M, Humaidan P, and Coetzee K. Concurrent oocyte retrieval and hysteroscopy: A novel approach in assisted reproduction freeze-all cycles. *Reprod Biomed Online.* 2016;33:206–13.
59. Hammadieh N, Coomarasamy A, Ola B, Papaioannou S, Afnan M, and Sharif K. Ultrasound-guided hydrosalpinx aspiration during oocyte collection improves pregnancy outcome in IVF: A randomized controlled trial. *EBM Reviews - Cochrane Central Register of Controlled Trials. Hum Reprod (Oxford, England).* 2008;23(5):1113–7.
60. Zhou Y, Jiang H, Zhang WX, Ni F, Wang XM, and Song XM. Ultrasound-guided aspiration of hydrosalpinx occurring during controlled ovarian hyperstimulation could improve clinical outcome of *in vitro* fertilization-embryo transfer. *J Obstet Gynaecol Res.* 2016;42(8):960–5.
61. Bennett SJ, Waterstone JJ, Cheng WC, and Parsons J. Complications of transvaginal ultrasound-directed follicle aspiration: A review of 2670 consecutive procedures. *J Assist Reprod Genet.* 1993;10:72–7.
62. Azem F, Wolf Y, Botchan A, Amit A, Lessing JB, and Kluger Y. Massive retroperitoneal bleeding: A complication of transvaginal ultrasonography-guided oocyte retrieval for *in vitro* fertilization–embryo transfer. *Fertil Steril.* 2000;74(2):405–6.
63. Nouri K, Walch K, Promberger R, Kurz C, Tempfer CB, and Ott J. Severe haematoperitoneum caused by ovarian bleeding after transvaginal oocyte retrieval: A retrospective analysis and systematic literature review. *Reprod Bio Med Online.* 2014;29:699–707.
64. Liberty G, Hyman JH, Eldar-Geva T, Latinsky B, Gal M, and Margalioth EJ. Ovarian hemorrhage after transvaginal ultrasonographically guided oocyte aspiration: A potentially catastrophic and not so rare complication among lean patients with polycystic ovary syndrome. *Fertil Steril.* 2010;93(3):874–9.
65. Siristatidis C, Chrelias C, Alexiou A, and Kassanos D. Clinical complications after transvaginal oocyte retrieval: A retrospective analysis. *J Obstet Gynaecol.* 2013;33(1):64–6.
66. Benaglia L, Somigliana E, Iemmello R, Colpi E, Nicolosi AE, and Ragni G. Endometrioma and oocyte retrieval–induced pelvic abscess: A clinical concern or an exceptional complication? *Fertil Steril.* 2008;89(5):1263–66.
67. Sharpe K, Karovitch AJ, Claman P, and Suh KN. Transvaginal oocyte retrieval for *in vitro* fertilization complicated by ovarian abscess during pregnancy. *Fertil Steril.* 2006;86(1):219e.11–13.

68. Zhen X, Qiao J, Ma C, Fan Y, and Liu P. Intraperitoneal bleeding following transvaginal oocyte retrieval. *Int J Gynecol Obstet*. 2010;108(1):31–4.
69. Nazar A. Debate: Potential health hazards of assisted reproduction, Problems facing the clinician. *Hum Reprod*. 1995;10(7):1628–30.
70. Hata T, Hata K, Senoh D et al. Doppler ultrasound assessment of tumor vascularity in gynecologic disorders. *J Ultrasound Med*. 1989;8:309–14.
71. Hata T, Hata K, Senoh D et al. Transvaginal Doppler colour flow mapping. *Gynecol Obstet Invest*. 1989;127(4):217–8.
72. Kurjak A, Jurkovic D, Alfirevic Z, and Zalud I. Transvaginal colour Doppler Imaging. *J Clin Ultrasound*. 1990;4:227–34.
73. Bhal PS, Pugh ND, Chui DK, Gregory L, Walzer SM, and Shaw RW. The use of transvaginal power Doppler ultrasonography to evaluate the relationship between per follicular vascular and outcome in *in-vitro* fertilization treatment cycles. *Hum Reprod*. 1999;14:939–45.
74. Bloechle M, Schreiner T, Küchler I, Schürenkämper P, and Lisse K. Colour Doppler assessment of ascendent uterine artery perfusion in an in-vitro fertilization-embryo transfer programme after pituitary desensitization and ovarian stimulation with human recombinant follicle stimulating hormone. *Hum Reprod*. 1997;12(8):1772–7.
75. Shalev J, Davidi O, and Fish B. Quantitative three-dimensional sonographic assessment of pelvic blood after transvaginal ultrasound-guided oocyte aspiration: Factors predicting risk. *Ultrasound Obstet Gynecol*. 2004;23(2):177–82.
76. Ng EHY, Chan CCW, Tang OS, Yeung WSB, and Ho PC. Factors affecting endometrial and subendometrial blood flow measured by three-dimensional power Doppler ultrasound during IVF treatment. *Hum Reprod*. 2006;21(4):1062–9.
77. Jayaprakasan K, Deb S, Sur S et al. Ultrasound and its role in assisted reproduction treatment. *Imaging Med*. 2010;2(2):135–50.
78. Paajanen H, Lahti P, and Nordback I. Sensitivity of transabdominal ultrasonography in detection of intraperitoneal fluids in human. *Eur J Radiol*. 1999;7:1423–5.
79. Dessole S, Rubattu G, Ambrosini G, Miele M, Nardelli GB, and Cherchi PL. Blood loss following noncomplicated transvaginal oocyte retrieval for *in vitro* fertilization. *Fertil Steril*. 2001;76:205–6.
80. Ragni G, Scarduelli C, Calanna G, Santi G, Benaglia L, and Somigliana E. Blood loss during transvaginal oocyte retrieval. *Gynecol Obstet Invest*. 2009;67:32–5.

10

Embryo Transfer

Julia Kopeika and Yacoub Khalaf

Brief History

In July 1978, the world celebrated the birth of the first baby conceived through *in vitro* fertilization (IVF). However, this achievement rested on the "shoulders of giants" after many years of trials and errors of scientific minds. Interestingly, the first successful embryo transfer was just a research tool to answer the scientific question of whether the uterine environment influences an embryo's phenotype and to define the mechanisms of the supposed phenomenon of telegony [1]. The first successful embryo transfer was achieved in rabbits in 1891: Walter Heape used a spear-headed needle to transport two fertilized eggs from an Angora doe rabbit into the fallopian tube of a Belgian Hare recipient [2]. This experiment resulted in a birth of six young offspring; two had Angora phenotypes and four had Belgian Hare phenotypes.

The field of embryology relied extensively on rabbits at the end of the nineteenth century. Other animals were also used to conquer this technique, but it was not until the 1930s when successful transfer in rats and mice was achieved. Originally such transfers in mice to the uterus rather than to the oviduct were rarely successful. Only one pregnancy was achieved from 70 experiments [1]. The high failure rate was due not only to the embryo transfer technique on its own, but also to a poor understanding at the time of what the optimal endocrine and embryo culture environment is. The beginning of the twentieth century was an active time in multiple aspects of relevance to embryo transfer: the relationship between the pituitary gland and ovaries was established, and considerable developments in artificial insemination and initial studies in the culture of oocytes *in vitro* occurred. By the late 1920s, the potential advantages of this knowledge were translated into advances in livestock breeding.

However, it took almost 50 years before some progress was made in humans. Work on the transfer of cleaving human embryos to the uterus was encouraged by the report of Marston et al. [3], who showed that a five-cell rhesus monkey embryo could develop into a newborn baby after transfer into the uterus of its mother [4]. However, despite positive experiences in the animal kingdom, there were multiple failures in humans. The one exception resulted in ectopic pregnancy [4]. One of the potential contributory causes of the failures in human patients was thought to be the trauma involved in transferring the embryos into the uterus.

It took 88 years until the first successful embryo transfer occurred in a human [5]. The main method of transfer in early animal studies was a surgical transfundal approach under anesthesia. Originally, the transcervical approach seemed to give the much more inferior pregnancy rate of 2%–4% [6] in comparison with the surgical transmyometrial approach (50%) in different animal species. The variety of techniques that were tried as nonsurgical methods in cattle is fascinating: besides cervical approaches with and without uterine insufflation, they included transrectal and transvaginal methods and the use of gelatin-embedded ova attached to the ovarian ligament by barbs [1].

However, refinement of the transcervical method soon became the mainstream technique in humans. In the next several years, incremental improvements were made to the embryo transfer process, to include using smaller-diameter transfer catheters, decreasing transfer fluid volume to 20–30 μL, and including a high proportion of serum in the transfer medium, resulting in increased pregnancy rates [7].

Patient Preparation Prior to Procedure

Patient Education

It is important to explain the process of embryo transfer in advance. Patients need to be reassured that even though it is one of the most important steps of their journey, it is a quite short and simple procedure with little or no discomfort. A positive attitude could help alleviate undue anxiety that has been shown to be associated with a higher frequency of uterine contractions [8]. Advance knowledge of additional risk factors such as difficulties during intimate examinations would ensure that necessary steps are undertaken to make the process less stressful and more straightforward.

Full Bladder

It is believed that a full bladder could straighten the uterocervical angle during embryo transfer and facilitate access into the uterine cavity with a soft catheter. In 2007, a systematic review [9] suggested that a full bladder could be associated with a higher pregnancy rate (odds ratio [OR] 1.44 95%; confidence interval [CI] 1.04–2.04). This review derived its conclusion from two studies [10,11]; the larger of the two studies was not a true randomized controlled trial (RCT), since allocation to the different treatment groups was performed on alternate days. A subsequent Cochrane review [12] showed no difference in pregnancy rates between a full or empty bladder (OR 0.98; CI 0.57–1.68), when only two small RCTs with no power calculation were included.

Hence, there is no good-quality evidence that a full bladder improves the pregnancy rate. However, a full bladder is known to improve visualization of the uterus during a transabdominal ultrasound scan (Figures 10.1 and 10.2) (Video 10.1). Visualization of catheter advancement and tip placement is shown to improve the pregnancy rate by 4%–8% [13–15].

The pitfall of an overfilled bladder, however, is patient discomfort, which arguably could increase uterine contractility. Therefore, the skill is to have an adequately full bladder that can make the procedure as easy as possible and could improve passage and visualization of the catheter without causing too much discomfort for patients. It is generally recommended that the patient should drink 500–1000 mL of fluid, 1 hour prior to the procedure, after emptying the bladder completely. It is also important to minimize

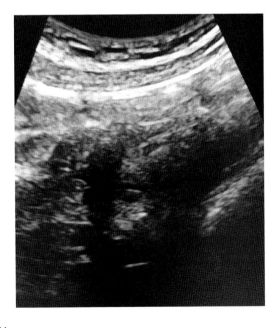

FIGURE 10.1   Empty bladder.

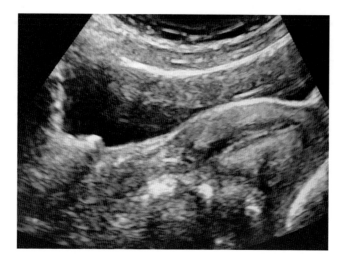

FIGURE 10.2   The same patient with full bladder.

VIDEO 10.1
Embryo transfer in axial uterus. This patient has a very full bladder that has straightened the uterus into axial position with an excellent view of the embryo transfer procedure. (https://youtu.be/sZ3SS69XYeI)

the waiting time prior to the procedure to avoid the patient getting more uncomfortable with her bladder and becoming more anxious.

Uterine Relaxants

Uterine contractility during embryo transfer has been thought to be associated with a lower implantation rate [16]. There is some evidence that uterine contractions are increased by sixfold during IVF in comparison with the natural cycle [17]. The frequency of subendometrial peristalsis has also been shown to be higher in ovarian stimulation cycles compared with natural cycles [18,19].

It was suggested that administration of pharmacological agents to reduce uterine contractility might have a positive effect on implantation rate [20,21]. There are several agents that may be able to accomplish this task:

- Oxytocin receptor antagonists that act by antagonizing naturally synthesized oxytocin as well as vasopressin at their receptors in the myometrium, promoting uterine relaxation [22].
- Prostaglandin synthetase (cyclooxygenase) inhibitors that reduce prostaglandins ($PGF_{2\alpha}$ and PGE2) and thromboxane A2, which are involved in myometrial contractions in nonpregnant and pregnant uteri [23–25].
- Nitric oxide that relaxes smooth muscle, helping with vasodilatation and possibly helping by inducing relaxation of the smooth muscles of the myometrium as shown in pregnancy [26,27].
- Beta-adrenergic receptor agonists that promote the relaxation of the smooth muscle in cases of preterm labor [28] and in the nonpregnant uterus [29].
- Anticholinergic agents that cause relaxation of the myometrial smooth muscles [30,31].
- Calcium channel blockers that inhibit the influx of calcium ions through the cell membranes of smooth muscle, inhibiting contractions. Their use has been reported for tocolysis [32].

Data from a prospective cohort study suggested that administration of atosiban (oxytocin/vasopressin receptor antagonist) at the time of embryo transfer was associated with a higher implantation rate [20]. However, when the same group conducted a multicenter RCT, they found no difference in live birth rates between atosiban and the placebo group in the general IVF population [33].

Beta-adrenergic receptor agonists, prostaglandin synthetase inhibitors, and nitric oxide donors also did not show any improvement in the clinical pregnancy rate in the systematic review [34]. The only exception was a single small study reporting on the use of the anticholinergic agent [21]; however, this study had significant methodological flaws.

Therefore, there is insufficient evidence to suggest that routine administration of uterine relaxants can improve IVF outcome after embryo transfer.

Visualization of the Cervix

Before commencing the procedure, patient identity should be confirmed according to the local protocols and, in the United Kingdom, Human Fertilisation and Embryology Authority (HFEA) guidelines. It is important that clinicians performing the procedure familiarize themselves with the history of the patient and understand all the underlying factors that may necessitate modifying the embryo transfer procedure.

Visualization of the cervix with a speculum in the setting of embryo transfer should be performed with utmost care to avoid initiating pain that could trigger uterine contractions. Undue stimulation of the cervix causes the release of oxytocin, thus increasing uterine contractility [35,36].

Two relatively old studies suggested that the uterus expels the fluid instilled into the cavity. This raises the possibility of expulsion of the embryo within the culture media after embryo transfer [37,38]. It has also been observed that after embryo transfer, the embryos can move as easily toward the cervical canal as toward the fallopian tubes [39]. The increased frequency of uterine contractions negatively correlated with the clinical pregnancy rate [40].

Cleaning of the Cervical Canal

Cervical mucus plays an important protective role against ascending bacterial infection. The consistency of mucus varies through the menstrual cycle and becomes very thin and watery at the time of ovulation to promote sperm access to the oocyte. However, during IVF, an excessive amount of mucus (from the effect of progesterone) may interfere with embryo transfer by blocking the tip of the catheter [41] or hindering embryo expulsion into the right place in the endometrial cavity. However, rigorous "cleaning" may cause trauma and bleeding to the cervical canal and may have a negative effect on implantation rate. Mucus cleaning has not been shown to confer any significant benefit [12,42].

Another risk is contamination of the catheter and uterus by cervical flora. Positive microbial growth in the embryo transfer catheter has been found in 49.1% of cases [43]. Bacterial contamination was thought to worsen treatment outcome, and a case was made for routine use of antibiotics [15]. However, a randomized study [44] found no improvement in pregnancy rate in patients treated with antibiotics, despite reducing genital tract microbial colonization.

Role of Ultrasound Scan in Embryo Transfer

Transabdominal ultrasound guided embryo transfer was first reported in 1985 [45]. However, despite the universal practice of transvaginal ultrasound guided oocyte retrieval, the role of the ultrasound guidance during the embryo transfer remained debatable. Some argued that the clinical touch method has the potential advantages of not needing the patient to have a very full bladder and not requiring a second operator [46] or extra equipment. But the use of ultrasound-guided embryo transfer has the potential benefit of visualization of the tip of the catheter allowing confirmation that the placement of

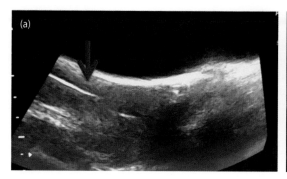
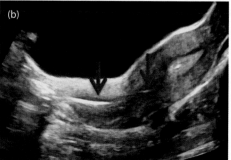

FIGURE 10.3   Visualization of catheter during advancement through the cervix. (a) Magnified image showing the catheter advancement through the cervical canal (red arrow). (b) Panoramic view of the cervix and uterus in midsagittal view showing the catheter inside the cervical canal (left arrow) and within the lower uterine body (right arrow).

the embryo has occurred beyond the internal os into the "optimal" place in the uterine cavity (Figure 10.3). Subsequent studies have demonstrated that ultrasound guidance is beneficial [13,47,48]. However, there was substantial heterogeneity among the included studies. A more recent systematic review [46] concluded that ultrasound guidance during embryo transfer improved the chance of achieving a live birth and the likelihood of a clinical pregnancy compared with clinical touch, when using the same catheters and techniques. It has been argued that ultrasound guidance should be used as a standard [49].

Transvaginal ultrasound guidance was also considered to aid embryo transfer. The potential advantages of this approach are obviating the need for a full bladder and obtaining better images of the details of anatomy.

VIDEO 10.2
Embryo transfer in a retroverted uterus. (https://youtu.be/B0NMT9_6D-4)

The challenge is how to simultaneously and adequately place the ultrasound probe, the speculum, and the catheter during embryo transfer. Several studies have assessed the benefit of transvaginal ultrasound guidance for embryo transfer [49–51] and reported comparable pregnancy rates with less pain reported by patients. There was also an attempt to explore the role of transrectal ultrasound in guiding embryo transfer, especially in the cases of retroverted uterus [52] (Video 10.2); however, this has not gained much utilization in current practice.

To date there is no RCT performed to assess the impact on effectiveness of the embryo transfer of transvaginal or transrectal ultrasound-guided access, so the transabdominal approach remains the most widely used.

Catheter

Types of Catheters

There is a wide variety of embryo transfer catheters available for clinical use. They differ in diameter, length, malleability, presence of an outer sheath, stiffness, material memory, and characteristics of the tip. The ideal catheter should cause as little trauma to the endometrium as possible but be firm enough to navigate the cervical canal. Several studies looked at the difference in pregnancy rates between different types of catheters. A systematic review [53] showed that the use of soft catheters was associated with a higher pregnancy rate (OR 1.49, 95% CI 1.26–1.77). There appears to be little variation in clinical pregnancy rates between the different types of soft catheters [54]. But some authors argue that it might be more difficult to pass a soft catheter only via the cervical canal [54]. To overcome this problem, a coaxial catheter system with more rigid outer sheath was introduced [55]. The full benefits of soft catheter are better appreciated if an outer sheath is minimally used and stopped just before the internal os [36], since irritation of the internal os is believed to trigger uterine contractions [56]. The inner soft catheter is better appreciated if it has air bubbles or an echogenic tip, since it is easier to visualize in real-time ultrasound and makes the transfer easier and quicker than with a nonechogenic catheter.

Two RCTs confirmed that the use of catheters with an echogenic tip simplifies ultrasound-guided embryo transfer and minimizes catheter movement to identify the tip [57,58] with no difference in pregnancy outcomes.

VIDEO 10.3
Embryo transfer in an anteverted uterus. Careful advancement of an inner embryo catheter into the uterine cavity. Once the tip has reached an upper third of the cavity, the embryo is expelled into the uterus. This appears as a sudden "flush" of a small white drop. (https://youtu.be/ONqFQGLIem4)

Mock Transfer under Ultrasound Guidance

Mock embryo transfer can be performed prior to an IVF cycle or just before actual embryo transfer. This is done in order to establish if there are any potential difficulties that could be addressed in a timely manner in order to reduce uterine trauma and avoid the risk of depositing the embryo in a suboptimal location. Mock embryo transfer may help to assess variables such as uterine cavity position, measurement, ease of access, and choice of catheter. However, since uterine and cervical anatomy have a great degree of variability, findings during mock embryo transfer may not be relevant by the time of the actual procedure. A previous study demonstrated that almost half of patients who had retroverted uterus during mock assessment were found to have anteverted uterus by the time of the actual procedure [59] (Video 10.3). However, for patients with previous surgeries on the cervix (i.e., previous cone biopsy, trachelectomy), it is imperative to establish if access to the uterine cavity is possible at all. If the mock procedure reveals complete stenosis of the passage, this patient may benefit from examination under anesthesia and cervical dilation prior to an IVF cycle commencement.

The mock embryo transfer just before the procedure has a different purpose. It serves as the first phase of the procedure. It involves negotiating the cervix and identifying difficulties that may arise with the ease of passage through the cervical canal before threading through a soft catheter containing the embryo. Introduction of an outer sheath to the internal os can pave a safer route for the soft catheter loaded with an embryo, making the passage of the latter as smooth and as atraumatic as possible.

However, a disadvantage of mock embryo transfer is the possibility of causing irritation, trauma, or increased contractility of the uterus. To date, there are no RCTs evaluating the advantages of mock embryo transfer.

A relatively small study of 135 patients randomly allocated to dummy embryo transfer before starting IVF showed that mock embryo transfer was associated with better implantation and pregnancy rate [60]. The timing of mock embryo transfer, whether before starting controlled ovarian stimulation, at the time of egg collection, or just before the actual embryo transfer, did not seem to influence IVF outcome [59–63.] Robust evidence in favor of routine performance of mock embryo transfer is still lacking. A recent Cochrane review failed to identify any eligible randomized studies for dummy transfer [12].

Location of Catheter Tip Placement and Loading Techniques

The optimal site of embryo placement has been the focus of research in many studies. An early study showed that in almost one in five embryo transfers, the embryo could be located in the fluid at the external os after completion of the procedure [64]. The site of embryo placement in the uterine cavity has been suggested to directly influence the implantation rate, with better outcome if the tip of the catheter

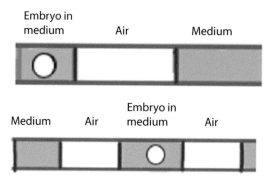

FIGURE 10.4   Scheme of catheter loading pattern.

is placed close to the middle area of the cavity [65,66] or 15–20 mm from the fundus [67] compared to 10 mm from the fundus. The issue is that an embryo is quite dynamic. A recent study demonstrated that even 1 hour after embryo transfer, more than 90% of "embryo flashes" (air bubbles with fluid seen at the time of embryo transfer) had changed their primary location and demonstrate significant migration assessed by three-dimensional (3D) scan [68]. One may argue that the location of the embryo 1 hour after transfer might be potentially more important than the location at the time of transfer. However, to date there are no studies to demonstrate that the direction of "embryo bubble" movement can be managed artificially. The other limitation of studies attempting to detect the optimal location of embryo placement is that most of them do not take into consideration the total volume of the uterine cavity, but focus on absolute distance from the fundus, which may not be relevant for all. However, to the best of the authors' knowledge, placement of embryo(s) in the mid to upper third of the cavity seems to result in a better pregnancy rate. Once the tip has reached the desired level in the cavity, the embryo(s) are deposited gently under ultrasound guidance (see Videos 10.1 through 10.3). Maximum effort should be exercised to avoid touching the fundus, since it can trigger uterine contractions. A recently developed mathematical model has also demonstrated the importance of a combination of factors, such as media viscosity, speed of injection, and catheter withdrawal, on subsequent embryo location [69]. These authors suggest that use of a transferred medium with similar viscosity to that of the uterine fluid and a slow injection and catheter withdrawal speed are crucial for optimal embryo placement.

The injected volume of media carrying the embryo(s) or loading technique may also affect the outcome [70]. Too small (under 10 μL) [71] or too large volumes are believed to account for a reduced implantation rate or an increased rate of ectopic pregnancy [72,73]. To date, there are no RCTs on optimal loading volume. Based on the available evidence in the literature, Sigalos et al. [70] recommended using less than 60 μL of culture media. However, this appears to be a very large volume, and with currently used catheters, the volume of media that is expelled is well under 10 μL. Several loading techniques have been described in the literature: one-drop, air brackets, and three-drop techniques with or without introduction of air bubble into the catheter (Figure 10.4). The logic behind introducing an air bubble was (1) to improve the ultrasonic visibility of the injected media into the cavity (Figure 10.5), (2) to improve embryo propulsion from the catheter and reduce the embryo retention rate, (3) to prevent transport of the embryo within the catheter, and (4) to protect the embryo from cervical mucus and accidental discharge before entering the cavity. The catheter is also filled with culture media before introducing bubbles and embryo(s) to minimize the capillary effect when the embryo is deposited into the uterine cavity.

Retained Embryo

Several factors were thought to be associated with embryo retention, namely, too small an amount of fluid loaded into the catheter, excessive cervical mucus, blood at the catheter tip, inadequate maintenance of pressure on the syringe or catheter, or withdrawal technique. Retained embryo is reported in 3%–4% of embryo transfers. However, it does not appear to negatively influence IVF outcome [74,75]. If an embryo was found to be retained in the catheter, the patient needs to be reassured and the procedure repeated.

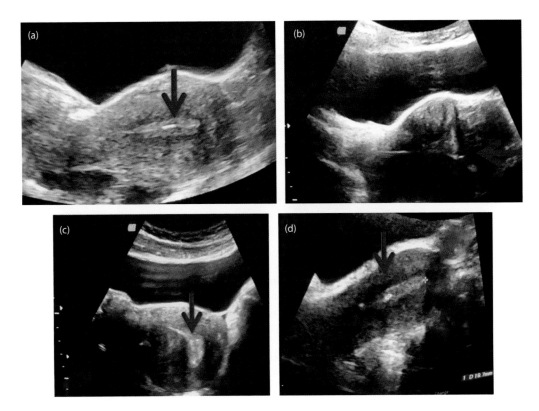

FIGURE 10.5 Distance of acoustic drop to uterine fundus. (a), (b), and (c) demonstrate the acoustic drops where the embryos are deposited inside the upper uterine cavity (red arrows). (d) Measurement of the distance between the acoustic drop (red arrow) and the upper end of the uterine cavity (calipers).

Difficult Transfer/Unable to Do the Transfer

A difficult embryo transfer can be defined as a procedure that may require additional maneuvers/instruments, force, and/or leading to the presence of blood at the catheter tip. The impact of difficult embryo transfer on pregnancy rate has also been studied.

It is important that the following conditions are identified at the beginning of the IVF process:

- Vaginismus or undue anxiety
- Pelvic endometriosis
- Multiple fibroids distorting anatomy and cervix visualization
- Previous cervical surgery
- Previous difficult embryo transfer

Patients with *severe vaginismus* will do better with continuity of care from the same clinician throughout the whole process. Once they establish rapport and trust, they could feel less anxious about examinations. Ongoing support of counselors could also be valuable in these cases. These patients could also be offered embryo transfer under sedation to minimize further distress.

Patients with *severe endometriosis* could also find examinations quite difficult, and it is not uncommon for them to have fixed retroverted uterus (Figure 10.6). It is helpful to assess the anatomy and possibility of gaining access to the uterine cavity causing minimal discomfort to a patient. These patients may benefit from either use of a smaller speculum or possibly also the procedure being performed under sedation.

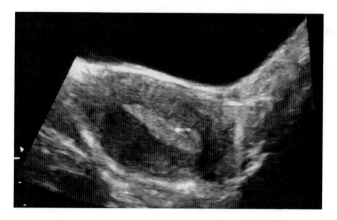

FIGURE 10.6 Retroverted uterus.

The majority of patients with uterine *fibroids* should have no problems with internal examination. However, low-lying fibroids could occasionally displace the cervix very anteriorly, hindering access to the uterine cavity and resulting in inevitable significant discomfort to patients. These patients need to be assessed prior to starting IVF. Other symptoms of fibroids should be taken into consideration, and myomectomy may need to be considered where appropriate.

Patients with previous *cervical surgery* could be very challenging when it comes to embryo transfer. In the first instance, it would be important for these patients to have examination and mock embryo transfer performed prior to commencing treatment. If there was difficulty in identifying the path to the uterus, and access to the uterine cavity proved impossible with both soft and rigid catheters, the next step would be to organize examination under anesthesia, during which hysteroscopy and dilatation of the isthmical canal should be attempted. Unfortunately, it is not uncommon that after successful access to the cavity under general anesthesia, by the time of embryo transfer, the entry could be impossible again. The insertion of slings (small tube) could be useful in these cases for at least 1 month after the procedure to reduce the chance of the canal being restenosed [76]. If all of the above fail, intramyometrial access should be considered. These patients also have a significant risk of premature delivery, so maximum effort needs to be put into minimizing the chances of multiple pregnancy.

If a patient had a *previous difficult procedure* secondary to some anatomical distortion of the cervical canal, it could often be useful to see the advice written by a previous clinician, who succeeded in gaining access to the cavity. Once understanding the nature of the distortion and how to overcome it is established, the rest of the procedure becomes easy.

A systematic review and meta-analysis of difficult transfer demonstrated that difficult embryo transfer was associated with reduced clinical pregnancy rate (OR 0.75, CI 0.66–0.86) [77]. However, the presence of blood was not shown to be associated with a drop in the clinical pregnancy rate. Once faced with difficulties in passing the catheter through the cervical canal, the operator should overcome the obstruction by using a malleable stylet catheter or very rarely a tenaculum. If all of the above failed, embryo freeze should be considered, while the patient could be offered cervical dilatation at another occasion [78], since the latter might improve access to the cavity at a later stage.

It is also important to understand the reason behind difficult transfers. A stenosed cervix [78] (natural or due to previous surgery) and extreme flexion of the uterus are commonly described as the main reasons for difficult access. However, a recent paper [79] systematically described anatomical causes of difficult transfers, the most common being abnormal crypts and tortuosity of the cervical canal. The same authors described internal os contractions. Not surprisingly, the most difficult cases occurred where several causes were present together.

Transmyometrial Access

In some cases, transmyometrial access needs to be gained. The transmyometrial access could be the only alternative when all other attempts failed despite using additional instruments and maneuvers. The patient needs to be sedated for this procedure, and the bladder should be emptied. Under transvaginal ultrasound

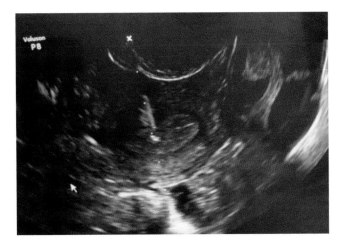

FIGURE 10.7   Transmyometrial insertion.

guidance, the uterus is visualized in the sagittal view, and the needle inserted through the needle-guide into the anterior myometrial wall until it reaches the cavity. The uterus is scanned so that the needle lies as perpendicular as possible to the endometrial cavity (Figure 10.7). Once the tip of the needle is clearly in the cavity, the stylet is withdrawn, and a thin embryo transfer catheter loaded with embryo(s) is advanced into the cavity. The embryo is deposited in the middle of the cavity, after which the catheter and needle are carefully withdrawn.

The pregnancy rate following transmyometrial embryo transfer is reported to be satisfactory and comparable to the difficult transvaginal access [80,81].

Post-Transfer Instructions

Historically, patients were encouraged to have bed rest following embryo transfer. However, evidence does not support this practice. Even in earlier studies, it was shown that embryo position was not affected by standing immediately after transfer [82]. Additionally, a meta-analysis concluded that there is no benefit of bed rest after embryo transfer for the ongoing pregnancy rate (OR 0.88; 95% CI 0.60–1.31) [83]. Some authors have even suggested that it might have a negative impact on implantation rate and cause more stress in patients [84].

Training and Quality Assurance

Embryo transfer, as any other medical procedure, requires proficiency that cannot be gained by just reading books or watching others and should be achieved through a systematic, structured training. This should include, in the first instance, theoretical explanation, observing senior clinicians, performing the procedure on simulators, and finally, performing procedures in real settings under supervision. Attempts to use intrauterine insemination (IUI) experience in a preparation for embryo transfer proficiency did not demonstrate any benefits [85]. Conversely, mock transfers before embryo transfers appear to have more benefits for future performance [86]. More simulator models are now on the market. Specifically, the American Society of Reproductive Medicine (ASRM) and VirtaMed developed a simulator for training in ultrasound-guided and ultrasound-unguided embryo transfer in IVF and IUI. TransferSim is another model that is also available for training and able to report for each student the simulation characteristic parameters, such as distance from uterine fundus, simulation timing, and total channel touches. Simulators are increasingly being used in the training of medical professionals. The evidence of a positive influence of simulation-based training on further patient-based setting performance has been established for surgical skills [87]. However, the evidence on its benefit for embryo transfer remains limited. The only retrospective study performed on a small number of trainees reported improved pregnancy rates from 31% to 46% when simulation training was utilized prior to embryo transfers [88].

Several studies confirmed that time to proficiency varies between individuals [89,90], and it is important to have a continuous monitoring of performance as well as an individualized approach to training [91]. Once competency was achieved, it was important to avoid breaks for more than 10 days to avoid a drop in performance [91].

As alluded to earlier, the outcome of embryo transfer depends on a number of optimal conditions. It is important not only to standardize the process within one clinic and have a robust system of training new doctors, but also to have continuous monitoring of the performance of each individual clinician. A statistical tool called the cumulative summative (CUSUM) test has been increasingly used in the health-care system. It is designed for continuous assessment of performance and has the power of early detection of when the process has become out of control [92]. This tool can reveal underperformance of all clinicians, new and established, and this may help them to improve. Dessole et al. [90] suggest that CUSUM can also be useful in evaluating the impact of new strategies that are implemented to improve pregnancy rates.

REFERENCES

1. Betteridge KJ. An historical look at embryo transfer. *J Reprod Fert.* 1981;62:1–13.
2. Heape W. Preliminary note on the transplantation and growth of mammalian ova within a uterine foster mother. *Proc R Soc Lond.* 1891;48:457–9.
3. Marston JH, Penn R, and Sivelle PC. Successful autotransfer of tubal eggs in the rhesus monkey (*Macaca mulatta*). *J Reprod Fertil.* 1977;49:175–6.
4. Biggers JD. IVF and embryo transfer: Historical origin and development. *Reprod Biomed Online.* 2012;25(2):118–27.
5. Buster J. Historical evolution of oocyte and embryo donation as a treatment for intractable infertility. In: Sauer MV (ed.) *Principals of Oocyte and Embryo Donation.* New York, NY: Springer; 1998, pp. 1–9.
6. Otsuki K, and Soma T. Transfer of fertilized ova through the cervix in goats. *Bull Natl Inst Anim Industry Chiba Japan.* 1964;6:27–32.
7. Healy MW, Hill MJ, and Levens ED. Optimal oocyte retrieval and embryo transfer techniques: Where we are and how we got here. *Semin Reprod Med.* 2015;33(2):83–91.
8. Fanchin R, Gellman S, Righini C, Ayoubi J-M, Olivennes F, and Frydman R. Uterine contraction frequency at the time of embryo transfer (ET) is correlated with anxiety levels. *Fertil Steril.* 2000;74:S252.
9. Abou-Setta AM. Effect of passive uterine straightening during embryo transfer: A systematic review and meta-analysis. *Acta Obstet Gynecol Scand.* 2007;86(5):516–22.
10. Lewin A, Schenker JG, Avrech O, Shapira S, Safran A, and Friedler S. The role of uterine straightening by passive bladder distension before embryo transfer in IVF cycles. *J Assist Reprod Genet.* 1997;14(1):32–4.
11. Lorusso F, Depalo R, Bettocchi S, Vacca M, Vimercati A, and Selvaggi L. Outcome of *in vitro* fertilization after transabdominal ultrasound-assisted embryo transfer with a full or empty bladder. *Fertil Steril.* 2005;84(4):1046–8.
12. Derks RS, Farquhar C, Mol BW, Buckingham K, and Heineman MJ. Techniques for preparation prior to embryo transfer. *Cochrane Database Syst Rev.* 2009;(4):CD007682.
13. Buckett WM. A meta-analysis of ultrasound-guided versus clinical touch embryo transfer. *Fertil Steril.* 2003;80(4):1037–41.
14. Mirkin S, Jones EL, Mayer JF, Stadtmauer L, Gibbons WE, and Oehninger S. Impact of transabdominal ultrasound guidance on performance and outcome of transcervical uterine embryo transfer. *J Assist Reprod Genet.* 2003;20(8):318–22.
15. Salim R, Ben-Shlomo I, Colodner R, Keness Y, and Shalev E. Bacterial colonisation of the uterine cervix and success rates in assisted reproduction: Results of a prospective survey. *Hum Reprod.* 2002;17:337–40.
16. Fanchin R, Righini C, Olivennes F, Taylor S, de Ziegler D, and Frydman R. Uterine contractions at the time of embryo transfer alter pregnancy rates after in-vitro fertilization. *Hum Reprod.* 1998;13(7):1968–74.
17. Ayoubi JM, Epiney M, Brioschi PA, Fanchin R, Chardonnens D, and De Ziegler D. Comparison of changes in uterine contraction frequency after ovulation in the menstrual cycle and in *in vitro* fertilization cycles. *Fertil Steril.* 2003;79:1101–5.

18. Lesny P, Killick SR, Tetlow RL, Robinson J, and Maguiness SD. Embryo transfer—Can we learn anything new from the observation of junctional zone contractions? *Hum Reprod*. 1998;13:1540–6.
19. Zhu L, Li Y, and Xu A. Influence of controlled ovarian hyperstimulation on uterine peristalsis in infertile women. *Hum Reprod*. 2012;27:2684–9.
20. Lan VT, Khang VN, Nhu GH, and Tuong HM. Atosiban improves implantation and pregnancy rates in patients with repeated implantation failure. *Reprod Biomed Online*. 2012;25(3):254–60.
21. Zargar M, Kajbaf S, and Hemadi M. The effect of administrating hyoscine bromide on pregnancy rate before embryo transfer in ART cycles. *Open J Obstet Gynaecol*. 2013;3:586–92.
22. Pierzynski P. Oxytocin and vasopressin V1A receptors as new therapeutic targets in assisted reproduction. *Reprod Biomed Online*. 2011;22:9–16.
23. Hagenfeldt K. The role of prostaglandins and allied substances in uterine haemostasis. *Contraception*. 1987;36:23–35.
24. Marjoribanks J, Proctor M, Farquhar C, and Derks RS. Non-steroidal anti-inflammatory drugs for dysmenorrhoea. *Cochrane Database Syst Rev*. 2010;(1):CD001751.
25. Olson DM, Zaragoza DB, Shallow MC et al. Myometrial activation and preterm labour: Evidence supporting a role for the prostaglandin F receptor—A review. *Placenta*. 2003;24(Suppl. A):S47–S54.
26. Bisits A, Madsen G, Knox M et al. The Randomized Nitric Oxide Tocolysis Trial (RNOTT) for the treatment of preterm labor. *Am J Obstet Gynecol*. 2004;191:683–90.
27. Lees CC, Lojacono A, Thompson C et al. Glyceryl trinitrate and ritodrine in tocolysis: An international multicenter randomized study. GTN Preterm Labour Investigation Group. *Obstet Gynecol*. 1999;94:403–8.
28. Leveno KJ, Klein VR, Guzick DS, Young DC, Hankins GD, and Williams ML. Single-centre randomised trial of ritodrine hydrochloride for preterm labour. *Lancet*. 1986;1:1293–6.
29. Fedorowicz Z, Nasser M, Jagannath VA, Beaman JH, Ejaz K, and Van Zuuren EJ. Beta2-adrenoceptor agonists for dysmenorrhoea. *Cochrane Database Syst Rev*. 2012;(5):CD008585.
30. Kido A, Togashi K, Hatayama H et al. Uterine peristalsis in women with repeated IVF failures: Possible therapeutic effect of hyoscine bromide. *J Obstet Gynaecol Can*. 2009;31:732–5.
31. Nakai A, Togashi K, Kosaka K et al. Do anticholinergic agents suppress uterine peristalsis and sporadic myometrial contractions at cine MR imaging? *Radiology*. 2008;246:489–96.
32. Flenady V, Wojcieszek AM, Papatsonis DN et al. Calcium channel blockers for inhibiting preterm labour and birth. *Cochrane Database Syst Rev*. 2014;(6):CD002255.
33. Ng EH, Li RH, Chen L, Lan VT, Tuong HM, and Quan S. A randomized double blind comparison of atosiban in patients undergoing IVF treatment. *Hum Reprod*. 2014;29(12):2687–94.
34. Khairy M, Dhillon RK, Chu J, Rajkhowa M, and Coomarasamy A. The effect of peri-implantation administration of uterine relaxing agents in assisted reproduction treatment cycles: A systematic review and meta-analysis. *Reprod Biomed Online*. 2016;32(4):362–76.
35. Dorn C, Reinsberg J, Schlebusch H, Prietl G, Van der Ven H, and Krebs D. Serum oxytocin concentration during embryo transfer procedure. *Eur J Obstet Gynecol Reprod Biol*. 1999;87:77–80.
36. Mansour RT, and Aboulghar MA. Optimizing the embryo transfer technique. *Hum Reprod*. 2002;17(5):1149–53.
37. Knutzen V, Stratton CJ, Sher G, McNamee PI, Huang TT, and Soto-Albors, C. Mock embryo transfer in early luteal phase, the cycle before *in vitro* fertilization and embryo transfer: A descriptive study. *Fertil Steril*. 1992;57:156–62.
38. Mansour RT, Aboulghar MA, Serour GI, and Amin YM. Dummy embryo transfer using methylene blue dye. *Hum Reprod*. 1994;9:1257–9.
39. Woolcott R, and Stanger J. Potentially important variables identified by transvaginal ultrasound-guided embryo transfer. *Hum Reprod*. 1997;12:963–6.
40. Zhu L, Che HS, Xiao L, and Li YP. Uterine peristalsis before embryo transfer affects the chance of clinical pregnancy in fresh and frozen-thawed embryo transfer cycles. *Hum Reprod*. 2014;29(6):1238–43.
41. Visschers BA, Bots RS, Peeters MF, Mol BW, and van Dessel HJ. Removal of cervical mucus: Effect on pregnancy rates in IVF/ICSI. *Reprod Biomed Online*. 2007;15(3):310–5.
42. Craciunas L, Tsampras N, and Fitzgerald C. Cervical mucus removal before embryo transfer in women undergoing in vitro fertilization/intracytoplasmic sperm injection: A systematic review and meta-analysis of randomized controlled trials. *Fertil Steril*. 2014;101(5):1302–7.

43. Egbase PE, al-Sharhan M, al-Othman S, al-Mutawa M, Udo EE, and Grudzinskas JG. Incidence of microbial growth from the tip of the embryo transfer catheter after embryo transfer in relation to clinical pregnancy rate following in-vitro fertilization and embryo transfer. *Hum Reprod.* 1996;11(8):1687–9.
44. Brook N, Khalaf Y, Coomarasamy A, Edgeworth J, and Braude P. A randomized controlled trial of prophylactic antibiotics (co-amoxiclav) prior to embryo transfer. *Hum Reprod.* 2006;21(11):2911–5.
45. Strickler RC, Christianson C, Crane JP, Curato A, Knight AB, and Yang V. Ultrasound guidance for human embryo transfer. *Fertil Steril.* 1985;43:54–61.
46. Teixeira DM, Dassunção LA, Vieira CV et al. Ultrasound guidance during embryo transfer: A systematic review and meta-analysis of randomized controlled trials. *Ultrasound Obstet Gynecol.* 201;45(2):139–48. doi:10.1002/uog.14639
47. Eskandar M, Abou-Setta AM, Almushait MA, El-Amin M, and Mohmad SE. Ultrasound guidance during embryo transfer: A prospective, single-operator, randomized, controlled trial. *Fertil Steril.* 2008;90:1187–90.
48. Brown J, Buckingham K, Abou-Setta AM, and Buckett W. Ultrasound versus 'clinical touch' for catheter guidance during embryo transfer in women. *Cochrane Database Syst Rev.* 2010;(1):CD006107.
49. Karavani G, Ben-Meir A, Shufaro Y, Hyman JH, and Revel A. Transvaginal ultrasound to guide embryo transfer: A randomized controlled trial. *Fertil Steril.* 2017;107(5):1159–65.
50. Hurley VA, Osborn JC, Leoni MA, and Leeton J. Ultrasound-guided embryo transfer: A controlled trial. *Fertil Steril.* 1991;55(3):559–62.
51. Kojima K, Nomiyama M, Kumamoto T, Matsumoto Y, and Iwasake T. Transvaginal ultrasound-guided embryo transfer improves pregnancy and implantation rates after IVF. *Hum Reprod.* 2001;16(12):2578–82.
52. Isobe T, Minoura H, Kawato H, and Toyoda N. Validity of trans-rectal ultrasound-guided embryo transfer against retroflexed uterus. *Reprod Med Biol.* 2004;2(4):159–163.
53. Abou-Setta AM, Al-Inany HG, Mansour RT, Serour GI, and Aboulghar MA. Soft versus firm embryo transfer catheters for assisted reproduction: A systematic review and meta-analysis. *Hum Reprod.* 2005;20(11):3114–21.
54. Buckett WM. A review and meta-analysis of prospective trials comparing different catheters used for embryo transfer. *Fertil Steril.* 2006;85(3):728–34.
55. Urbina MT, Benjamin I, Medina R, and Lerner J. Echogenic catheters and embryo transfer standardization. *JBRA Assist Reprod.* 2015;19(2):75–82.
56. Fraser IS. Prostaglandin inhibitors and their roles in gynecological disorders. *Baillieres Clin Obstet Gynecol.* 1992;6:829–57.
57. Coroleu BA, Barri P, Carreras O et al. Effect of using an echogenic catheter for ultrasound-guided embryo transfer in an IVF programme: A prospective, randomized, controlled study. *Hum Reprod.* 2006;21:1809–15.
58. Karande V, Hazlett D, Vietzke M, and Gleicher N. A prospective randomized comparison of the Wallace catheter and the Cook Echo-Tip catheter for ultrasound-guided embryo transfer. *Fertil Steril.* 2002;4:826–30.
59. Henne MB, and Milki AA. Uterine position at real embryo transfer compared with mock embryo transfer. *Hum Reprod.* 2004;19(3):570–2.
60. Mansour R, Aboulghar M, and Serour G. Dummy embryo transfer: A technique that minimizes the problems of embryo transfer and improves the pregnancy rate in human *in vitro* fertilization. *Fertil Steril.* 1990;54(4):678–81.
61. Sharif K, Afnan M, and Lenton W. Mock embryo transfer with a full bladder immediately before the real transfer for *in-vitro* fertilization treatment: The Birmingham experience of 113 cases. *Hum Reprod.* 1995;10(7):1715–8.
62. Katariya KO, Bates GW, Robinson RD, Arthur NJ, and Propst AM. Does the timing of mock embryo transfer affect in vitro fertilization implantation and pregnancy rates? *Fertil Steril.* 2007;88(5):1462–4.
63. Yoldemir T, and Erenus M. Does the timing of mock embryo transfer trial improve implantation in intracytoplasmic sperm injection cycles? *Gynecol Endocrinol.* 2011;27(6):396–400.
64. Ghazzawi IM, Al-Hasani S, Karaki R, and Souso S. Transfer technique and catheter choice influence the incidence of trans-cervical embryo expulsion and the outcome of IVF. *Hum Reprod.* 1999;14(3):677–82.
65. Oliveira JB, Martins AM, Baruffi RL et al. Increased implantation and pregnancy rates obtained by placing the tip of the transfer catheter in the central area of the endometrial cavity. *Reprod Biomed Online.* 2004;9(4):435–41.

66. Kwon H, Choi DH, and Kim EK. Absolute position versus relative position in embryo transfer: A randomized controlled trial. *Reprod Biol Endocrinol*. 2015;13:78.
67. Coroleu B, Barri PN, Carreras O et al. The influence of the depth of embryo replacement into the uterine cavity on implantation rates after IVF: A controlled, ultrasound-guided study. *Hum Reprod*. 2002;17(2):341–6.
68. Saravelos SH, Wong AW, Chan CP et al. Assessment of the embryo flash position and migration with 3D ultrasound within 60 min of embryo transfer. *Hum Reprod*. 2016;31(3):591–6.
69. Ding D, Shi W, and Shi Y. Numerical simulation of embryo transfer: How the viscosity of transferred medium affects the transport of embryos. *Theor Biol Med Model*. 2018;15:20.
70. Sigalos G, Triantafyllidou O, and Vlahos N. How do laboratory embryo transfer techniques affect IVF outcomes? A review of current literature. *Hum Fertil (Camb)*. 2017;20(1):3–13.
71. Ebner T, Yaman C, Moser M, Sommergruber M, Polz W, and Tews, G. The ineffective loading process of the embryo transfer catheter alters implantation and pregnancy rates. *Fertil Steril*. 2001;76:630–2.
72. Leeton J, Trounson A, Jessup D, and Wood C. The technique for human embryo transfer. *Fertil Steril*. 1982;38:156–61.
73. Poindexter AN, 3rd, Thompson DJ, Gibbons WE, Findley WE, Dodson MG, and Young RL. Residual embryos in failed embryo transfer. *Fertil Steril*. 1986;46:262–7.
74. Nabi A, Awonuga A, Birch H, Barlow S, and Stewart B. Multiple attempts at embryo transfer: Does this affect *in-vitro* fertilization treatment outcome? *Hum Reprod*. 1997;12(6):1188–90.
75. Vicdan K, Işik AZ, Akarsu C et al. The effect of retained embryos on pregnancy outcome in an *in vitro* fertilization and embryo transfer program. *Eur J Obstet Gynecol Reprod Biol*. 2007;134(1):79–82.
76. Aust TR, Herod JJ, and Gazvani R. Placement of a Malecot catheter to enable embryo transfer after radical trachelectomy. *Fertil Steril*. 2005;83(6):1842.
77. Phillips JA, Martins WP, Nastri CO, and Raine-Fenning NJ. Difficult embryo transfers or blood on catheter and assisted reproductive outcomes: A systematic review and meta-analysis. *Eur J Obstet Gynecol Reprod Biol*. 2013;168(2):121–8.
78. Arora P, and Mishra V. Difficult embryo transfer: A systematic review. *J Hum Reprod Sci*. 2018;11(3):229–35.
79. Larue L, Keromnes G, Massari A et al. Anatomical causes of difficult embryo transfer during *in vitro* fertilization. *J Gynecol Obstet Hum Reprod*. 2017;46(1):77–86.
80. Ferreri J, Portillo EG, Peñarrubia J, Vidal E, and Fábregues F. Transmyometrial embryo transfer as a useful method to overcome difficult embryo transfers—A single-center retrospective study. *JBRA Assist Reprod*. 2018;22(2):134–8.
81. Khairy M, Shah H, and Rajkhowa M. Transmyometrial versus very difficult transcervical embryo transfer: Efficacy and safety. *Reprod Biomed Online*. 2016;32(5):513–7.
82. Woolcott R, and Stanger J. Ultrasound tracking of the movement of embryo-associated air bubbles on standing after transfer. *Hum Reprod*. 1998;13:2107–9.
83. Abou-Setta AM, Peters LR, D'Angelo A, Sallam HN, Hart RJ, and Al-Inany HG. Post-embryo transfer interventions for assisted reproduction technology cycles. *Cochrane Database Syst Rev*. 2014;(8):CD006567.
84. Craciunas L, and Tsampras N. Bed rest following embryo transfer might negatively affect the outcome of IVF/ICSI: A systematic review and meta-analysis. *Hum Fertil (Camb)*. 2016;19(1):16–22.
85. Shah DK, Missmer SA, Correia KFB, Racowsky C, and Ginsburg E. Efficacy of intrauterine inseminations as a training modality for performing embryo transfer in reproductive endocrinology and infertility fellowship programs. *Fertil Steril*. 2013;100:386–91.
86. Bishop L, Brezina PR, and Segars J. Training in embryo transfer: How should it be done? *Fertil Steril*. 2013;100(2):351–2.
87. Dawe SR, Pena GN, Windsor JA et al. Systematic review of skills transfer after surgical simulation-based training. *Br J Surg*. 2014;101(9):1063–76.
88. Heitmann RJ, Hill MJ, Csokmay JM, Pilgrim J, DeCherney AH, and Deering S. Embryo transfer simulation improves pregnancy rates and decreases time to proficiency in reproductive endocrinology and infertility fellow embryo transfers. *Fertil Steril*. 2017;107(5):1166–72.
89. Papageorgiou TC, Hearns-Stokes RM, Leondires MP et al. Training of providers in embryo transfer: What is the minimum number of transfers required for proficiency? *Hum Reprod*. 2001;16:1415–9.

90. Dessolle L, Fréour T, Barrière P, Jean M, Ravel C, Daraï E, and Biau DJ. How soon can I be proficient in embryo transfer? Lessons from the cumulative summation test for learning curve (LC-CUSUM). *Hum Reprod.* 2010;25(2):380–6.
91. López MJ, García D, Rodríguez A, Colodrón M, Vassena R, and Vernaeve V. Individualized embryo transfer training: Timing and performance. *Hum Reprod.* 2014;29(7):1432–7.
92. Wohl H. The CUSUM plot: Its utility in the analysis of clinical data. *N Engl J Med.* 1977;296:1044–5.

11

Ultrasound Features of Ovarian Hyperstimulation Syndrome

Arianna D'Angelo, Rudaina Hassan, and Nazar N. Amso

Pathophysiology

Ovarian hyperstimulation syndrome (OHSS) is a potentially life-threatening systemic complication caused by ovarian stimulation treatment. Rarely, it may also occur as a spontaneous event in pregnancy. The syndrome is estimated to occur in approximately 5% of patients undergoing *in vitro* fertilization (IVF)/intracytoplasmic sperm injection (ICSI). It is characterized by massive cystic ovarian enlargement and fluid shift from the intravascular compartment into the third space, resulting in profound intravascular depletion and hemoconcentration. The factors leading to this syndrome have not been completely elucidated. It seems likely that the release of vasoactive substances, for example, vascular endothelium growth factor (VEGF) secreted by the ovaries under human chorionic gonadotropin (hCG) stimulation, play a key role in triggering this syndrome. As more follicles are recruited in response to gonadotropin stimulation, the mass of the granulosa cells increases, while at the same time, the cells gain functional maturation. These two factors, acting synergistically, cause a concomitant increase in serum estradiol levels and vasoactive substances. The vascular fluid leakage is thought to result from an increased capillary permeability of mesothelial surfaces under the action of one or several vasoactive ovarian factors produced by multiple corpus lutea under hCG stimulation. Risk factors for OHSS include younger age, low body mass index, black race, polycystic ovarian syndrome (PCOS), establishment of pregnancy during assisted reproduction treatment (ART), hCG supplementation of the luteal phase, and high serum estradiol [1].

Clinical Presentation and Classification

The clinical picture may vary from abdominal distension and discomfort to potentially life-threatening extravascular accumulation of fluid leading to varying degrees of ascites, pleural effusion, and oliguria. Pain, abdominal distention, nausea, and vomiting are frequently seen as symptoms.

OHSS was originally classified as mild, moderate, and severe and subsequently modified to incorporate ultrasonographic measurement of the stimulated ovaries (Tables 11.1 and 11.2) [2–4].

OHSS is classified into four categories based on the severity of symptoms, signs, and laboratory and radiological findings:

1. *Mild OHSS*: It is defined by the enlargement of bilateral ovaries with multiple follicular and corpus luteal cysts, measuring up to 8 cm and accompanied by abdominal bloating and mild abdominal pain.
2. *Moderate OHSS*: It is characterized by the enlargement of the ovaries up to 12 cm, accompanied by abdominal bloating due to an increase in ovarian size and gastrointestinal symptoms (e.g., nausea, vomiting, and diarrhea) as well as ultrasound evidence of ascites.
3. *Severe OHSS*: About 2% of OHSS cases are classified as severe. The severe form is described by the presence of large ovarian cysts (greater than 12×12 cm), clinical ascites with or without hydrothorax, hyperkalemia (potassium greater than 5 mmol/L), hyponatremia (sodium less than

TABLE 11.1

Golan Classification of Ovarian Hyperstimulation Syndrome

Classification	Size of Ovaries	Grade	Symptoms
Mild	5–10 cm	Grade 1:	Abdominal tension and discomfort
		Grade 2:	Grade 1 signs plus nausea, vomiting, and/or diarrhoea
Moderate	>10 cm	Grade 3:	Grade 2 signs plus ultrasound evidence of ascites
Severe	>12 cm	Grade 4:	Grade 3 signs plus clinical evidence of ascites and/or pleural effusion and dyspnoea
		Grade 5:	Grade 4 signs plus hemoconcentration increased blood viscosity, hypovolemia, decreased renal perfusion, oliguria

Source: Golan A, Ron-El R, Herman A, Soffer Y, Wainraub Z, and Caspi E. *Obstet Gynaecol Surv.* 1989;44:430–40. With permission.

TABLE 11.2

Navot Classification of Severe Ovarian Hyperstimulation Syndrome (OHSS)

Severe OHSS	Critical OHSS
Variably enlarged ovary	Variably enlarged ovary
Massive ascites ± hydrothorax	Tense ascites ± hydrothorax
Hct >45% (>30% increment over baseline value)	Hct >55%
WBC >15,000	WBC >35,000
Oliguria	
Creatinine 1.0–1.5	Creatinine >1.6
Creatinine clearance >50 mL/min	Creatinine clearance <50 mL/min
Liver dysfunction	Renal failure
Anasarca	Thromboembolic phenomena
	ARDS

Source: Navot D, Bergh PA, and Laufer N. *Fertil Steril.* 1992;58:249–61. With permission.
Abbreviations: ARDS, adult respiratory distress syndrome; Hct, hematocrit; WBC, white blood cells.

135 mmol/L), hypo-osmolarity (osmolarity less than 282 mOsm/kg), hypoproteinemia (serum albumin less than 35 g/L), oliguria (less than 300 mL/d or less than 30 mL/h), creatinine 1.1–1.5 mg/dL, and hypovolemic shock. Hemoconcentration with hematocrit greater than 45%, white cell count greater than 15,000 μL, liver dysfunction, increased blood viscosity, and thromboembolic events occurs in the most severe cases.

4. *Critical OHSS*: It is diagnosed when there is severe ascites or hydrothorax, hematocrit greater than 55%, white cell count greater than 25,000/mL, oliguria or anuria, creatinine greater than or equal to 1.6 mg/dL, creatinine clearance less than 50 mL/min, thromboembolism, or acute respiratory distress syndrome (ARDS).

Ultrasound

Ultrasound Features

Ultrasound is key in the diagnosis and classification of OHSS. It is also used to confirm the underlying etiology and monitor the course of the disease. Ultrasound identifies the degree of ovarian enlargement, presence and volume of free fluid in the peritoneal, pleural, and pericardial cavity. The sonographic findings typically include bilateral symmetric enlargement of ovaries with multiple cysts of varying sizes, giving the classic spoke-wheel appearance (Figure 11.1). The multiple cysts seen may be simple or hemorrhagic with no abnormal solid component or vascularity within the cystic areas [5].

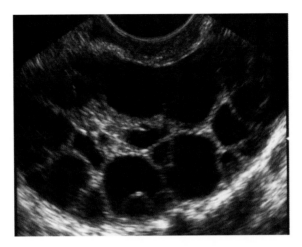

FIGURE 11.1 Ultrasound appearance of enlarged ovary.

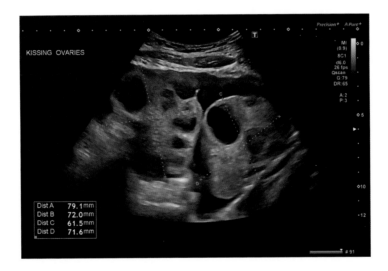

FIGURE 11.2 Ultrasound appearance of "kissing ovaries."

Mild OHSS: The only sonographic characteristic of mild OHSS may be enlarged ovaries (5–12 cm) often described as "kissing ovaries" (Figure 11.2).

Moderate OHSS: Enlarged ovaries of up to 12 cm are seen (see Figure 11.1) with abdominal or pelvic ascites (Figure 11.3).

Severe OHSS: Enlarged ovaries over 12 cm with abdominal or pelvic ascites with or without hydrothorax (Figure 11.4a and b).

Critical OHSS: Enlarged ovaries over 12 cm with severe ascites or hydrothorax.

Ultrasound in Prevention of Ovarian Hyperstimulation Syndrome

There are strategies aimed at reducing the risk of OHSS for women undergoing ART who are at high risk of OHSS. These include coasting (withholding gonadotropins) [6]; elective embryo freezing, originally described in 1990 [7], then further evaluated by Cochrane systematic review and comparison with other strategies [8,9]; gonadotropin-releasing hormone (GnRH) antagonist cycles with GnRH agonist trigger; intravenous albumin infusion; and cabergoline [10,11]. None of these strategies eliminate OHSS but may reduce its risk. They are not further described in this book.

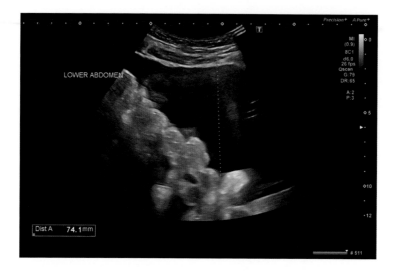

FIGURE 11.3   Ultrasound appearance of fluid collection in the lower abdomen (ascites).

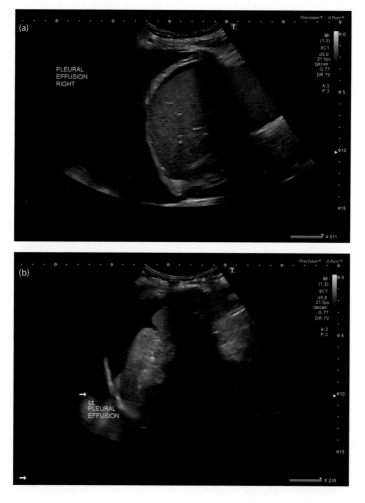

FIGURE 11.4   (a) Ultrasound appearance of right pleural effusion (RT hydrothorax). (b). Ultrasound appearance of left pleural effusion (LT hydrothorax).

Ultrasound also plays a role in prevention by predicting cases that are at high risk of developing OHSS and therefore allowing caution in initial gonadotropin dosing and choice of stimulation protocol [1].

A high antral follicle count (AFC) has been reported to be associated with an increased risk of developing OHSS. The cut-off for AFC used to predict OHSS varies within studies depending on the definition of antral follicle and operator technique used in follicle counting the AFC. Various studies have found that if the AFC is found to be greater than 14, there is an increased risk of OHSS.

Women with polycystic ovarian syndrome (PCOS) have an increased risk of developing OHSS. They have a high AFC, and ultrasound assessment of ovarian morphology is one of the key criteria for the diagnosis of PCOS. However, in patients with irregular menstrual cycles and hyperandrogenism, an ovarian ultrasound is not necessary for PCOS diagnosis. According to the international evidence-based guideline for the assessment and management of PCOS (2018) [4], the current threshold for PCOS should be on either ovary, a follicle number per ovary of 20 or greater, and/or an ovarian volume 10 mL or greater, ensuring no corpora lutea, cysts, or dominant follicles are present. This is different than the old sonographic findings highlighted by the Rotterdam criteria, which were either 12 or more follicles in each ovary measuring 2–9 mm in diameter and/or increased ovarian volume greater than 10 mL. Women with polycystic appearing ovaries on ultrasound who do not meet the diagnostic criteria for PCOS have also been found to have increased risk of OHSS.

A large number of growing follicles seen on ultrasound during ovarian stimulation is also associated with an increased risk of OHSS. Studies have reported if there are 13 or more follicles measuring 11 mm or greater, there is an increased risk of developing OHSS. Additionally, the value of serum estradiol for preventing OHSS was evaluated in a retrospective case control study [12]. The authors concluded that a serum E2 level of 12,315 pmol/L (3354 pg/mL) on day 11 of ovarian stimulation gave a sensitivity and specificity of 85% for the detection of women at risk for OHSS.

There are other ultrasound features that have been investigated including ovarian volume and vascular flow analysis [13], but they have not been proven to be useful clinically in the prediction of OHSS.

Management

The syndrome is usually self-limiting, and in most cases, management of mild to moderate OHSS is mainly supportive in outpatient settings. In severe and critical OHSS, fatal cases have been reported; therefore, prompt diagnosis and treatment are required with hospitalization and close monitoring of the hematocrit, liver function, renal function, serum electrolytes, and oxygen saturation. In some cases, treatment involves drainage of ascites (Figure 11.5) and pleural effusion. Critical cases require admission to high dependency units and intensive care.

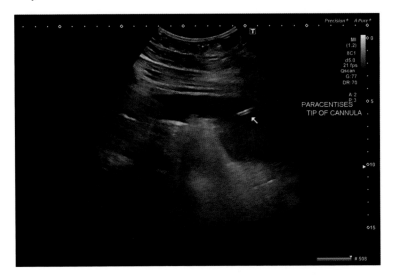

FIGURE 11.5 Ultrasound appearance of paracentesis cannula tip inside abdominal cavity.

REFERENCES

1. Nastri C, Teixeira D, Moroni R, Leitao V, and Martins W. Ovarian hyperstimulation syndrome: Pathophysiology, staging, prediction and prevention, *Ultrasound Obstet Gynecol.* 2015;45(4):377–93.
2. Golan A, Ron-El R, Herman A, Soffer Y, Wainraub Z, and Caspi E. Ovarian hyperstimulation syndrome: An update review. *Obstet Gynaecol Surv.* 1989;44:430–40.
3. Navot D, Bergh PA, and Laufer N. Ovarian hyperstimulation syndrome in novel reproductive technologies: Prevention and treatment. *Fertil Steril.* 1992;58:249–61.
4. Teede HJ, Misso ML, Costello MF et al. Recommendations from the international evidence-based guideline for the assessment and management of polycystic ovary syndrome. *Fertil Steril.* 2018;110(3):364-379. doi:10.1016/j.fertnstert.2018.05.004
5. Kim IY, and Lee BH. Ovarian hyperstimulation syndrome. US and CT appearances. *Clin Imaging.* 1997;21(4):284–6.
6. D'Angelo A, Amso NN, and Hassan R. Coasting (withholding gonadotrophins) for preventing ovarian hyperstimulation syndrome. *Cochrane Database Syst Rev.* 2017;(5):CD002811.
7. Amso N, Ahuja K, Morris N, and Shaw RW. The management of predicted ovarian hyperstimulation involving gonadotropin releasing hormone analogue with elective cryopreservation of all embryos. *Fertil Steril.* 1990;53:1087–90.
8. D'Angelo A, and Amso NN. Embryo freezing for preventing ovarian hyperstimulation syndrome. *Cochrane Database Syst Rev.* 2007;(3):CD002806.
9. D'Angelo A. OHSS prevention strategies: Cryopreservation of all embryos. *Semin Reprod Med.* 2010;28(6):513–8.
10. Rizk B, and Aboulghar MA. Classification, pathophysiology and management of ovarian hyperstimulation syndrome. In: Brinsden P (ed.) *A Textbook of In Vitro Fertilization and Assisted Reproduction.* 2nd ed. London, UK: Parthenon Publishing; 1999, pp. 131–55.
11. Smith V, Osianlis T, and Vollenhoven B. Prevention of ovarian hyperstimulation syndrome: A review. *Obstet Gynecol Int.* 2015;2015:514159.
12. D'Angelo A, Davies R, Salah E, Nix BA, and Amso NN. Value of the serum estradiol level for preventing ovarian hyperstimulation syndrome: A retrospective case control study. *Fertil Steril.* 2004;81(2):332–6.
13. Jayaprakasan K, Jayaprakasan R, Al-Hasie HA et al. Can quantitative three-dimensional power Doppler angiography be used to predict ovarian hyperstimulation syndrome? *Ultrasound Obstet Gynecol.* 2009;33(5):583–91.

12

Ultrasound-Guided Intervention in Assisted Reproductive Technology

Candice Cheung and Andrew Sizer

Introduction

Ultrasound scan (USS) assessment plays a significant role in patients undergoing assisted reproductive technology (ART) treatment. A baseline USS should be performed in all women prior to starting treatment. This allows screening for any pelvic pathology such as congenital uterine malformations, presence of fibroids, polyps, intrauterine adhesions, ovarian cysts, and hydrosalpinx that are associated with adverse outcomes in ART. Certain interventions such as aspiration of hydrosalpinx and ovarian cysts and follicle reduction can also be performed under USS guidance.

In this chapter, we focus on how these conditions are diagnosed on USS. We discuss their impact on subfertility and ART treatment and the various treatment options available.

Hydrosalpinx

Tubal factor accounts for 25%–30% of female factor infertility, and 30% of these patients have hydrosalpinx identified on USS [1]. Hydrosalpinx is an accumulation of fluid in a distally occluded fallopian tube and appears on USS as a fluid-filled, cystic structure with the "beads of string" sign due to the presence of hyperechoic mural nodules (Figure 12.1) [2]. The sensitivity and specificity of transvaginal ultrasound (TVUS) in diagnosing hydrosalpinx are 84.6 and 99.7%, respectively [3].

It has been demonstrated that patients with hydrosalpinx having IVF have a 50% decrease in live birth rate (LBR) when compared to other women who do not [4]. Studies have also found that the presence of hydrosalpinx could lead to an increase in spontaneous miscarriage rate, ectopic pregnancies, preterm birth, and low birth weight [5].

Pathophysiology

The major cause of tubal occlusion is pelvic inflammatory disease secondary to ascending infection from sexually transmitted diseases such as *Chlamydia trachomatis* or *Neisseria gonorrhoeae*. It can also be due to adhesions formation from endometriosis and previous operations [6].

Multiple theories have suggested why the presence of hydrosalpinx can contribute to poor ART outcomes. First, hydrosalpinx can be associated with impairment of ovarian function, follicular development, and oocyte quality [7]. Also, fluid from the hydrosalpinx contains cytokines and endotoxins that can be harmful to the developing embryos [8]. Moreover, when collected in the uterine cavity, the fluid can lead to decreased endometrium receptivity demonstrated by reduced receptivity markers [9], the fluid can cause mechanical washout of the embryos or can prevent implantation due to poor apposition with the endometrium [10].

If hydrosalpinx is identified on baseline USS of patients who are about to receive ART treatment, surgical intervention should be offered prior to starting IVF due to the deleterious effect of hydrosalpinx on outcomes.

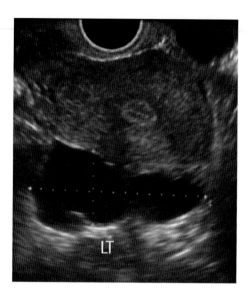

FIGURE 12.1   Ultrasound appearance of hydrosalpinx (LT, left tube). (Reproduced from Na ED et al. *Clin Exp Reprod Med.* 2012;39[4]:182–6 under Open Access.)

Treatment Options

The main treatment options for hydrosalpinx prior to IVF treatment are laparoscopic salpingectomy, laparoscopic or hysteroscopic proximal tubal occlusion, and transvaginal aspiration of hydrosalpingeal fluid with or without sclerotherapy. We discuss the pros and cons of each method in the following sections.

Laparoscopic Salpingectomy

Laparoscopic salpingectomy involves complete removal of the diseased fallopian tube. A prospective randomized controlled trial (RCT) demonstrated that in women undergoing their first IVF cycle with hydrosalpinges identified on USS, salpingectomy prior to IVF is associated with a significant increase in clinical pregnancy rates (CPRs) (45.7% versus 22.5%) and LBR (40% versus 17.5%, $P = 0.038$) compared to the group without treatment [11].

Subsequent meta-analysis has confirmed the effectiveness of laparoscopic salpingectomy, demonstrating ongoing pregnancy rates in the intervention group to be 31% compared to 17.6% of the control group [12].

The main advantage of performing salpingectomy is that the chronically infected tissue is completely removed and the future risk of abscess formation or torsion is eliminated [6]. It also allows better accessibility of the ovary during oocyte retrieval [13].

Despite the promising results of salpingectomy and the National Institute for Health and Care Excellence (NICE) recommendation that "women with hydrosalpinges should be offered salpingectomy, preferably by laparoscopy, before IVF treatment because this improves the chance of a live birth," there are certain disadvantages with regard to salpingectomy, including the operative risks, difficulty in accessing the fallopian tube in the presence of dense adhesions, and increased risk of interstitial pregnancy [14]. Studies have also suggested a possible adverse effect on ovarian blood supply leading to subsequent reduction of ovarian response to gonadotropin stimulation [15,16].

Proximal Tube Occlusion

Proximal occlusion of the fallopian tube isolates the hydrosalpingeal fluid from the uterine cavity and is an alternative to salpingectomy. It is technically faster and easier to perform and theoretically does not compromise the ovarian blood supply [6]. It can be done laparoscopically, or more recently, hysteroscopic occlusion has been introduced with the use of Essure with promising results [17].

Studies have demonstrated comparable treatment outcomes in terms of CPR between proximal tubal occlusion and laparoscopic salpingectomy [18].

The disadvantages with regard to tubal occlusion include risk of recurrent infection and development of pyosalpinx leading to further surgery of the diseased tube at a later date; also, patients can experience residual pain due to the pressure of the affected tube.

In patients where laparoscopic treatment is contraindicated, an alternative treatment modality may be considered such as TVUS-guided aspiration of hydrosalpinx.

Ultrasound-Guided Aspiration and Sclerotherapy

Transvaginal aspiration of hydrosalpinx is done usually at the time of oocyte collection under USS guidance when the patient is under sedation. An aspiration needle is introduced into the hydrosalpinx and suction applied to aspirate the fluid completely.

Ultrasound-guided aspiration has the advantage of being less invasive, being cheaper, and avoiding hospitalization and risks for surgery and general anesthesia. It also allows treatment in patients who wish to avoid surgery or when hydrosalpinges are detected after commencement of the IVF procedure.

Studies have been inconsistent with regard to the efficacy of this procedure. While some concluded that aspiration of hydrosalpinx fluid offered no benefit in terms of IVF outcomes [19], others show a higher CPR with treatment [20]. A recent RCT reported that implantation, clinical, and ongoing pregnancy rates were significantly higher in the aspiration group compared with no intervention [21].

In conclusion, although ultrasound-guided aspiration is not as effective when compared to both salpingectomy and proximal tubal occlusion, it is associated with better outcomes when compared with no intervention [1], and clinicians should consider aspirating the fluid from the tube, particularly when diagnosis is made during IVF treatment.

A major disadvantage of aspiration of hydrosalpinx is the rapid reaccumulation of fluid being reported as high as 30.8% within a 2-week interval [20]. It was noted that the implantation and pregnancy rates were higher in the subgroup of patients with no reaccumulation of hydrosalpingeal fluid compared to those with reaccumulation [21].

It has been proposed that applying sclerotherapy during ultrasound-guided aspiration of hydrosalpinx can prevent rapid reaccumulation of fluid. After aspirating the hydrosalpingeal fluid, the fallopian tube is then washed with 98% of ethanol with gentamicin [22] or tetracycline [2] added to the solution.

The contact of the sclerosing agent and the epithelial lining of the tube cause activation of coagulation cascade and production of mediators for inflammation and fibrosis, which leads to hardening of the tube and decreased secretion. This stops substances that inhibit implantation from formation and backflow into the endometrial cavity. Sclerotherapy has also been shown to improve blood flow of the uterine arcuate artery and hence leads to better perfusion to the endometrium leading to better implantation rates [22].

There have been promising study results with regard to the use of sclerotherapy. Multiple studies have demonstrated significantly higher implantation and CPRs compared to an untreated control group [22,23]. The clinical pregnancy and miscarriage rates of sclerotherapy were comparable to salpingectomy [24]. There are no reports of any adverse effect on perinatal outcomes in relation to sclerotherapy [25].

The most common complication from sclerotherapy is the leakage of alcohol into the abdominal cavity causing severe pain; however, this tends to resolve within a short period of time with conservative management. There are no other reports of serious complications, and it is considered to be a safe, effective, alternative approach in the management of hydrosalpinx [2].

Ovarian Cysts

Ovarian cysts are common findings in women of reproductive age and are often incidentally found during the investigations for ART treatment. The majority of ovarian cysts are benign, including the following:

- Functional cysts
- Dermoid cysts

- Serous cystadenoma
- Mucinous cystadenoma
- Endometrioma

We discuss the management of endometrioma in more detail owing to the fact of the causal relationship between subfertility and endometriosis.

Endometrioma

The prevalence of endometriosis is as high as 50% among infertile women [26]. Ovarian endometrioma is found in 17%–44% of cases of endometriosis [27] and is often indicative of a more severe spectrum of the disease. On USS, endometriomas have diffuse low-level echoes with a typical "ground glass" appearance (Figure 12.2).

Pathophysiology

There are a number of possible theories of how endometrioma contributes to infertility. The pelvic adhesions caused by endometriosis can lead to distortion of the tubo-ovarian anatomy. Endometriomas can cause increased oxidative stress to the ovarian tissue leading to fibrosis, loss of cortex specific stroma, vascularization defect, and reduced follicle maturation [28] leading to a significant reduction in the primordial follicle. The presence of endometrioma alters the follicular environment as evident by increased progesterone and interleukin-6 and decreased vascular endothelial growth factor. This can impact on the quality of the oocytes and embryos, leading to lower fertilization and implantation rates, respectively [29].

Treatment Options

Laparoscopic Cystectomy

Despite the association between endometrioma and infertility, meta-analyses and systemic reviews showed that there was no significant difference in CPRs, LBRs, and miscarriage rates between women who had surgery for endometrioma compared to those who did not [30]. The findings of such have led to much controversy with regard to the "gold-standard" management of endometriomas.

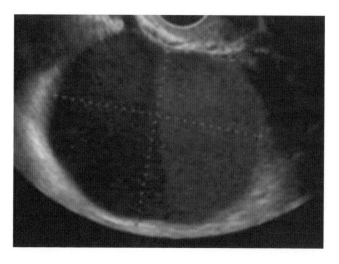

FIGURE 12.2   Ultrasound appearance of endometrioma.

Surgical excision of endometriosis and endometrioma before ART is traditionally practiced. One of the major benefits of surgery is the relief of symptoms secondary to endometriosis [31]. Another argument for surgical excision of endometrioma is due to the potential complications in expectant management, such as cyst rupture, torsion, progression of the disease, and risk of missing underlying malignancy. The presence of endometriomas can also complicate oocyte retrieval due to difficult access and development of pelvic infection secondary to accidental puncture of the endometrioma [32].

Women with endometrioma already have a higher baseline follicle-stimulating hormone level and a lower mean number of oocytes retrieved compared to women who do not have the condition [30], surgical excision of endometrioma carries the risk of further compromising ovarian reserve. This is evident by the decreased antimüllerian hormone (AMH) levels by 30%, which can be sustained for 9 months postoperatively [33]. Women who had undergone surgical treatment also had a lower antral follicle count and required a higher dosage of gonadotropin for stimulation compared to those with untreated endometrioma [30].

The current guideline from the European Society of Human Reproduction and Embryology (ESHRE) stated that laparoscopic ovarian cystectomy of endometriomas before ART may not improve cycle outcome. It is therefore recommended that the decision to treat endometrioma should be individualized, taking into account the patient's symptoms, ovarian reserve, age, and the patient's choice [34].

Transvaginal Ultrasound Guided Aspiration and Sclerotherapy

Ultrasound-guided aspiration of endometrioma has been used as an alternative treatment modality with the proposed advantage of being less invasive and the ability to preserve healthy ovarian tissue.

One of the major drawbacks of aspiration is the technical challenge of complete aspiration of the cyst content due to the thick nature of endometriosis debris [35]. Also, as the cyst capsule is not removed, the recurrence rate is reported to be as high as 83.3% within a 3-month period [36]. Monthly reaspiration of endometrioma reduces the recurrence rate to 27.9% [37]. A more efficient way to reduce recurrence is to infiltrate a sclerosis agent such as ethanol, tetracycline, methotrexate, and recombinant interleukin-2 [38] after aspiration. With sclerotherapy, the recurrence rate at 1 year ranges from 8% to 15%; this is significantly lower compared to aspiration only [39] but is still higher when compared to laparoscopic treatment.

Study results are conflicting with regard to the ART outcomes of USS-guided aspiration of endometriomas. Some studies have shown promising outcomes including higher fertilization rates [40] and clinical and cumulative pregnancy rates [41] when compared to patients who had laparoscopic treatment. Other studies did not demonstrate any benefit of aspiration and showed similar fertilization rates, implantation rates (IRs), and CPRs compared with the control group who received no treatment [42]. Neither surgical resection nor aspiration of endometrioma improve ART outcomes when compared to conservative management [43]. Meta-analysis also concluded that the total gonadotropin dosage, mean number of oocytes retrieved, CPRs, LBRs, and miscarriage rates were similar [30] between laparoscopic cystectomy and aspiration.

Another major concern with aspiration of endometrioma is the risk of infection—the bloody content endometriomas act as an excellent medium for bacteria. Development of pelvic abscess, and in extreme cases, requiring salpingo-oophorectomy, following aspiration of endometrioma has been reported [44].

Most of these studies included a small number of patients; further large RCTs are needed to ascertain the indication, efficacy, and safety before offering aspiration of endometriomas routinely to patients undergoing ART treatment.

Dermoid Cysts

Dermoid cysts account for 70% of ovarian cysts in women younger than 30 years. USS findings of a dermoid cyst include areas of focal acoustic impedance with bright echoes and hyperechoic lines and dots, a "Rokitansky protuberance" seen as a dense echogenic nodule, with posterior acoustic shadowing projecting into the lumen of the cyst. Other pathognomonic features are the presence of fine, echogenic bands representing hair within the cystic area and the presence of a fat-fluid level [3].

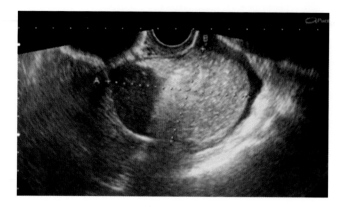

FIGURE 12.3 Dermoid cyst with a "fat-fluid" level. (Adapted from Abdusamad K, Hamoudi R, and Maiti S. *BMJ Case Rep*. 2013;2013:bcr2012007909.)

In terms of management, laparoscopic cystectomy is generally performed due to the risk of torsion of dermoid cysts. However, surgical excision also carries the risk of compromising ovarian reserve, as it has been evident that the ovarian volume is decreased by 40% with a reduction in the number of dominant follicles [45] and AMH levels [46]. There is no role in aspiration of a dermoid cyst due to the content of the cysts and the risk of chemical peritonitis [47].

The presence of a dermoid cyst does not seem to affect AMH levels [48] or the number of oocytes retrieved [49]. Also, there is evidence to suggest that dermoid cysts less than 6 cm can be followed up with minimal risks [50]; it is therefore reasonable to defer surgical removal of the cyst until after IVF treatment.

Functional Cysts

Simple ovarian cysts appear on USS as thin-walled, anechoic lesion with no intracystic structures (Figure 12.4). They are benign and often physiological and will spontaneously regress over a few menstrual cycles [51]. Ovarian cysts can also develop during pituitary downregulation as part of the IVF treatment cycle.

It has been suggested that the presence of these ovarian cysts can disrupt folliculogenesis by reducing the area available for follicle development and by altering local blood supply [52], which could possibly lead to negative impact on IVF outcomes [53].

Cochrane review compared IVF outcomes of aspiration versus conservative management of functional ovarian cysts and concluded that there is insufficient evidence to determine whether drainage of these

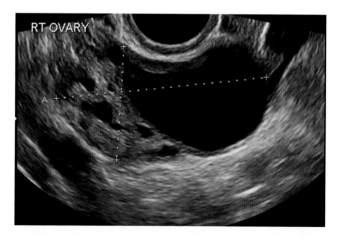

FIGURE 12.4 Simple ovarian cyst. (Adapted from Schwarzler P et al. *Ultrasound Obstet Gynecol*. 1998;11(5):337–42.)

cysts prior to IVF improves LBR, CPR, number of follicles recruited, or number of oocytes collected [54]. Aspiration of cysts that developed with the use of GnRH agonist did not increase the quantity and quality of retrieved oocytes [55]. Although aspiration does not improve IVF outcomes, it can be considered if the ovarian cyst interferes with oocyte retrieval.

Ovarian cysts that persist or increase in size after several menstrual cycles may require surgical intervention due to the risk of rupture and torsion. Other indications for surgery include patients who are symptomatic, who have large cysts (greater than 70 mm), or when tissue diagnosis is required [51].

Follicle Reduction

Intrauterine insemination (IUI) refers to the introduction of sperm directly into the uterus during ovulation with or without controlled ovarian stimulation. It can be offered to people who have difficulty with vaginal intercourse due to physical disability or psychosexual problems, same-sex relationship couples, and people with conditions that require specific consideration in relation to methods of conception (e.g., sperm washing where the man is HIV positive) [56]. IUI combined with ovarian stimulation is associated with a higher CPR [57] but also increases the risk of multiple pregnancies, which is reported to be 21%–29% [58].

In IVF/ICSI treatment, single embryo transfer (SET) has lowered the rate of multiple pregnancies. However, there is much less control over the risk of multiple pregnancies with IUI. One way to reduce the incidence of multiple pregnancies is to aspirate the excess follicles under ultrasound guidance with a single lumen needle.

Studies have shown that TVUS-guided aspiration of supernumerary follicles after ovulation induction can reduce multiple pregnancies without compromising the CPR [59]. With the development of vitrification in recent years, matured oocytes obtained from follicle aspiration can be vitrified to potentially achieve future pregnancies [60].

Role of Perioperative Ultrasound in Assisted Reproductive Technology

Uterine cavity abnormalities such as fibroids, polyps, intrauterine adhesions, and congenital uterine anomalies are common findings in the subfertile population. The prevalence is reported to be as high as 45% [61]. Some of these pathologies can contribute to subfertility and are also associated with adverse pregnancy outcomes such as miscarriage and preterm delivery. These uterine abnormalities are often diagnosed with USS. Surgical corrections can be offered to patients to improve the chance of successful ART outcome.

Fibroids

Fibroids are the most common gynecological tumors and are diagnosed with TVUS, combined with abdominal US if necessary. Fibroids typically appear as well-defined, solid masses with a whorled appearance; they are often homogenous and blend in with the surrounding myometrium but can also appear hypoechoic [62]. Uterine fibroids cause increased uterine contractility, a deranged cytokine profile, abnormal vascularization, and chronic endometrial inflammation, all of which can contribute to implantation failure [63].

Submucous fibroids (Figure 12.5) distort the endometrial cavity and are associated with lower IR, LBR, CPR, and higher miscarriage rate [64]. Multiple studies have demonstrated that resection of these fibroids improves CPRs [64,65]. Hysteroscopic resection of submucous fibroids has shown to double the CPR compared to expectant management [66].

While study results are supportive of the removal of submucosal fibroids in women undergoing fertility treatment, there is controversy over the role of myomectomy in intramural fibroids (Figure 12.6), particularly the smaller (less than 4 cm) ones that are not distorting the cavity. Meta-analysis demonstrated that intramural fibroids reduce LBRs by 21% and CPRs by 15% [67]. However, it is unclear whether

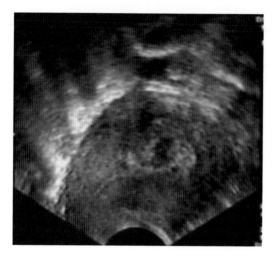

FIGURE 12.5   Submucosal fibroid. (From Schwarzler P et al. *Ultrasound Obstet Gynecol* 1998;11[5]:337–42. With permission.)

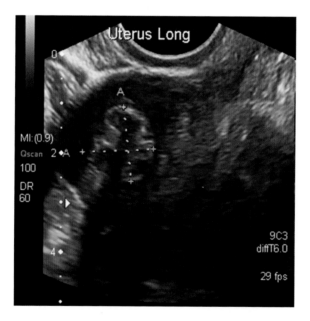

FIGURE 12.6   Intramural fibroid.

myomectomy improves the outcome [64]. Patients should be carefully counseled about the benefits and risks of myomectomy, and the final decision should be individualized.

Ultrasound assessment of the fibroid should include the number, size, location, and relation with the endometrial cavity to determine the necessity and mode of surgery prior to ART. If there are any uncertainties, magnetic resonance imaging should be considered for further evaluation to guide the next step in the management plan.

Endometrial Polyp

Endometrial polyps are defined as overgrowth of the endometrial glands and stroma covered by endometrial epithelium [68]. They appear as pedunculated endometrial masses and usually demonstrate an intact overlying endometrial stripe [62]. The presence of endometrial polyps causes decreased uterine

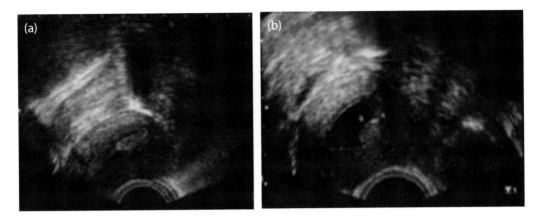

FIGURE 12.7 (a) Endometrial polyp on conventional ultrasound. (b) Endometrial polyp clearly delineated with saline infusion sonography.

receptivity, possibly secondary to an inflammatory process caused by the polyp. These polyps can also cause anatomical distortion of the endometrial cavity, hence affecting implantation [68].

Endometrial polyps are seen on TVUS as a hyperechogenic endometrial mass that is best visualized during the early proliferative phase of the menstrual cycle. The diagnostic accuracy of TVUS is relatively poor. Saline infusion sonography (SIS) provides better visualization of an endometrial polyp compared to conventional USS. The saline allows delineation of the polyp to facilitate more accurate assessment of the size and position of the polyp (Figure 12.7a and b).

Hysteroscopy is the gold standard in the diagnosis of endometrial polyps. It also allows removal of the polyp during the procedure. Hysteroscopic polypectomy resulted in higher spontaneous pregnancy rates [69] and doubles the CPR in patients undergoing ART treatment [70]. It is estimated that one in every three subfertile women with endometrial polyps will achieve a clinical pregnancy after polypectomy [71].

Congenital Uterine Anomalies

The prevalence of congenital uterine anomalies is higher in women who are subfertile and in those who suffer from recurrent miscarriages when compared to the general population. Uterine anomalies occur due to a defect in the development or fusion of the Müllerian ducts during embryogenesis.

Congenital uterine anomalies appear on USS as a double endometrial echo complex seen on the transverse plane (Figure 12.8). However, it is not possible to accurately distinguish the type of uterine

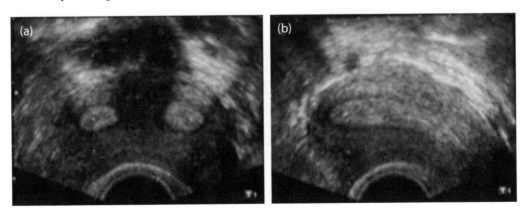

FIGURE 12.8 (a) Double endometrial echo complex seen on transverse view with (b) an otherwise unremarkable longitudinal view.

anomaly, as such a finding is observed with arcuate, bicornuate, didelphic, and septate uteri. A three-dimensional scan is needed to confirm and classify the anomaly.

A septate uterus accounts for over half of all congenital Müllerian anomalies [72] and is associated with decreased CPRs and LBRs in IVF/ICSI [73] and higher rates of miscarriages and preterm birth. These adverse reproductive outcomes are thought to be attributive to the disturbance of the regularity of the uterine cavity and also inadequate blood supply to the septum [74].

Hysteroscopic resection of the uterine septum should be considered in women undergoing ART treatment. Studies have demonstrated that septoplasty improves LBRs in IVF/ICSI. It also reduces miscarriage rates from 80% to 30% [75].

Intrauterine Adhesions

Adhesions can develop secondary to previous intrauterine surgery or infection. It can lead to subfertility due to complete or partial blockage of tubal ostia, uterine cavity, or the cervical canal, thus preventing the migration of sperm. Disruption of the endometrial lining can also prevent the implantation of embryos [70].

Adhesions are seen as bands of myometrial tissue traversing the endometrial cavity and adjoining the opposite uterine walls in USS. Typical USS findings demonstrate hypoechoic areas with interruptions of the endometrial layer. The cavity may also be distended with uterine secretions or blood if the adhesions obliterate the internal os (Figure 12.9). The sensitivity of detecting adhesions on USS varies significantly and is largely dependent on the skill of the operator and the quality of the USS equipment [76]. SIS can detect intrauterine adhesions better than conventional ultrasound. Adhesions appear as echogenic bands bridging a normally distensible endometrial cavity with pockets of fluid trapped between them [77] (Figure 12.10).

Hysteroscopic adhesiolysis is the main treatment for intrauterine adhesions. Removal of adhesions allows the uterine cavity and endometrium to be restored prior to ART treatment and should particularly be considered in those with recurrent implantation failure [63]. However, the reported recurrence rate varies from 3.1% to 23.5% and can be as high as 62.5% in severe adhesions [76]. In some cases, multiple surgeries are required. Adhesiolysis should be performed by an experienced reproductive surgeon under ultrasound guidance to reduce complications. Postoperatively, estrogen supplements are given to encourage regeneration of the endometrium.

In conclusion, USS plays a significant role in the diagnosis and subsequent management of various pelvic pathology, which can greatly impact fertility outcomes.

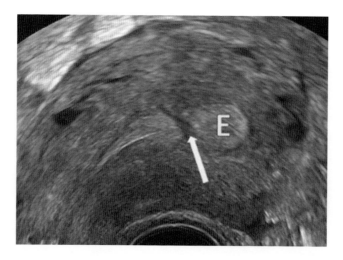

FIGURE 12.9   Endometrium (E) with a thick band of adhesion (white arrow). (From Amin TN et al. *Ultrasound Obstet Gynecol*. 2015;46[2]:131–9. With permission.)

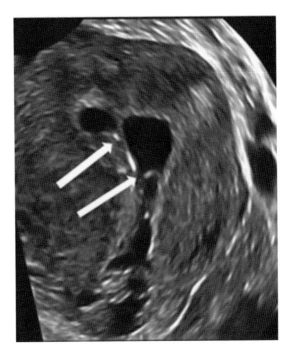

FIGURE 12.10   Intrauterine adhesions clearly highlighted by saline infusion sonography. (From Amin TN et al. *Ultrasound Obstet Gynecol.* 2015;46[2]:131–9. With permission.)

REFERENCES

1. Tsiami A, Chaimani A, Mavridis D, Siskou M, Assimakopoulos E, and Sotiriadis A. Surgical treatment for hydrosalpinx prior to *in-vitro* fertilization embryo transfer: A network meta-analysis. *Ultrasound Obstet Gynecol.* 2016;48(4):434–45.
2. Na ED et al. Comparison of IVF-ET outcomes in patients with hydrosalpinx pretreated with either sclerotherapy or laparoscopic salpingectomy. *Clin Exp Reprod Med.* 2012;39(4):182–6.
3. Walker KF, Jayaprakasan K, and Raine-Fenning N. Ultrasound in benign gynaecology. *Obstet Gynaecol Reprod Med.* 2007;17:33–44.
4. Zeyneloglu HB, Arici A, and Olive DL. Adverse effects of hydrosalpinx on pregnancy rates after *in vitro* fertilization-embryo transfer. *Fertil Steril.* 1998;70(3):492–9.
5. Kawwass JF et al. Tubal factor infertility and perinatal risk after assisted reproductive technology. *Obstet Gynecol.* 2013;121(6):1263–71.
6. D'Arpe S et al. Management of hydrosalpinx before IVF: A literature review. *J Obstet Gynaecol.* 2015;35(6):547–50.
7. Freeman MR, Whitworth CM, and Hill GA. Permanent impairment of embryo development by hydrosalpinges. *Hum Reprod.* 1998;13(4):983–6.
8. Mukherjee T et al. Hydrosalpinx fluid has embryotoxic effects on murine embryogenesis: A case for prophylactic salpingectomy. *Fertil Steril.* 1996;66(5):851–3.
9. Meyer WR, Lessey BA, and Castelbaum AJ. Hydrosalpinx and altered uterine receptivity. *Fertil Steril.* 1997;68(5):944–5.
10. Vejtorp M et al. [Fertilization *in vitro* in the presence of hydrosalpinx and in advanced age]. *Ugeskr Laeger.* 1995;157(29):4131–4.
11. Strandell A et al. Hydrosalpinx and IVF outcome: A prospective, randomized multicentre trial in Scandinavia on salpingectomy prior to IVF. *Hum Reprod.* 1999;14(11):2762–9.
12. Johnson N et al. Surgical treatment for tubal disease in women due to undergo *in vitro* fertilisation. *Cochrane Database Syst Rev.* 2010;2010(1):CD002125.
13. Kontoravdis A et al. Proximal tubal occlusion and salpingectomy result in similar improvement in *in vitro* fertilization outcome in patients with hydrosalpinx. *Fertil Steril.* 2006;86(6):1642–9.

14. Herman A et al. The dilemma of the optimal surgical procedure in ectopic pregnancies occurring in *in-vitro* fertilization. *Hum Reprod.* 1991;6(8):1167–9.
15. Orvieto R et al. Does salpingectomy affect the ipsilateral ovarian response to gonadotropin during *in vitro* fertilization-embryo transfer cycles? *Fertil Steril.* 2011;95(5):1842–4.
16. Friedman O et al. Possible improvements in human ovarian grafting by various host and graft treatments. *Hum Reprod.* 2012;27(2):474–82.
17. Ozgur K et al. ICSI pregnancy outcomes following hysteroscopic placement of Essure devices for hydrosalpinx in laparoscopic contraindicated patients. *Reprod Biomed Online.* 2014;29(1):113–8.
18. Zhang Y et al. Salpingectomy and proximal tubal occlusion for hydrosalpinx prior to *in vitro* fertilization: A meta-analysis of randomized controlled trials. *Obstet Gynecol Surv.* 2015;70(1):33–8.
19. Sowter MC et al. Is the outcome of *in-vitro* fertilization and embryo transfer treatment improved by spontaneous or surgical drainage of a hydrosalpinx? *Hum Reprod.* 1997;12(10):2147–50.
20. Hammadieh N et al. Ultrasound-guided hydrosalpinx aspiration during oocyte collection improves pregnancy outcome in IVF: A randomized controlled trial. *Hum Reprod.* 2008;23(5):1113–7.
21. Fouda UM, and Sayed AM. Effect of ultrasound-guided aspiration of hydrosalpingeal fluid during oocyte retrieval on the outcomes of *in vitro* fertilisation-embryo transfer: A randomised controlled trial (NCT01040351). *Gynecol Endocrinol.* 2011;27(8):562–7.
22. Jiang H et al. A prospective clinical study of interventional ultrasound sclerotherapy on women with hydrosalpinx before *in vitro* fertilization and embryo transfer. *Fertil Steril.* 2010;94(7):2854–6.
23. Song XM et al. Ultrasound sclerotherapy pretreatment could obtain a similar effect to surgical intervention on improving the outcomes of *in vitro* fertilization for patients with hydrosalpinx. *J Obstet Gynaecol Res.* 2017;43(1):122–7.
24. Cohen A, Almog B, and Tulandi T. Hydrosalpinx sclerotherapy before *in vitro* fertilization: Systematic review and meta-analysis. *J Minim Invasive Gynecol.* 2018;25(4):600–7.
25. Zhang WX et al. Pregnancy and perinatal outcomes of interventional ultrasound sclerotherapy with 98% ethanol on women with hydrosalpinx before *in vitro* fertilization and embryo transfer. *Am J Obstet Gynecol.* 2014;210(3):250 e1–5.
26. Meuleman C et al. High prevalence of endometriosis in infertile women with normal ovulation and normospermic partners. *Fertil Steril.* 2009;92(1):68–74.
27. The effect of surgery for endometriomas on fertility: Scientific Impact paper no. 55. *BJOG.* 2018;125(6):e19–28.
28. Sanchez AM et al. The distinguishing cellular and molecular features of the endometriotic ovarian cyst: From pathophysiology to the potential endometrioma-mediated damage to the ovary. *Hum Reprod Update.* 2014;20(2):217–30.
29. Garrido N et al. Follicular hormonal environment and embryo quality in women with endometriosis. *Hum Reprod Update.* 2000;6(1):67–74.
30. Hamdan M et al. The impact of endometrioma on IVF/ICSI outcomes: A systematic review and meta-analysis. *Hum Reprod Update.* 2015;21(6):809–25.
31. Hart RJ et al. Excisional surgery versus ablative surgery for ovarian endometriomata. *Cochrane Database Syst Rev.* 2008;(2):CD004992.
32. Keyhan S et al. An update on surgical versus expectant management of ovarian endometriomas in infertile women. *Biomed Res Int.* 2015;2015:204792.
33. Somigliana E et al. Surgical excision of endometriomas and ovarian reserve: A systematic review on serum antimullerian hormone level modifications. *Fertil Steril.* 2012;98(6):1531–8.
34. *Guideline on the Management of Women with Endometriosis.* 2013. https://www.eshre.eu/Guidelines-and-Legal/Guidelines/Endometriosis-guideline.aspx
35. Fisch JD, and Sher G. Sclerotherapy with 5% tetracycline is a simple alternative to potentially complex surgical treatment of ovarian endometriomas before *in vitro* fertilization. *Fertil Steril.* 2004;82(2):437–41.
36. Chan L. Rapid recurrence of endometrioma after transvaginal ultrasound-guided aspiration. *Eur J Obstet Gynecol Reprod Biol.* 2004;114(2):242.
37. Zhu W et al. Repeat transvaginal ultrasound-guided aspiration of ovarian endometrioma in infertile women with endometriosis. *Am J Obstet Gynecol.* 2011;204(1):61.e1–6.
38. Garcia-Velasco JA, and Somigliana E. Management of endometriomas in women requiring IVF: To touch or not to touch. *Hum Reprod.* 2009;24(3):496–501.
39. Koike T et al. Reproductive performance after ultrasound-guided transvaginal ethanol sclerotherapy for ovarian endometriotic cysts. *Eur J Obstet Gynecol Reprod Biol.* 2002;105(1):39.

40. Suganuma N et al. Pretreatment for ovarian endometrial cyst before *in vitro* fertilization. *Gynecol Obstet Invest.* 2002;54(Suppl 1):36–40; discussion 41–2.

41. Yazbeck C et al. Ethanol sclerotherapy: A treatment option for ovarian endometriomas before ovarian stimulation. *Reprod Biomed Online.* 2009;19(1):121–5.

42. Aflatoonian A, Rahmani E, and Rahsepar M. Assessing the efficacy of aspiration and ethanol injection in recurrent endometrioma before IVF cycle: A randomized clinical trial. *Iran J Reprod Med.* 2013;11(3):179–84.

43. Lee KH et al. Surgical resection or aspiration with ethanol sclerotherapy of endometrioma before *in vitro* fertilization in infertile women with endometrioma. *Obstet Gynecol Sci.* 2014;57(4):297–303.

44. Wei CF, and Chen SC. Pelvic abscess after ultrasound-guided aspiration of endometrioma: A case report. *Zhonghua Yi Xue Za Zhi (Taipei).* 1998;61(10):603–7.

45. Somigliana E et al. Does laparoscopic removal of nonendometriotic benign ovarian cysts affect ovarian reserve? *Acta Obstet Gynecol Scand.* 2006;85(1):74–7.

46. Chang HJ et al. Impact of laparoscopic cystectomy on ovarian reserve: Serial changes of serum anti-Mullerian hormone levels. *Fertil Steril.* 2010;94(1):343–9.

47. Legendre G et al. Relationship between ovarian cysts and infertility: What surgery and when? *Fertil Steril.* 2014;101(3):608–14.

48. Kim JY et al. Preoperative serum anti-mullerian hormone level in women with ovarian endometrioma and mature cystic teratoma. *Yonsei Med J.* 2013;54(4):921–6.

49. Caspi B et al. Ovarian stimulation and *in vitro* fertilization in women with mature cystic teratomas. *Obstet Gynecol.* 1998;92(6):979–81.

50. Hoo WL et al. Expectant management of ultrasonically diagnosed ovarian dermoid cysts: Is it possible to predict outcome? *Ultrasound Obstet Gynecol.* 2010;36(2):235–40.

51. Rofe G, Auslender R, and Dirnfield M. Benign ovarian cysts in reproductive-age women undergoing assisted reproductive technology treatment. *Open J Obstet Gynaecol.* 2013;3:17–22.

52. Segal S et al. Effect of a baseline ovarian cyst on the outcome of *in vitro* fertilization-embryo transfer. *Fertil Steril.* 1999;71(2):274–7.

53. Qublan HS et al. Ovarian cyst formation following GnRH agonist administration in IVF cycles: Incidence and impact. *Hum Reprod.* 2006;21(3):640–4.

54. McDonnell R, Marjoribanks J, and Hart RJ. Ovarian cyst aspiration prior to *in vitro* fertilization treatment for subfertility. *Cochrane Database Syst Rev.* 2014;2014(12):CD005999.

55. Firouzabadi RD, Sekhavat L, and Javedani M. The effect of ovarian cyst aspiration on IVF treatment with GnRH. *Arch Gynecol Obstet.* 2010;281(3):545–9.

56. National Institute for Health and Care Excellence (NICE). *NICE Guideline: Fertility: For People with Fertility Problems*; 2013.

57. Veltman-Verhulst SM et al. Intra-uterine insemination for unexplained subfertility. *Cochrane Database Syst Rev.* 2012;(9):CD001838.

58. Medical Advisory Secretariat. *In vitro* fertilization and multiple pregnancies: An evidence-based analysis. *Ont Health Technol Assess Ser.* 2006;6(18):1–63.

59. De Geyter C et al. Experience with transvaginal ultrasound-guided aspiration of supernumerary follicles for the prevention of multiple pregnancies after ovulation induction and intrauterine insemination. *Fertil Steril.* 1996;65(6):1163–8.

60. Stoop D et al. Offering excess oocyte aspiration and vitrification to patients undergoing stimulated artificial insemination cycles can reduce the multiple pregnancy risk and accumulate oocytes for later use. *Hum Reprod.* 2010;25(5):1213–8.

61. Seshadri S et al. Diagnostic accuracy of saline infusion sonography in the evaluation of uterine cavity abnormalities prior to assisted reproductive techniques: A systematic review and meta-analyses. *Hum Reprod Update.* 2015;21(2):262–74.

62. Wilde S, and Scott-Barrett S. Radiological appearances of uterine fibroids. *Indian J Radiol Imaging.* 2009;19(3):222–31.

63. Coughlan C et al. Recurrent implantation failure: Definition and management. *Reprod Biomed Online.* 2014;28(1):14–38.

64. Pritts EA, Parker WH, and Olive DL. Fibroids and infertility: An updated systematic review of the evidence. *Fertil Steril.* 2009;91(4):1215–23.

65. Fernandez H et al. Hysteroscopic resection of submucosal myomas in patients with infertility. *Hum Reprod.* 2001;16(7):1489–92.

66. Shokeir T et al. Submucous myomas and their implications in the pregnancy rates of patients with otherwise unexplained primary infertility undergoing hysteroscopic myomectomy: A randomized matched control study. *Fertil Steril.* 2010;94(2):724–9.
67. Sunkara SK et al. The effect of intramural fibroids without uterine cavity involvement on the outcome of IVF treatment: A systematic review and meta-analysis. *Hum Reprod.* 2010;25(2):418–29.
68. Tiras B et al. Management of endometrial polyps diagnosed before or during ICSI cycles. *Reprod Biomed Online.* 2012;24(1):123–8.
69. Shokeir TA, Shalan HM, and El-Shafei MM. Significance of endometrial polyps detected hysteroscopically in eumenorrheic infertile women. *J Obstet Gynaecol Res.* 2004;30(2):84–9.
70. Bosteels J et al. The effectiveness of hysteroscopy in improving pregnancy rates in subfertile women without other gynaecological symptoms: A systematic review. *Hum Reprod Update.* 2010;16(1):1–11.
71. Bosteels J et al. The effectiveness of reproductive surgery in the treatment of female infertility: Facts, views and vision. *Facts Views Vis Obgyn.* 2010;2(4):232–52.
72. Grimbizis GF et al. Clinical implications of uterine malformations and hysteroscopic treatment results. *Hum Reprod Update.* 2001;7(2):161–74.
73. Tomazevic T et al. *Septate,* subseptate and arcuate uterus decrease pregnancy and live birth rates in IVF/ICSI. *Reprod Biomed Online.* 2010. 21(5):700–5.
74. Fedele L et al. Urinary tract anomalies associated with unicornuate uterus. *J Urol.* 1996;155(3):847–8.
75. Ban-Frangez H et al. The outcome of singleton pregnancies after IVF/ICSI in women before and after hysteroscopic resection of a uterine septum compared to normal controls. *Eur J Obstet Gynecol Reprod Biol.* 2009;146(2):184–7.
76. Amin TN, Saridogan E, and Jurkovic D. Ultrasound and intrauterine adhesions: A novel structured approach to diagnosis and management. *Ultrasound Obstet Gynecol.* 2015;46(2):131–9.
77. Abdusamad K, Hamoudi R, and Maiti S. Simultaneous bilateral torsion of the adnexae in an adult female without any history of ovarian stimulation. *BMJ Case Rep.* 2013;2013:bcr2012007909.
78. Schwarzler P et al. An evaluation of sonohysterography and diagnostic hysteroscopy for the assessment of intrauterine pathology. *Ultrasound Obstet Gynecol.* 1998;11(5):337–42.

13

Implantation and In Utero *Growth*

Kugajeevan Vigneswaran and Ippokratis Sarris

Physiology of Implantation

Human conception begins at fertilization, after which the tiny fertilized egg positioned at the oviduct of the uterus has to undertake a journey of mammoth proportions. Upon reaching the uterus, the embryo engages in a complex process of interaction with the maternal interface. This two-way communication results in the physical contact of the embryo with the endometrium and subsequent implantation. Without implantation, the embryo, unable to sustain its nutritional requirements, will arrest its growth.

Progestogenic domination is necessary for implantation to occur. Rising progesterone levels results in a transition from little growth to a secretory phase endometrium contributing to the creation of a nutritionally rich glandular support network for the arrival of the embryo. Following implantation, the embryo is able to establish its own circulation as well as provoke maternal circulatory changes.

Long-range signaling to the pituitary-ovarian axis of the implanted embryo results in maintenance of the corpus luteum and a sustained progestogen environment. The implanted embryo, now at the blastocyst stage, induces ongoing epithelial and stromal changes within the endometrium, which results in the development of the maternal component of the placenta.

The Implantation Window

Successful embryo implantation can only take place within a receptive uterus. During the midsecretory phase of the menstrual cycle, a functional window opens, signaling a receptive period. The endometrium undergoes significant histological changes as this window of implantation opens. Apical protrusions known as "pinopodes" begin to cover much of the epithelial surface of the endometrium as well as within the lumen of the endometrial glands, and this increases absorption of uterine fluids, resulting in a reduction of the uterine cavity volume [1]. In normal fertile women, pinopode formation and regression are closely related to serum progesterone levels.

The resulting apposition of the uterine cavity walls, along with an edematous uterine stroma, pushes the trophoblast closer to the uterine epithelium. At a molecular level, there is recruitment of specialized natural killer cells, vascular remodeling, and transformation of stromal fibroblasts into rounded decidual cells.

Failure of the embryo to attach leads to a refractory period as the window closes. Beyond this point, the uterus will resist any further attempts at attachment. For an embryo to thrive, early development and transport to reach the uterus at the point of receptivity are paramount. Providing the necessary endocrine conditions are maintained, the uterus will continue to provide a suitable environment for the embryo. Upon securing a stable physical and nutritional grounding, the embryo will prevent corpus luteal regression. Eventually the placental unit will assume ongoing support for the implanted pregnancy.

Ultrasound in the Role of Assessing Implantation Potential

Evaluation of the endometrium and its implantation potential focuses on identification of the "window of receptivity" to establish and predict chances of successful pregnancy. Under the influence of increasing

Zaidi et al. analyzed several parameters in relation to this vascular network to the endometrium on the day of hCG administration during IVF cycles and pregnancy outcomes. There were no statistical differences in subendometrial peak systolic velocity or PI when comparing pregnant cycles with nonpregnant cycles. In cases where there was an absence of both subendometrial and intraendometrial vascularization, there was a lower likelihood of implantation [12].

An alternative method of assessing vascularization called intraendometrial power Doppler area (EDPA) was proposed by Yang et al., looking at power Doppler sonography of vascular signals within the endometrial borders. Although once again the overall predictive value of EDPA was limited, the higher the EDPA, the more likely implantation was to take place [13].

It would appear that on the whole, the higher the degree of endometrial perfusion as shown by the various methods proposed, the greater the degree of endometrial receptivity. A consensus has not been reached on the most accurate method to assess this; however, the literature would point to the combination of both endometrial and subendometrial flow parameters to determine vascularity and thereby assess perfusion.

A correlation with intraendometrial vascular penetration and endometrial thickness has been shown. In addition, patients with no detectable endometrial-subendometrial flow demonstrated a higher uterine arterial resistance than those with the presence of flow.

In conclusion, transvaginal color Doppler examination of the endometrial-subendometrial blood flow distribution can offer a possible method to assess endometrial receptivity. The absence of adequate flow when assessing these parameters may reflect a less receptive endometrial environment, although current data are lacking to implement this into routine practice.

Three-Dimensional Endometrial Assessment of Volume and Blood Flow

Calculation of endometrial volume can be achieved using three-dimensional (3D) ultrasound. This has been shown to have a low intra- and interobserver variability. It is also possible to assess endometrial vascularity by merging 3D ultrasound and power Doppler (3D power Doppler). By combining measures of uterine size, morphology, and vascularity, it is possible to correlate patterns according to the cyclical changes of the menstrual cycle.

Endometrial volume is found to increase throughout the follicular phase and plateaus in the luteal phase. The subendometrial region is considered to be the 5 mm shell around the defined endometrial contour. Both endometrial and subendometrial 3D power Doppler indices have good reproducibility and can be useful in endometrial assessment of function (Figure 13.2). Vascularity of both the endometrial and subendometrial areas increases from the mid-follicular phase and appears to peak at 3 days prior to ovulation [14]. There is then a gradual fall seen over the next 5 days, until the process starts over again in the next menstrual cycle.

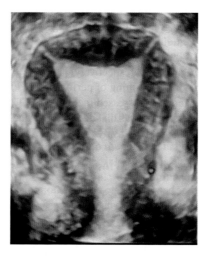

FIGURE 13.2   Three-dimensional image of uterus.

Raine-Fenning et al. found that in women with unexplained subfertility, there was a reduction in both endometrial and subendometrial vascularity as measured by 3D during the mid to late follicular phase, even when controlling for estradiol and progesterone levels [15].

Despite these results, the literature does not conclusively support the concept that endometrial vascularity directly impacts on implantation potential. Ng et al. found that when assessing endometrial vascularity in 451 IVF pregnancies, there was no distinction made in the indices between pregnant and nonpregnant cycles [16]. In a later study, the same authors found in a further 161 patients that there was an increased vascularity in cycles that resulted in a live birth when compared to cycles that ended in a miscarriage.

Uterine Contractility

An evolving area of study of endometrial physiology is subendometrial contractility, which has been described as endometrial "waves" seen on transvaginal ultrasound. Without the use of invasive uterine pressure catheters, ultrasound may provide insight into the frequency and direction of uterine activity. It is thought that these waves are the result of hormonal-directed contractions of the subendometrial myometrium, more specifically from the junctional zone.

The uterine junctional zone (JZ) is the transitional zone between the endometrium and the outer myometrium, also referred to as the endometrial-myometrial junction. Irregular thickening of the JZ can be seen in patients with diffuse adenomyosis.

Studies have been conducted into the patterns and behaviors of these waves and correlated with cycle-related variations. In the early follicular phase, there is predominantly a fundus to cervix directional pattern observed, and this is reversed in the late follicular/peri-ovulatory phase of the cycle [17]. In addition, as ovulation approaches, there is an increase in both amplitude and frequency of the contractions. Following ovulation, the influence of progesterone causes a reduction in uterine contractions.

With respect to human reproduction, it only stands to reason that these waves may play a role in sperm and embryo transportation and therefore generate interest in their role in implantation potential. It is likely that as a result of supraphysiological estradiol levels, there is an exaggerated wave pattern observed in IVF cycles. A greater deviation from physiological behavior has been shown to negatively correlate with cycle outcome [18]. The clinical applicability of this potential marker of uterine function has yet to be clearly outlined.

Assessment of the frequency of uterine waves at the time of embryo transfer may be associated with a reduced chance of implantation in both fresh and frozen embryo transfers, when more than two to three contractions per minute are seen [19]. It has been postulated that this may be due to aforementioned supraphysiological levels of hormones found in IVF cycles, thus increasing peristalsis or mechanical stimuli such as touching the top of the fundus with the embryo transfer catheter, inducing bleeding, or using a rigid catheter and/or a tenaculum in the case of difficult embryo transfers. Such factors may add weight to the argument for segmented embryo transfers in some IVF cycles and reinforces the need for ultrasound-guided embryo transfer.

Possible Impediments to Implantation

Congenital Uterine Anomalies

The infertile population has a 3.4%–8% prevalence of uterine abnormalities, which is not dissimilar to the fertile population. The prevalence of uterine abnormalities rises to approximately 12.6% in women who have suffered recurrent pregnancy loss [20]. This is also reflected in women undergoing ART. It is thought that abnormal musculature, vascularity, and reduced cavity size along with increased rates of cervical incompetence may all contribute to the rise in pregnancy loss.

The most common uterine abnormality found on imaging is the arcuate and septate uterus. The arcuate uterus is found in both the fertile and infertile populations in equivalent prevalences (3.9%) [21]. Given the lack of reduction in reproductive potential in these cases, surgical intervention is not warranted.

The septate uterus is the most frequent uterine abnormality found in the population suffering from both infertility and recurrent pregnancy loss (3%–15.4% in a recent meta-analysis). It is thought that a septate uterus consists of a hypovascular region of muscle that may also affect the overlying endometrium, thus

(a)   (b)   (c)

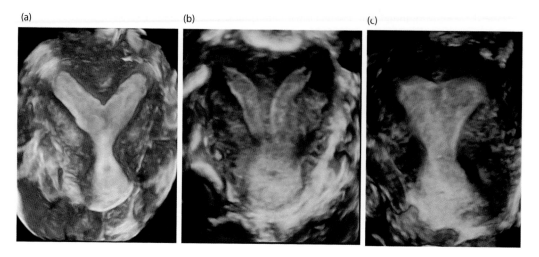

FIGURE 13.3   (a) Subseptate uterus; (b) septate uterus; (c) post resection.

resulting in a possible impairment in both implantation as well as early *in utero* development. When examining the studies showing the reproductive outcomes of women with untreated septate uteri, there appears to be an increased miscarriage rate (41.1% versus 12.1%) [22]. However, there is a large degree of heterogeneity within the studies conducted and a tendency to put forth the worst-case scenarios. That being said, a septate uterus can be corrected relatively easily via the hysteroscopic route (Figure 13.3) and may improve reproductive outcomes in some women.

Other uterine abnormalities that can be detected with ultrasound include unicornuate, didelphys, and bicornuate uteri. All have been shown to increase the risk of adverse reproductive outcomes, however not to the degree of impact that the septate uterus would cause [23]. Other factors such as the severity of the uterine abnormality can determine impact on outcomes. One such example would be bicornuate uteri. A complete bicornuate uterus can result in a 66% chance of a preterm delivery as opposed to a partial bicornuate uterus, which carries a risk of approximately 29% [24].

Uterine Fibroids

Uterine fibroids are growths arising from the myometrium consisting of fibrovascular cells. They develop under the influence of estrogen and progesterone, as evidenced by the presence of hormone receptors on their surface. Fibroids invariably are coated in a vascular pseudo-capsule and develop a gradually increasing vascular supply with increasing mass (Figure 13.4).

Since fibroids are found to increase in frequency with age, this confounds data assessing the impact of fibroids on implantation and fertility. Although pregnancy is entirely possible despite the presence of fibroids in some women, fibroid location dictates the extent to which symptoms result from their presence. In general, the greater the degree of endometrial distortion, the more likely there is compromised fertility.

Submucous fibroids can distort the uterine cavity, alter the biomechanics of the endometrium, and impact an embryo's ability to implant and develop. Changes to the vascular supply and changes in endometrial proliferation in addition to alterations in inflammatory substances and growth factors in the presence of fibroids may all contribute to a decline in implantation potential [25]. Recent data have found that changes in signaling molecules produced by fibroids have adverse effects on receptivity throughout the endometrium, and as a result, removal of these fibroids can be expected to improve not only local endometrial receptivity immediately overlying the fibroid, but also the entire endometrium.

Submucosal fibroids have been shown uniformly to have a negative impact on rates of implantation, clinical pregnancy, miscarriage, and live birth/ongoing pregnancy, although available studies are few and small. Much of the data is derived from IVF cycle results. There is evidence that submucous fibroids reduce IVF pregnancy and live birth rates and that hysteroscopic myomectomy significantly improves outcomes, bringing results in line with women with normal uterine cavities [25].

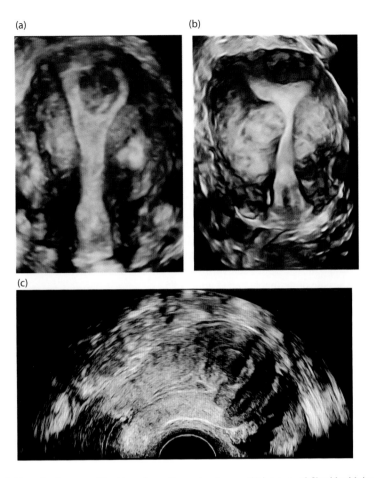

FIGURE 13.4 (a) Type 0 submucous fibroid on three-dimensional scan; (b) intramural fibroid with impingement of the cavity; (c) Type 0 submucous fibroid on two-dimensional scan.

There is also increasing data that suggest that sizable intramural fibroids can reduce fertility, especially when intramural myomas are 4 cm or larger, and myomectomy appears to restore fertility [26]. However, this is not conclusive as a recent meta-analysis found only a nonsignificant trend of slightly lower pregnancy rates in women with intramural myomas and a nonsignificant trend of improved pregnancy rates after myomectomy in women during assisted reproduction procedures [27]. Therefore, currently there is no clearly proven benefit that myomectomy enhances fertility in women with intramural myomas. The possible complications of fibroid surgery, with their subsequent negative iatrogenic impact on fertility, must be considered in these cases. Subserosal fibroids found on the external surface of the uterus do not appear to affect fertility.

Adenomyosis

Adenomyosis is regarded to be a disease originating from the endomyometrial junction and is defined by the presence of endometrial glands and stroma within the myometrium. The condition occurs when there is a disruption of the boundary between the endometrial basal layer and myometrium, allowing for invasion and migration of endometrial cells, giving rise to ectopic intramyometrial glands. These glands subsequently cause hypertrophy and hyperplasia of adjacent myometrium [28].

As our understanding of the features associated with adenomyosis as well as diagnostic modalities continues to improve, detection rates have risen, and the condition is more frequently diagnosed within the subfertile population and those undergoing IVF treatment.

In general, the detrimental effect of adenomyosis on fertility outcomes appears to be related to reduced rates of implantation and pregnancy, increased risk of early pregnancy loss, and as a result, a decrease in live birth rate. A recent meta-analysis estimated a 41% decrease in live birth rate in the presence of adenomyosis (OR 0.59; 95% CI 0.42–0.82) [29].

Several theories have been put forth to explain this effect of adenomyosis on implantation, including altered uterine peristaltic activity, altered endometrial-myometrial vascular growth, and increased levels of prostaglandins in the ectopic endometrial epithelium.

Multiple attempts to outline ultrasound features of adenomyosis and their significance have been proposed, although no consensus has been reached on diagnostic criteria. Further information on the ultrasonographic features of adenomyosis can be found in Chapter 3.

Endometrial Polyps

Endometrial polyps are localized overgrowths of endometrial glandular and stromal tissue formed around a vascular core projecting into the uterine cavity. Histologically, polyps can exhibit functional (cyclical changes), atrophic, or even hyperplastic changes. Polyps can be located throughout the uterine cavity or the cervix and can range in size from a few millimeters to several centimeters. Morphologically, polyps can be described as sessile or pedunculated (Figure 13.5).

The incidence of polyps gradually increases with age, peaking within the age range of 40 to 50 years, and then a steady decline following menopause [30]. There is no evidence to suggest that the subfertile population has a greater prevalence of polyps in comparison to an age-matched control population.

As already established, adequate endometrial thickness and quality are indicative of uterine receptivity; therefore, any structural disruption of this may lead to implantation failure.

Endometrial polyps are the most common intracavity finding on ultrasound, and although the exact cause for possible impaired function is not known, various hypotheses have been postulated. Polyps may cause a physical barrier to adequate sperm or embryo transport within the uterine cavity, as well as obstruct the steps involved in implantation. Alternatively, there may be an exaggerated inflammatory response because of the polyp, altering receptivity on a molecular level.

Data demonstrate a decreased pregnancy rate in spontaneous conception as well as in intrauterine insemination cycles [31]. However, in the absence of hyperplasia or malignancy, there is no randomized trial data available to guide treatment of asymptomatic polyps. In the case of symptomatic polyps, resolution of symptoms, which was predominantly intermenstrual bleeding, can be observed in up to 75% of patients who underwent polypectomy [32]. Hysteroscopically guided polypectomy, using microscissors or a resectoscope, has been shown to be superior to blind curettage.

Stamatellos et al. reported the fertility outcomes in 83 women with endometrial polyps and otherwise unexplained subfertility who underwent hysteroscopic polypectomy in a retrospective study [33]. The mean size of the polyps was 19 mm. A normal menstrual pattern was achieved in 91.6% of patients postoperatively, and spontaneous pregnancy rates increased to 61.4%, with a live birth rate at term of 54.2%. Interestingly, the group found no statistical difference in the outcomes when the patients were grouped according to size or number of polyps. They therefore concluded from their cohort that in women with otherwise unexplained subfertility, there may be a role for hysteroscopic polypectomy to improve chances of implantation and pregnancy.

This cohort seems to represent most of the data published indicating that in a subfertile population, a polypectomy improves fertility. This may well be the case for both spontaneous pregnancies as well as assisted reproductive cycles.

Intrauterine Adhesions

Joseph Asherman presented the first description of intrauterine adhesions (IUAs; Figure 13.6) in 1948, as an organic amenorrhea and inactive endometrium due to stenosis of the internal os of the cervix [34]. A follow-up paper in 1950, entitled "Traumatic Intra-uterine Adhesions," also by Asherman, discussed total obliteration of the cavity as a result of these adhesions.

The true incidence of Asherman syndrome is unclear. Estimates range from 6% to 40% after dilatation and curettage [35]. The American Society for Reproductive Medicine estimates IUA to be the cause of

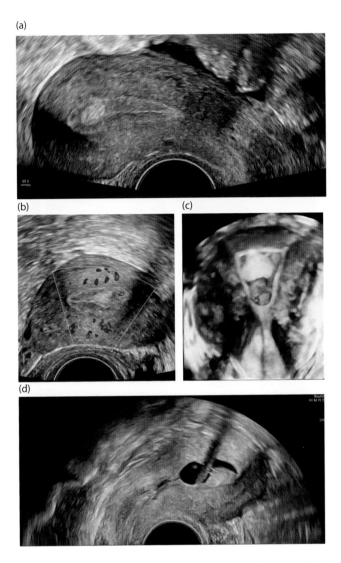

FIGURE 13.5 (a) Endometrial polyp; (b) endometrial polyp on transverse view; (c) endometrial polyp on three-dimensional saline infusion (balloon noted below polyp); (d) endometrial polyp on saline infusion.

approximately 7% of all cases of secondary amenorrhea [36]. Uterine adhesions are almost exclusively caused by injury to the basal layer of the endometrium. This most commonly occurs during uterine curettage for miscarriages, terminations, or removal of retained products of conception. Evidence of association with cesarean section, myomectomy, removal of septae, and other intrauterine operations is also increasing [37].

Several classification systems exist for intrauterine adhesions; however, there is not one universally accepted or validated method to follow. Amenorrhea and infertility are the most common presenting symptoms that result in the diagnosis of IUA, and the history of menstrual disorders following the curettage of the pregnancy should prompt the question of IUA.

Asherman syndrome has significant reproductive implications for patients. In most case series, the rate of fertility and full-term birth directly correlates to extent of disease. However, there does not seem to be a connection between number of prior curettages or the etiology of adhesions in predicting outcome. Fertility following hysteroscopic treatment of adhesions is possible provided there is adequate residual normal endometrial tissue, although gonadotropins, intrauterine insemination, or IVF is sometimes necessary.

Although hysteroscopy remains the gold standard test for diagnosis of IUA as well as offering a means to therapeutic interventions, there is also a place for diagnostic imaging. There are currently no

(a)   (b)

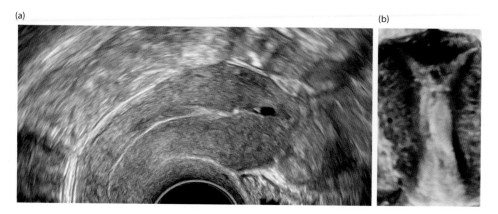

FIGURE 13.6   (a) Intrauterine adhesions—Ashermen syndrome; (b) intrauterine adhesions—Ashermen syndrome on three-dimensional ultrasound scan.

randomized data comparing the use of imaging with hysteroscopy; however, the literature would suggest several ultrasound techniques exist, such as transvaginal two-dimensional (2D) ultrasound, SIS, and 3D ultrasound, to aid in the diagnosis in a comparatively less invasive way.

Ultrasound features suggestive of IUA include visualization of an irregular endometrium that is thinner and more echogenic than would be otherwise expected for the day of the cycle. In addition, cystic anechoic pockets within the endometrium are suggestive of IUA. The addition of saline in a SIS may further reveal adhesions that characteristically appear as "bridging bands" of tissue that distort the cavity. Filmy adhesions are described as thin, undulating membranes that are most easily seen on real-time scanning.

Three-dimensional ultrasound allows for greater visualization and provides more accurate assessment than traditional 2D ultrasound imaging. Three-dimensional ultrasound can provide useful information on the location and extent of adhesions, therefore assisting with grading of severity. This additionally allows for more accurate prediction of prognosis and fertility outcomes. This can be done in combination with a SIS (3D-SIS) to further improve diagnostic accuracy.

Hysterosalpingography (HSG) is a commonly used first-line investigation of uterine abnormalities and infertility. It involves injection of a radiopaque dye into the uterine cavity and x-ray evaluation of the uterus and fallopian tubes. Adhesions are seen as filling defects that do not change with positioning.

The high sensitivity of HSG has made it a useful screening tool for intrauterine abnormalities. Compared with hysteroscopy, HSG is a relatively safe, cheaper, and less-invasive test. However, it does result in exposure to ionizing radiation as well as has the potential to cause a great deal of patient discomfort. It also produces a high number of false positives and can overestimate the severity of disease.

A case series by Knopman and Copperman studied 54 women with a primary diagnosis of Asherman syndrome and compared 3D ultrasound to HSG for evaluation of diagnostic accuracy. Sensitivity was calculated using hysteroscopy as the gold standard. One hundred percent of preoperative 3D imaging was found to be consistent with hysteroscopy results in assessing severity of disease, compared to 66.7% for HSG. It provided a more precise map of intrauterine adhesions and also enabled differentiation between severe intrauterine disease and outflow tract obstruction [38].

Tubal Factor: Hydrosalpinx

The fallopian tubes, which derive their name from the sixteenth-century Italian anatomist Gabriel Fallopius, are essential for oocyte pickup, sperm transport, fertilization, and early embryonic development.

Due to the indirect connection with the lower genital tract, the fallopian tubes are at risk of exposure to sexually transmitted infections. At the distal end of the tubes, delicate structures known as fimbriae are particularly susceptible to damage following infection and abdominal or pelvic surgery. This injury

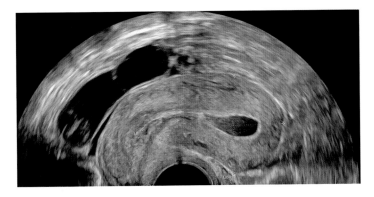

FIGURE 13.7   Hydrosalpinx resulting from accumulation of fluid within the uterine cavity.

can result in tubal occlusion and subsequent accumulation of fluid within the lumen of the tubes. This process results in the formation of a hydrosalpinx (Figure 13.7). The natural history of hydrosalpinges is poorly understood. It is unclear how rapidly they develop within the fallopian tube after exposure to an insult, or indeed how many resolve or recur.

The incidence of hydrosalpinges as well as more on causes can be found in Chapter 12.

Several retrospective studies have shown a reduction in successful outcomes in IVF when a hydrosalpinx is present. Meta-analyses suggest that in the presence of a hydrosalpinx, the probability of pregnancy after IVF is reduced by half, and the rate of miscarriage doubles [39]. Surgical intervention to interrupt the communication of the hydrosalpinx and the uterus has also demonstrated a restoration of pregnancy rates. This is particularly the case in patients with hydrosalpinges large enough to be visible on ultrasound examination.

The underlying mechanism for impaired implantation in the presence of a hydrosalpinx has not yet been established. Theories have suggested a dual pathology: a direct impact on the embryo as well as an impact on the endometrium and its receptivity.

Beyler et al. studied the contents of tubal fluid from the hydrosalpinges from infertile women and compared several parameters with normal human tubal fluid. Hydrosalpinx fluid was found to have lower concentrations of potassium, calcium, phosphate, glucose, and protein. They concluded that the reflux of lipophilic embryotoxic factors into the uterine cavity may play a role in the reduction in implantation [40].

The "cross-talk" between the embryo and endometrium is mediated by the secretion and expression of certain cytokines and other substances present during the implantation window. The presence of hydrosalpinx fluid may impair expression of cytokines such as IL-1 (interleukin-1), LIF (leukemia inhibitory factor), colony-stimulating factor (CSF)-1, and integrin. In respect to integrin, Meyer et al. were able to show reduced α-V β-3 integrin levels in women with hydrosalpinges, possibly suggesting reduced endometrial receptivity. There was a restoration of the markers following surgery [41].

With the aid of transvaginal ultrasound, it is possible to detect a hydrosalpinx, as a cystic hypoechoic adnexal mass. Several distinguishing sonographic features have been suggested in the literature. Patel described the following: incomplete septation, short linear projections, tubular shape, and the "waist sign" [42]. The waist sign refers to directly opposing indentations within the cystic structure possibly representing distended rugae noted within the lumen of the tube. This is also known as the "cogwheel" sign. The combination of a tubal structure and the waist sign results in a likelihood ratio (LR) of 18.9. However, the highest LR was noted when there were short linear projections seen within a tubular structure (LR = 22.1). In the absence of any solid-appearing areas or other features denoting the likelihood of ovarian pathology, the previously mentioned features allow for the diagnosis of a hydrosalpinx with a high degree of confidence.

It is important to consider alternative diagnoses for the appearance of fluid-filled structures within the pelvis. Peritoneal inclusion cysts caused by adhesions are complex cystic adnexal masses consisting of a normal ovary entrapped in multiple fluid-filled adhesions. The cysts usually develop in women of reproductive age who have a history of previous pelvic surgery or pelvic infection.

Fluid normally produced by the ovaries during ovulation is absorbed by the peritoneum. However, if the peritoneum has been disrupted by previous surgery, inflammation, or infection, its absorptive properties diminish, thus trapping this physiologic fluid. Although often a sign of, and coexisting with, other pelvic pathology such as previously described, as there is no connection in these cases to the endometrial cavity, there is no known impact on implantation potential, per se.

Beyond Implantation

Following on from the successful "breaching" of the endometrium by the embryo, the stromal compartment undergoes decidualization. The degree of decidualization correlates with the depth of trophoblastic invasion. In humans, the formation of the placenta also relies on further invasion of the trophoblast into the junctional zone, the highly specialized area found in the inner layer of the myometrium. Thus, the ability of the junctional zone and the decidua to form a functional unit, with low resistance and high-capacity spiral vessels, helps to determine the likelihood of a successful pregnancy outcome.

It was thought previously that the trophoblast is the invader of a somewhat passive endometrium; however, more recent observations have shown the decidual cells themselves develop an invasive phenotype of their own. The fetal-maternal interaction is now thought of as a process by which the decidua actively encapsulates the embryo once it has breached the luminal epithelium. Additionally, the decidua is also thought to play a "biosensor" role in the selection of embryos, limiting implantation to those that demonstrate greater potential to result in an ongoing pregnancy. Deviation of this screening process may allow a prolonged window of implantation and allow a compromised embryo to get through, thus resulting in a possible reason for recurrent miscarriages.

Miscarriage rates vary depending on maternal age, previous obstetric history, and a multitude of other factors. It is thought that most of these miscarriages are due to chromosomal abnormalities and occur during the embryonic period of development. Ultrasound is often the first method of determining the risk and indeed diagnosing a miscarriage; therefore, it is important to understand the sonographic features of both a healthy ongoing pregnancy as well as that of a failing one.

Gestational Sac

The gestational sac (GS) is the first sonographic visualization of the conceptus. It is denoted by a spherical, fluid-filled cavity located within the endometrium surrounded by an echogenic rim. With the advent of a high-resolution transvaginal ultrasound, it is possible to visualize this structure as early as 2 weeks after fertilization and is the earliest sign of an intrauterine pregnancy.

The anechoic appearance of the early GS represents the exocelomic fluid of the blastocyst, and the echogenic rim is trophoblastic tissue comprising chorionic villi. The rim that represents these chorionic villi should have a greater echodensity than the surrounding myometrium, and once it reaches a thickness of beyond 2 mm, it indicates a possible intrauterine pregnancy.

The location of the GS is generally found eccentrically buried within the endometrium and in its early stages does not appear to distort the endometrial lining interface. The size of the GS directly correlates with trophoblastic function, as well as rising hCG levels. Beyond a level of between 1000 and 2000 mIU/mL, the GS should always be visible on transvaginal ultrasound in the case of an intrauterine pregnancy, and the levels are expected to rise by at least 53% within 48 hours [43]. This logarithmic rise in hCG levels is predictable from the fourth to the tenth weeks of gestation, after which there is wide biological variation. The mean sac diameter (MSD) is measured using an average of anteroposterior, transverse, and cephalocaudal dimensions and is thought to grow approximately 1.1 mm per day once visualized on ultrasound [44].

Although the GS cannot be relied on to calculate precise gestational age, features such as appearance, location, and growth rate may provide useful indicators of the health of the ongoing pregnancy. A reduced choriodecidual reaction to the GS, irregular contour of the GS, and its appearance low down in the uterine cavity may all signal an abnormally developing pregnancy.

Bromley et al. found that when the difference in size between the crown rump length and the MSD was less than 5 mm, there was a greater risk of embryonic demise, and if the pregnancy did progress despite this finding, there was a greater risk of preterm delivery and low birth weight [45].

Yolk Sac

The first structure to appear within the GS is the yolk sac (YS). Its appearance denotes a true GS and increases the positive predictive value of an intrauterine pregnancy to 100% [46]. It is often seen at the periphery of the chorionic cavity and has a spherical echogenic appearance with a sonolucent center, giving rise to a ring-like formation. The YS represents the embryological secondary YS and develops at the same time as the amniotic membrane; however, it is more readily visible owing to its echogenicity. Once the MSD reaches between 5 and 13 mm, indicating a gestational age of 5–6 weeks, the YS should be visible on transvaginal ultrasound [47].

The function of the YS is primarily nutritional support of the developing embryo, providing a metabolic transport system across the maternal-embryo interface until placental function is established. It is also the site for primordial germ cell formation. Therefore, its adequate growth is essential for the health of the ongoing pregnancy. This growth is a steady rise to a maximal diameter of 6 mm usually reached at 11 weeks of gestation, at which point there is spontaneous regression and disappearance by the end of the first trimester.

Given the significance of YS function, deviation from normal development may signal a poor pregnancy outcome. Mara et al. found that premature regression of the YS can signal impending embryonic demise [48]. Other predictors that have been studied include absence of the YS in the presence of an embryonic pole, distortion of the shape and contour of the YS, opacification, and a floating central location within the GS. It is important to note that these findings can all be transient, and regular surveillance is warranted. The finding that has been shown to have the greatest weight in predictive value is the YS size. Any significant variation below or above the reported mean may indicate a greater chance of pregnancy loss.

Embryo

Following on from the appearance of the YS, the next structure that becomes visible within the chorionic sac is the early embryo. Ultrasound can detect the presence of an embryo from 5 to 6 weeks of gestational age, where it is first seen as a linear echogenic structure measuring 2–3 mm lying alongside the YS. From the gestational age of 5 to 9 weeks, there is rapid embryonic development and organogenesis, and the "fetal pole" can be measured along its long axis. The term *crown-rump length* had been used to denote the size of the embryo at this stage; however, these anatomical structures are not possible to differentiate until 10 weeks of gestation.

The cardiovascular system is the first embryonic system to develop, with the functional heartbeat being observed as early as 5 weeks of gestational age. In fact, cardiac pulsations may be more prominent than the fetal pole on sonographic examination. Certainly, by the time the fetal pole has reached 7 mm, there should be a fetal heartbeat; the absence of such has shown a 100% positive predictability for embryonic demise [49].

Once a fetal heartbeat is detected, the rate of pregnancy loss drops to approximately 5%, but there are several confounding factors such as advanced maternal age, obstetric history, and signs or symptoms of threatened miscarriage [49]. A slow fetal heartbeat observed in the first trimester, particularly in cases where it is found to be less than or equal to 90 beats per minute, has been shown to increase the chance of miscarriage [8]. In cases of ongoing pregnancy with this finding, additional ultrasound surveillance should be performed owing to the possibility of increased fetal anomalies.

KEY MESSAGES

As the content within this chapter has demonstrated, human conception is indeed an inefficient process. The advent of ultrasound, and in particular transvaginal ultrasound, has allowed a great deal of insight into physiology of implantation and early *in utero* development. As evident throughout this chapter, the use of ultrasound has enabled the diagnosis and subsequent treatment of factors that have been shown to impede implantation and early growth. As technology develops, ultrasound is further likely to enhance our understanding of these intricate processes and remain at the frontier of our practice.

REFERENCES

1. Amso NN, Crow J, Lewin J, and Shaw RW. Physiology: A comparative morphological and ultrastructural study of endometrial gland and Fallopian tube epithelia at different stages of the menstrual cycle and the menopause. *Hum Reprod.* 1994;9(12):2234–41.

2. Friedler S, Schenker JG, Herman A, and Lewin A. The role of ultrasonography in the evaluation of endometrial receptivity following assisted reproductive treatments: A critical review. *Hum Reprod Update.* 1996;2:323–35.

3. Kasius A, Smit JG, Torrance HL et al. Endometrial thickness and pregnancy rates after IVF: A systematic review and meta-analysis. *Hum Reprod Update.* 2014;20:530–41.

4. Gingold JA, Lee JA, Rodriguez-Purata J et al. Endometrial pattern, but not endometrial thickness, affects implantation rates in euploid embryo transfers. *Fertil Steril.* 2015;104:620–8.e5.

5. Zhao J, Zhang Q, Wang Y, and Li Y. Endometrial pattern, thickness and growth in predicting pregnancy outcome following 3319 IVF cycle. *Reprod Biomed Online.* 2014;29(3):291–8.

6. Khalifa E, Brzyski RG, Oehninger S, Acosta AA, and Muasher SJ. Sonographic appearance of the endometrium: The predictive value for the outcome of *in-vitro* fertilization in stimulated cycles. *Hum Reprod.* 1992;7:677–80.

7. Grunfeld L, Walker B, Bergh PA, Sandler B, Hofmann G, and Navot D. High-resolution endovaginal ultrasonography of the endometrium: A noninvasive test for endometrial adequacy. *Obstet Gynecol.* 1991;78(2):200–4.

8. Chittacharoen A, and Herabutya Y. Slow fetal heart rate may predict pregnancy outcome in first-trimester threatened abortion. *Fertil Steril.* 2004;82(1):227–9.

9. Goswamy RK, Williams G, and Steptoe PC. Decreased uterine perfusion—A cause of infertility. *Hum Reprod.* 1988;3:955–9.

10. Steer CV, Tan SL, Dillon D, Mason BA, and Campbell S. Vaginal color Doppler assessment of uterine artery impedance correlates with immunohistochemical markers of endometrial receptivity required for the implantation of an embryo. *Fertil Steril.* 1995;63:101–8.

11. Dechaud H, Bessueille E, Bousquet PJ, Reyftmann L, Hamamah S, and Hedon B. Optimal timing of ultrasonographic and Doppler evaluation of uterine receptivity to implantation. *Reprod Biomed Online.* 2008;16:368–75.

12. Zaidi J, Campbell S, Pittrof R, and Tan SL. Endometrial thickness, morphology, vascular penetration and velocimetry in predicting implantation in an *in vitro* fertilization program. *Ultrasound Obstet Gynecol.* 1995;6(3):191–8.

13. Yang JH, Wu MY, Chen CD, Jiang MC, Ho HN, and Yang YS. Association of endometrial blood flow as determined by a modified colour Doppler technique with subsequent outcome of *in-vitro* fertilization. *Hum Reprod.* 1999;14(6):1606–10.

14. Raine-Fenning NJ, Campbell BK, Kendall NR, Clewes JS, and Johnson IR. Quantifying the changes in endometrial vascularity throughout the normal menstrual cycle with three-dimensional power Doppler angiography. *Hum Reprod.* 2004;19:330–8.

15. Raine-Fenning NJ, Campbell BK, Kendall NR, Clewes JS, and Johnson IR. Endometrial and subendometrial perfusion are impaired in women with unexplained subfertility. *Hum Reprod.* 2004;19(11):2605–14.

16. Ng EH, Chan CC, Tang OS, Yeung WS, and Ho PC. The role of endometrial and subendometrial blood flows measured by three-dimensional power Doppler ultrasound in the prediction of pregnancy during IVF treatment. *Hum Reprod.* 2006;21:164–70.

17. Naftalin J, and Jurkovic D. The endometrial–myometrial junction: A fresh look at a busy crossing. *Ultrasound Obstet Gynecol.* 2009;34:1–11.

18. Fanchin R, and Ayoubi JM. Uterine dynamics: Impact on the human reproduction process. *Reprod Biomed Online.* 2009;18:57–62.

19. Zhu L, Che HS, Xiao L, and Li YP. Uterine peristalsis before embryo transfer affects the chance of clinical pregnancy in fresh and frozen-thawed embryo transfer cycles. *Hum Reprod.* 2014; 29(6):1238–43.

20. Grimbizis GF, Camus M, Tarlatzis BC, Bontis JN, and Devroey P. Clinical implications of uterine malformations and hysteroscopic treatment results. *Hum Reprod Update.* 2001;7:161–74.

21. Saravelos SH, Cocksedge KA, and Li TC. Prevalence and diagnosis of congenital uterine anomalies in women with reproductive failure: A critical appraisal. *Hum Reprod Update.* 2008; 14:415–29.
22. Kupesic S, Kurjac A, Skenderovic S, and Bjelos D. Screening for uterine abnormalities by three-dimensional ultrasound improves perinatal outcomes. *J Perinat Med.* 2002;30:9–17.
23. Reichman DE, and Laufer MR. Congenital uterine anomalies affecting reproduction. *Best Pract Res Clin Obstet Gynaecol.* 2010;24:193–208.
24. Heinonen PK, Saarikoski S, and Pystynen P. Reproductive performance of women with uterine anomalies: An evaluation of 182 cases. *Acta Obstet Gynecol Scand.* 1982;61:157–62.
25. Olive DL, and Pritts EA. Fibroids and reproduction. *Semin Reprod Med.* 2010;28:218–27.
26. Oliveira FG, Abdelmassih VG, Diamond MP, Dozortsev D, Melo NR, and Abdelmassih R. Impact of subserosal and intramural uterine fibroids that do not distort the endometrial cavity on the outcome of *in vitro* fertilization-intracytoplasmic sperm injection. *Fertil Steril.* 2004;81:582–7.
27. Wallach EE, and Vlahos NF. Uterine myomas: An overview of development, clinical features, and management. *Obstet Gynecol.* 2004;104:393–406.
28. Vercellini P, Cortesi I, Giorgi O, De Merlo D, Carinelli SG, and Crosignani PG. Transvaginal ultrasonography versus uterine needle biopsy in the diagnosis of diffuse adenomyosis. *Hum Reprod Update.* 1998;13:2884–7.
29. Younes G, and Tulandi T. Effects of adenomyosis on *in vitro* fertilization treatment outcomes: A meta-analysis. *Fertil Steril.* 2017;108(3):483–90.e3.
30. Van Bogaert LJ. Clinicopathologic findings in endometrial polyps. *Obstet Gynecol.* 1988;71:771–3.
31. Perez-Medina T, Bajo-Arenas J, Salazar F et al. Endometrial polyps and their implication in the pregnancy rates of patients undergoing intrauterine insemination: A prospective, randomized study. *Hum Reprod.* 2005;20:1632–5.
32. Nathani F, and Clark TJ. Uterine polypectomy in the management of abnormal uterine bleeding: A systematic review. *J Minim Invasive Gynecol.* 2006;13:260.
33. Stamatellos I, Apostolides A, Stamatopoulos P, and Bontis J. Pregnancy rates after hysteroscopic polypectomy depending on the size or number of polyps. *Arch Gynecol Obstet.* 2008;277:395–9.
34. Berman JM. Intrauterine adhesions. *Semin Reprod Med.* 2008;26(4):349–55.
35. Salzani A, Yela DA, Gabiatti JR, Bedone AJ, and Monteiro IM. Prevalence of uterine synechia after abortion evacuation curettage. *Sao Paulo Med J.* 2007;125(5):261–4.
36. Practice Committee of the American Society for Reproductive Medicine. Current evaluation of amenorrhea. *Fertil Steril.* 2006;86:S148–55.
37. Adoni A, Palti Z, Milwidsky A, and Dolberg M. The incidence of intrauterine adhesions following spontaneous abortion. *Int J Fertil.* 1982;27:117–8.
38. Knopman J, and Copperman AB. Value of 3D ultrasound in the management of suspected Asherman's syndrome. *J Reprod Med-Chicago.* 2007;52(11):1016.
39. Zeyneloglu HB, Arici A, and Olive DL. Adverse effects of hydrosalpinx on pregnancy rates after *in vitro* fertilization embryo transfer. *Fertil Steril.* 1998;70:492–9.
40. Beyler SA, James KP, Fritz MA, and Meyer WR. Hydrosalpingeal fluid inhibits *in-vitro* embryonic development in a murine model. *Hum Reprod.* 1997;12(12):2724–8.
41. Meyer WR, Castelbaum AJ, Somkuti S et al. Hydrosalpinges adversely affect markers of endometrial receptivity. *Hum Reprod.* 1997;12(7):1393–8.
42. Patel MD. Likelihood ratio of sonographic findings in discriminating hydrosalpinx from other adnexal masses. *AJR Am J Roentgenol.* 2006;186:1033–8.
43. Barnhart KT, Sammel MD, Rinaudo PF, Zhou L, Hummel AC, and Guo W. Symptomatic patients with an early viable intrauterine pregnancy: HCG curves redefined. *Obstet Gynecol.* 2004;104(1):50–5.
44. Nyberg DA, Mack LA, Laing FC, and Patten RM. Distinguishing normal from abnormal gestational sac growth in early pregnancy. *J Ultrasound Med.* 1987;6(1):23–7.
45. Bromley B, Harlow BL, Laboda LA, and Benacerraf BR. Small sac size in the first trimester: A predictor of poor fetal outcome. *Radiology.* 1991;178(2):375–7.
46. Nyberg DA, Mack LA, Harvey D, and Wang K. Value of the yolk sac in evaluating early pregnancies. *J Ultrasound Med.* 1988;7(3):129–35.

47. Rowling SE, Langer JE, Coleman BG, Nisenbaum HL, Horii SC, and Arger PH. Sonography during early pregnancy: Dependence of threshold and discriminatory values on transvaginal transducer frequency. *Am J Roentgenol.* 1999;172(4):983–8.

48. Mara E, and Foster GS. Spontaneous regression of a yolk sac associated with embryonic death. *J Ultrasound Med.* 2000;19(9):655–6.

49. Brown DL, Emerson DS, Felker RE, Cartier MS, and Smith WC. Diagnosis of early embryonic demise by endovaginal sonography. *J Ultrasound Med.* 1990;9(11):631–6.

14

Sonoembryology

Veronika Frisova

Stages of Development of Human Embryo

The most widely used method for the classification of human embryos is the Carnegie staging system, which divides the embryonic period into 23 developmental stages, starting with fertilization at stage 1 and finishing with the onset of marrow formation in the humerus at stage 23 (approximately 56–57 postovulatory days, 10 gestational weeks, crown-rump length [CRL] 30 mm). From the end of stage 23 onward, the term *embryo* is replaced by term *fetus* [1–4]. The staging system has its origin in the work of Franklin P. Mall, who established the Carnegie Collection of human embryos and categorized 266 human embryos from 2 to 25 mm on the basis of photographs of their external form [5]. George L. Streeter provided the definitive classification of human embryos into stages, called "horizons," based on both the external and the internal morphological states (using the light microscope) of development. This classification was later modified by O'Rahilly and Müller and has now become accepted as the effective Carnegie staging system for human embryos [1].

Age and size of embryo alone have been demonstrated to be of limited value in the Carnegie staging system. The difficulties in assigning the size and age to an embryo after fixation derive from the possibility of embryonic growth retardation and also from the effects of postmortem changes as well as the materials used for the preservation of specimens [4]. A stage should therefore never be assigned merely on the basis of embryonic length and age. A 20 mm embryo, for example, could belong to any of three stages [2]. It is believed that the development of a discrete structure is a more reliable marker of the stage of embryonic development than the size or putative age [4].

Age of Human Embryo

The description of age in traditional embryology is different from that used in obstetrics [1,3,4]. Gestational (menstrual) age in obstetrics and fetal medicine represents embryonic age plus 14 days [1,3,4]. In this chapter, the term *menstrual (gestational) age* is used, because this is the parameter widely used in clinical medicine.

Estimation of gestational age was originally derived from the date of the last menstrual period (LMP) or from the date of conception in IVF pregnancies. However, in a high proportion of women, the date of LMP cannot be used for estimation of gestational age because of irregular menstrual cycles, uncertain LMP, or conception within 3 months of previous pregnancy, or stopping the contraceptive pills [3]. Therefore, the performance of several ultrasound parameters (size and volume of gestational, amniotic and yolk sac, CRL, biparietal diameter [BPD], and head circumference [HC]) was tested in the dating of pregnancy [3,6,7]. Many parameters are related closely to gestational age, but CRL was found to be the most precise [3,7]. It is known that in about 15% of women with a certain date of LMP and regular 28-days cycle, considerable variations in the day of ovulation occur causing wrong dating of pregnancy; hence, measurement of CRL in the first trimester was decided to be the best tool for pregnancy dating [3,7,8] in both singleton and multiple pregnancies [3,9].

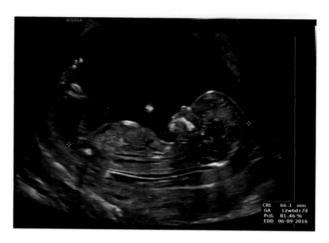

FIGURE 14.1   Correct measurement of crown-rump length at 12 weeks. The image is magnified, with fetus oriented horizontally on the screen in neutral position. Calipers mark the correct measurement.

Ultrasound CRL measurements can be carried out transabdominally or transvaginally. A midline sagittal section of the whole embryo should be obtained, ideally with the embryo or fetus oriented horizontally on the ultrasound screen. An image should be magnified sufficiently to fill most of the width of the screen, so that the measurement line between crown and rump is at about 90° to the ultrasound beam. The embryo should be measured in a neutral position (i.e., neither flexed nor hyperextended) (Figure 14.1). The neutral position may be difficult to achieve at earlier gestations (around 6–9 weeks) when the embryo is typically hyperflexed. In this situation, the actual measurement represents the neck-rump length, but it is still referred to as the CRL [3].

Several charts and normograms for dating of the pregnancy by CRL were produced; the most commonly recommended formula is that of Robinson and Fleming [2,7,10]. Although the original formula was derived in 1975 from a study of 334 singleton pregnancies in women with regular menstrual cycles and certain LMP, several subsequent studies have confirmed the accuracy of its prediction [2,7,11–14].

An exception represents very early pregnancies, in which the formula of Robinson and Fleming underestimates the gestation by 1 day for CRL 7–10 mm, exponentially increasing to an underestimation of 9 days for a CRL of 1 mm [7].

Modern Imaging Technologies

A major limitation to define human embryonic anatomy noninvasively has been the resolution of available tools. The development of experimental magnetic resonance (MR) microscopy and its application to the studies of embryos [15] coupled with the application of computer graphics [16] have allowed acquisition of microscopic three-dimensional (3D) images, thus offering another new insight into early human development. Still, due to the long acquisition time of MR, this technology has not allowed the acquisition of data from living human embryos [17].

In 1990, the term *sonoembryology* was coined, following the introduction of high-frequency transvaginal transducers, which resulted in remarkable progress in ultrasound visualization of living human embryos and fetuses and ultimately the development of this field [18]. Moreover, in 2003, transvaginal 3D sonography expanded the depth of inquiry and allowed development of 3D sonoembryology [19]. Three-dimensional sonoembryology improved visualization of embryonic and fetal body and face appearance by using 3D rendered images in surface mode and assessing the embryonic and fetal brain simultaneously in all three orthogonal planes by multiplanar mode [19–23]. Inversion rendering switches anechoic into echo-filled spaces and therefore is particularly useful in displaying developing embryonic and fetal brain [20,21]. Tomographic ultrasound imaging (TUI) (GE Healthcare) or multislice mode (SAMSUNG; Korea) (see further Figures 14.13 and 14.19). allow demonstration of embryonic and fetal brain structures in several parallel sections through a selected cardinal plane [20,21]. Maximum intensity mode (x-ray mode) eliminates weaker echoes originating from the soft tissues of the fetus, thus allowing emphasis of fetal bony structures. It is particularly helpful for the assessment of the sutures and fontanels on the skull and of the spine [19,20,22,24]. During the embryonic period, the VOCAL software (Virtual Organ Computer-Aided Analysis; GE Healthcare and SAMSUNG) enables the operator to trace the periphery of a region of interest on-screen, and by repeating the process through a stepwise rotation of the organ, to recognize its actual shape, and subsequently, to "cut-out" and display the organ. After this, the volume of the "cut-out" organ like gestational, amniotic, and yolk sac, can be measured [20]. Newer 3D technologies like 3D HDlive silhouette (GE Healthcare) or HDVI (High-Definition-Volume-Imaging) with Crystal and Realistic View (SAMSUNG) improve the 3D image quality to even more realistic views of embryonic and fetal body and organ appearance [25] (see further Figures 14.3, 14.5, 14.10, 14.12, 14.15, and 14.18). Fetal movements can be observed by four-dimensional (4D) ultrasonography [19,22].

Ultrasound Assessment of Normal Embryonic Development

Four Gestational Weeks

Two-Dimensional Sonoembryology

At 4 weeks and 1 day, an intrauterine gestational sac can be visualized by a transvaginal transducer as a small spherical anechoic structure that is placed between endometrial leafs. Its diameter is very small, only about 2 mm [18] (Figure 14.2).

Three-Dimensional Sonoembryology

The presence of a gestational sac between the endometrial leafs can be demonstrated in planar mode with 3D rendering [24].

Five Gestational Weeks

Two-Dimensional Sonoembryology

At 5 weeks and 0 days, the gestational sac measures 5 or 6 mm in diameter [18]. At the beginning of the fifth week, a small secondary yolk sac is visible as the earliest sign of the developing embryo [19,22]. At the end of the fifth week, an embryo measuring 2–3 mm in length can be seen as a small straight line

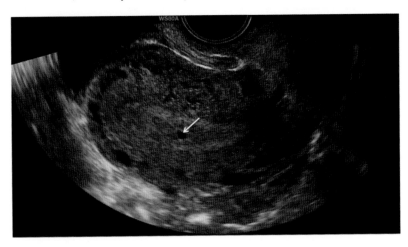

FIGURE 14.2   An arrow points to a small anechogenic gestational sac (diameter of only 3 mm) placed eccentric within the uterine cavity. This sac can be displayed as the first sign of intrauterine pregnancy at 4 gestational weeks.

adjacent to the yolk sac [18,19,22]. As the connecting stalk is short, the embryonic pole is found near the wall of the gestational sac. Even though the embryo is so small, heartbeats at a rate of about 100 bpm can frequently be detected within the embryonic pole [18,26] (Video 14.1).

VIDEO 14.1

A 3 mm long embryo with heartbeats at 5 gestational weeks; the embryo has a shape of tiny lines and is adjacent to the ovoid yolk sac. (https://youtu.be/_3TcHqL3MD0)

Three-Dimensional Sonoembryology

Planar mode can help in distinguishing an early intraendometrial gestational sac from a collection of free fluid between the endometrial leafs (pseudogestational sac) [19] (Figure 14.3). Moreover, VOCAL and other 3D ultrasound techniques enable precise measurement of the exponentially expanding gestational sac and yolk sac volume [6,27–29].

Six Gestational Weeks

Two-Dimensional Sonoembryology

At the sixth week, the CRL is about 4–8 mm, and the developing embryonic plate (the trilaminar embryo) is adjacent and tangential to the yolk sac [10,18,21,26] (Figure 14.4). The heartbeat should always be detectable, with heart rate increasing to 130 bpm [18,26]. At the end of the sixth week, the first sign of the rhombencephalic central nervous system (CNS) cavity can be seen as a tiny hypoechogenic area in the cranial pole of the embryo [21,26].

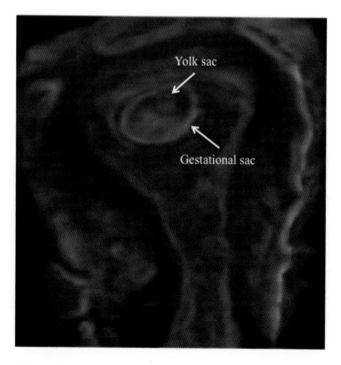

FIGURE 14.3 This three-dimensional rendered image shows early (5 weeks) pregnancy. Ovoid structures—gestational sac containing smaller yolk sac—are displayed within the uterine cavity.

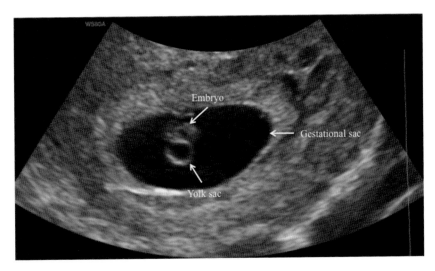

FIGURE 14.4 An arrow points to a 6-week embryo (crown-rump length 5 mm) still adjacent to the ovoid yolk sac.

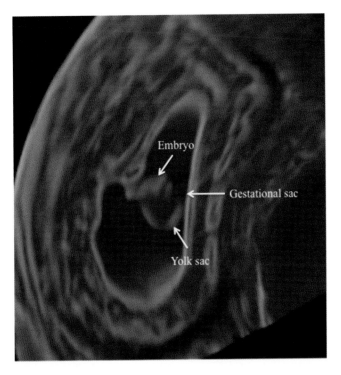

FIGURE 14.5 Rendered three-dimensional image of 6-week embryo with yolk sac placed within the gestational sac. The embryo typically has a rounded bulky head and a thinner body at this time.

Three-Dimensional Sonoembryology

Typical characteristics of the surface-rendered 3D image of the embryo at the sixth gestational week include a rounded bulky head and a thinner body (Figure 14.5). The head is prominent due to the developing forebrain. Limb buds are already present [18]; however, they are rarely visible by ultrasound at this stage of pregnancy. The umbilical cord and vitelline duct are always clearly visible.

Seven Gestational Weeks

Two-Dimensional Sonoembryology

At the seventh week, the CRL is about 9 to 14 mm [10,14], and for the first time, it is possible to distinguish the amnion separately from the embryo [21]. The mean diameter of the amniotic cavity is nearly the same as the corresponding CRL [26]. The yolk sac, which is situated in the extra-embryonic coelom, can be seen outside the amnion, between the amnion and the chorion. The chorion is the most peripheral structure lining the uterine cavity [18].

The embryonic body is slender in the coronal plane and has a triangular shape in sagittal section. The sides consist of the back, the roof of the rhombencephalon, the frontal part of the head, the base of the umbilical cord, and the embryonic tail [18,26] (Figure 14.6). The head is acutely flexed anteriorly, being in contact with the chest [19,22]. The short umbilical cord shows a large coelomic cavity at its insertion, where the primary intestinal loop can be identified. The first sign of herniation of the gut occurs during week 7 as a thickening of the cord, showing a slight echogenic area at the abdominal insertion. Within a few days, this echogenic structure becomes more distinct [26]. Although the limbs start to develop in the craniocaudal direction already at the second half of the sixth gestational week [18], the limb buds can be seen from the seventh week onward like short, paddle-shaped outgrowths [26]. The tail section usually protrudes caudally and exceeds the lower limbs in length at this time [18] (Figure 14.7).

The heart can be recognized as a beating, large, and bright structure below the embryonic head. The heart rate increases from 130 to 160 bpm [7,26]. Details of the heart anatomy are not visible; however, the movements of the cardiac walls can already be observed in M-mode [18,26].

During the seventh week of pregnancy, rapid development of the embryonic brain takes place. In the midsagittal section of the fetal head, the developing vesicles of the brain can be depicted as anechoic structures. The biggest—and in the beginning usually the only one visible—is the rhombencephalon placed on the top of the head (vertex). The diencephalon cavity (future third ventricle with surrounding structures) becomes visible a few days later [19,22]. It is situated anteriorly in the flexed embryonic head and continues posteriorly into the mesencephalon (future Sylvian aqueduct) and rhombencephalon. The curved tube-like mesencephalic cavity is located at the most anterior part of the embryo, its height being slightly smaller than the height of the cavity of the diencephalon. Thus, the wide border between the

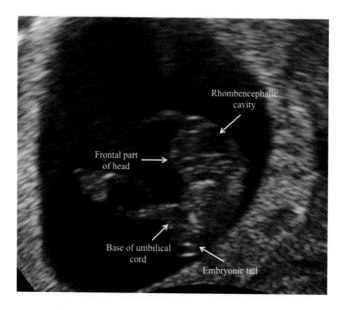

FIGURE 14.6 Sagittal section of an embryo at 7 gestational weeks (crown-rump length 14 mm). At this stage, the embryo has a triangular shape, which consists of the back, the roof of the rhombencephalon (on the top of the head), the frontal part of the head, the base of the umbilical cord, and the embryonic tail. The head is strongly flexed anteriorly in contact with the chest.

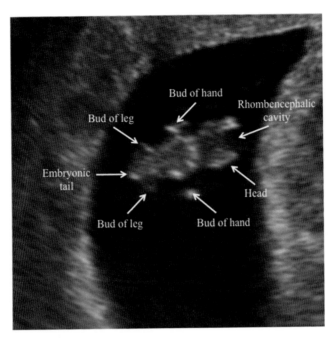

FIGURE 14.7   Coronal image of an embryo at 7 gestational weeks (crown-rump length 14 mm). Head, body, limb buds, and tail protruding caudally can clearly be distinguished.

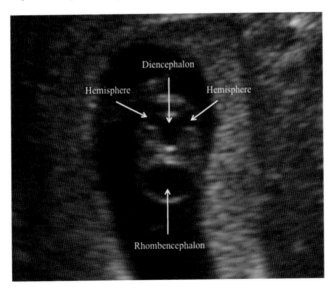

FIGURE 14.8   Axial/oblique section through fetal head in the embryo of 14 mm, in which it is possible to distinguish cerebral hemispheres (telencephalic vesicles), diencephalon, and rhombencephalon. The future foramina of Monro are wide during the seventh week.

cavities of the diencephalon and the mesencephalon is clearly indicated [26]. In the axial/oblique section through the fetal head, it is possible from a CRL of 12 mm onward to visualize cerebral hemispheres (telencephalic vesicles), diencephalon, and rhombencephalon [21]. The future foramina of Monro are wide during the seventh week [26] (Figure 14.8). Figure 14.9 illustrates normal embryological development of the brain from 25 to 100 days (6–17 postmenstrual weeks) and the ensuing structural changes to the forebrain, midbrain, and hindbrain.

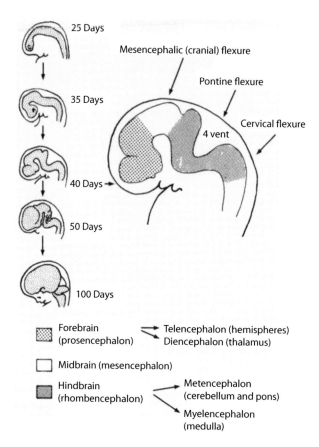

FIGURE 14.9   Normal embryological development of the brain from 25 to 100 days (6–17 postmenstrual weeks) and the ensuing structural changes to the forebrain, midbrain, and hindbrain. (From Nyberg DA et al., *Diagnostic Imaging of Fetal Anomalies*, Philadelphia, PA: Lippincott Williams & Wilkins; 2002, with permission.)

Three-Dimensional Sonoembryology

Surface-rendered 3D images of the embryo at the seventh gestational week show a prominent head that is acutely flexed anteriorly, in contact with the chest. Limb buds are often visible on either side of the body (Figure 14.10). With the use of multiplanar mode, developing vesicles of the brain can be depicted as anechoic structures inside the head. The biggest—and usually the only visible—one is the rhombencephalon placed on the top of the head (vertex). The diencephalon and its cavity continuing into mesencephalon become visible a few days later [19,22,26].

Eight Gestational Weeks

Two-Dimensional Sonoembryology

At 8 gestational weeks, the CRL is about 15 to 22 mm [10,14]. The amnion and yolk sac are yet to be clearly visible. The extra-embryonic coelom is still larger in volume and more echogenic than the amniotic sac [22]. The embryonic body gradually grows thicker and becomes cuboidal [26]. Both upper and lower extremities can be seen in the whole length [18,19,26]. The arms are no longer parallel with the body and are seen at an angle, and the fingers can be distinguished [18,26].

Structures of the viscerocranium (facial skeleton) and brain structures are not visible due to their small size. The insertion of the umbilical cord can be clearly recognized on the anterior abdominal wall, with developing intestine being physiologically herniated into the proximal umbilical cord [18,19,22,26].

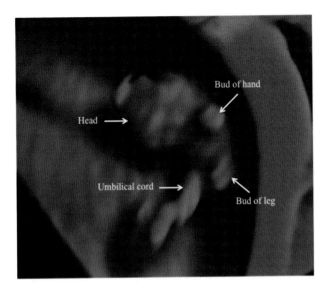

FIGURE 14.10 Surface-rendered three-dimensional image of a 7-week embryo (crown-rump length 14 mm). At this stage, the embryo has a prominent head that is strongly flexed anteriorly in contact with the chest. Limb buds are visible on either side of the body.

The heart rate has increased to 160 bpm [7,26]. At the end of the eighth week, it is occasionally possible to identify the atrial and ventricular walls [26].

The embryonic brain continues to develop. The increased growth of the rostral brain structures and the deepening of the pontine flexure lead to the deflection of the brain, thus moving the mesencephalon to the top of the head. Structures of embryonic brain become clearer and two main flexures of the brain can be located—the mesencephalic flexure between diencephalon and mesencephalon, and the pontine flexure between metencephalon and myelencephalon. The mesencephalic flexure is nearly in line with the longitudinal body axis [21]. At 8 weeks and 5 days (CRL 20 mm), it is possible to observe in the midsagittal plane in the anteroposterior direction the diencephalon (future third ventricle), mesencephalon (future aqueduct), metencephalon (future cerebellum and pons), and myelencephalon (future medulla oblongata) (Figure 14.11). In the axial/oblique section through the fetal head, cerebral hemispheres (telencephalic vesicles), rhombencephalon, and diencephalon are much better defined than at the seventh week, with ventricular foramina (Monro) getting smaller and thus more easily defined than a week earlier [21]. In the coronal section leading through the posterior part of the fetal head, three cavities, namely, mesencephalon, metencephalon, and myelencephalon can be clearly identified at the end of the eighth week [21]. In addition to these structures, the choroids fold, and slightly later, at 8 weeks and 5 days, the first sighting of choroid plexus was reported [21]. As for the spine, it is possible to detect the parallel echogenic lines marking the neural tube. However, due to the curled position of the embryo at this age, it is possible to see only parts of the neural tube in single coronal sections [18].

Three-Dimensional Sonoembryology

Surface-rendered 3D images of the embryo at the eighth gestational week allow for the first time visualization of the upper and lower extremities throughout its whole length. Abdominal insertion of the umbilical cord remains wide due to the herniation of the developing bowel [19,22] (Figure 14.12). With the multiplanar mode, it is possible to observe the development of fetal brain anatomy simultaneously in all three orthogonal planes. Moreover, several consecutive parallel sections through the sagittal or other plane of brain can be displayed by the use of TUI (GE Healthcare ultrasound systems, Austria) or multislice (SAMSUNG ultrasound systems, Korea) [21,30] (Figure 14.13). The spinal cord can be seen on the back of the embryo and has the appearance of two lines running parallel to each other [4,24].

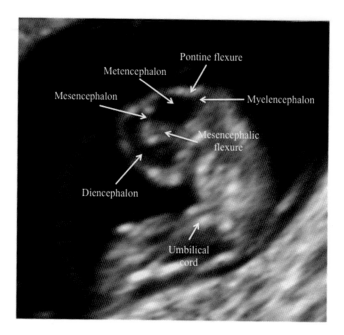

FIGURE 14.11 Midsagittal section of embryonic brain at 8 weeks (crown-rump length 17 mm). In the anteroposterior direction of the embryo, it is possible to observe the diencephalon (future third ventricle), mesencephalon (future aqueduct), metencephalon (future cerebellum and pons), and myelencephalon (future medulla oblongata).

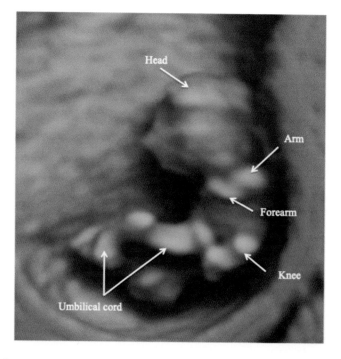

FIGURE 14.12 Surface-rendered three-dimensional image of an embryo at 8 gestational weeks (crown-rump length 19 mm). Note the earliest appearance of the upper and lower extremities along the whole length. Abdominal insertion of the umbilical cord remains wide due to persistent bowel herniation.

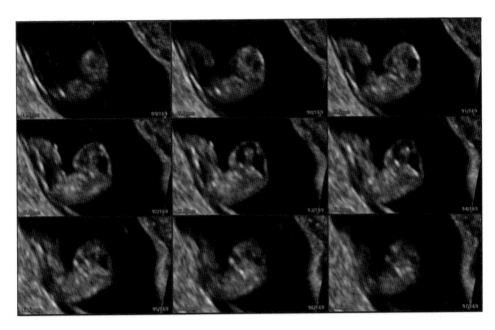

FIGURE 14.13 Three-dimensional image volume postprocessed in multislice view (SAMSUNG ultrasound systems, Korea) displays shows several consecutive parallel sections through the sagittal plane of embryonic brain at 8 gestational weeks (crown-rump length 17 mm).

Nine Gestational Weeks

Two-Dimensional Sonoembryology

At the ninth gestational week, the CRL is about 22 to 29 mm [10], and the body of the embryo develops into an ellipsoid shape with a large head [26]. This gestational age marks the end of the embryonic stage (Carnegie stage 23) and the beginning of the fetal stage. The fetus assumes a more natural state compared to the extreme flexion of earlier gestation; hence, the crown becomes the endpoint of the fetal head, and the true CRL can be measured reliably [21]. The head starts to be clearly divided from the body by the neck [19,22]; thus, it becomes possible to obtain acceptable images of the embryonic profile (Figure 14.14).

Whole extremities with fingers on hands can be seen [18]. The arm bends at the elbow and rotates 90° laterally [18]. The soles of the feet touch in the midline at the end of this week [26] (Video 14.2).

The ventral body wall is well defined, with developing intestine still physiologically herniated into the umbilical cord. The stomach can be detected in 75% of the embryos before 10 weeks [26].

Heartbeats are clearly visible, and the heart rate reaches around 175 bpm at this stage [7,26].

From the ninth week, there is significant change in the image of embryonic brain. Because of the gradual development and increase in size, more structures can be seen. The development of the tortuous, fluid-filled ventricular system is clearly visible in midsagittal plane. More consecutive sections of brain can now be generated in almost all three orthogonal planes [21]. The different parts of the ventricular system are visible. In the midsagittal plane, the anechoic chain of the ventricular system winds itself around the two most prominent solid structures—the echogenic pontine and mesencephalic flexures. The first rostral (anterior) anechoic structure in the brain is the diencephalon, followed by mesencephalon, metencephalon, myelencephalon, and the part of the medulla that contains the central canal. In the parasagittal section, the relatively large choroid plexus nearly fills the whole lateral (telencephalic) ventricle. On coronal and axial sections, the falx is seen as an echogenic structure. It is in the ninth week when falx together with choroid plexuses can be visualized for the first time [21] (see Video 14.2). As for the spine, it is possible to obtain images of spinal structures in dorsal coronal sections in all fetuses at the ninth week [18].

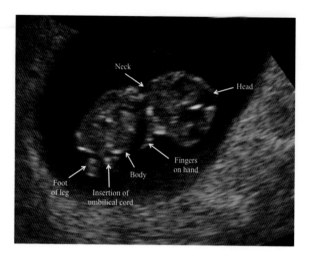

FIGURE 14.14   Midsagittal section of embryo at 9 gestational weeks (crown-rump length 24 mm). At this stage, the head starts to be clearly divided from the body by the neck; thus, it becomes possible to obtain acceptable profile images.

VIDEO 14.2
Axial section of an embryo at 9 gestational weeks (crown-rump length 24 mm). In the axial section of embryonic brain, the division by falx cerebri into two halves is visible. Choroid plexuses fill the whole lateral ventricles. In axial sections through the embryonic body, it is possible to observe the beating heart, wide insertion of umbilical cord containing herniated bowel, and both hands and legs in the full length. It is possible to count fingers on hands and see soles of the feet touching in the midline. (https://youtu.be/11_qcEoBouI)

Three-Dimensional Sonoembryology

Surface-rendered three-dimensional image of an embryo in the ninth gestational week shows the head to be clearly divided from the body by the neck. External ears can sometimes be depicted [19,22]. The umbilical cord remains thicker in the part close to the abdominal wall due to persistent herniation of the midgut [19,22,26]. The dorsal column—the early spine—can be examined in its whole length [4,19,22]. The arms with elbows and legs with knees are clearly visible (Figure 14.15). Feet can be seen approaching the midline [19,22].

As for imaging the embryonic brain, the multiplanar mode enables the depiction of all three orthogonal planes (Figure 14.16), TUI or multislice and rendered 3D imaging of cerebral cavities in inversion mode makes examination of the brain easier and more understandable than conventional 2D images [4,19,21,22,31].

The spinal cord appearance changes to a thin line, compared with two lines at 8 weeks of gestation [4,24].

Ultrasound Assessment of Normal Fetal Development

Ten Gestational Weeks

Two-Dimensional Sonoembryology

With CRL of 30 mm and gestational age of 10 weeks and 0 days, the embryonic period finishes, and the term *embryo* is replaced by the term *fetus*. At 10 weeks, CRL is between 30 and 41 mm [10,14]. The human features of the fetus become clearer. The fetal body elongates, the arms develop into upper and

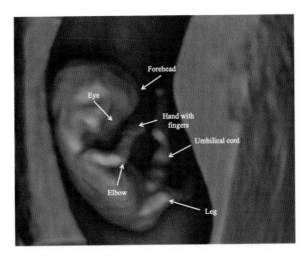

FIGURE 14.15   Surface-rendered three-dimensional image of the embryo at 9 gestational weeks (crown-rump length 29 mm). The head is clearly divided from the body by the neck, and the arms with elbows, and legs with knees are clearly visible.

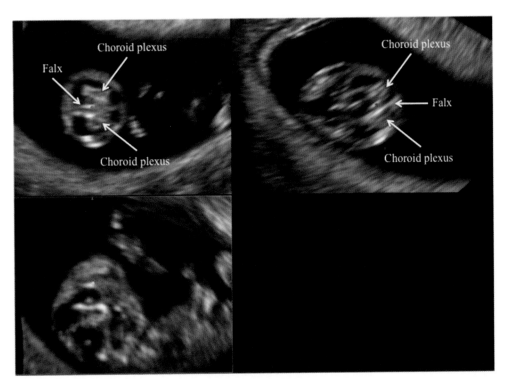

FIGURE 14.16   Three-dimensional image of all three cardinal orthogonal planes of embryonic brain (crown-rump length 29 mm) displayed in multiplanar mode. A-plane (upper left image) shows the axial plane with falx in the middle and choroid plexuses filling lateral ventricles. Falx with choroid plexus can be observed also in the coronal section of brain in B-plane (upper right image). C-plane (lower left image) represents the midsagittal section of the embryonic brain.

lower arms, hands, and fingers, and the legs develop into upper and lower legs, feet, and toes [26]. Fetal knees rotate ventrally [18], and feet are approaching the midline [19,22] (Video 14.3). The head is still relatively large with a prominent forehead and a flat occiput [26]. Moreover, the orbital area, maxilla, and mandible can be distinguished in midsagittal plane images [18] (Figure 14.17).

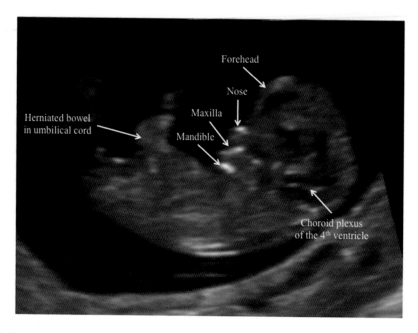

FIGURE 14.17   Sagittal section of the head and body of the fetus at 10 weeks, 5 days (crown-rump length 35 mm). The fetal head profile, neck, and abdominal wall with herniated bowel in the cord insertion are clearly demonstrated. In the brain, choroid plexus of the fourth ventricle is clearly apparent.

Midgut herniation has its maximal extension at the beginning of the tenth week and returns into the abdominal cavity between 10 weeks, 4 days and 11 weeks, 5 days. A filled stomach can be seen in the majority of fetuses [26] (see Video 14.3).

VIDEO 14.3

Axial section of an embryo at 10 gestational weeks (crown-rump length 33 mm). In axial section of fetal brain, it is possible to see falx cerebri dividing the brain into two halves and choroid plexuses filling lateral ventricles. Moving down, it is possible to see both arms with elbows, hands, and fingers. In the axial sections through fetal thorax, the four-chamber view of the fetal heart can be observed. Moving more down to abdomen, it is possible to see the stomach (black bubble), which is placed below the heart, the wide insertion of umbilical cord containing herniated bowel, and legs in the full length approaching the midline. (https://youtu.be/Ej2SP8PIg1s)

The heart rate starts to decrease at this time from around 175 bpm at the beginning to around 170 at the end of the tenth week [32]. The atria and ventricles can already be identified (see Video 14.3).

From the tenth gestational week onward, it is possible to obtain up to four parallel images or sections of all three orthogonal cardinal planes of the brain (sagittal, coronal, and axial) [21]. The thick crescent-shaped lateral ventricles fill the anterior part of the head and conceal the diencephalic cavity. The diencephalon lies between the hemispheres, and the mesencephalon gradually moves toward the center of the head [26]. Lateral ventricles are fully filled with choroid plexuses, and the falx is clearly visible [21]. After 10 weeks, 3 days, the choroid plexuses of the fourth ventricle can always be visualized [26]. As for the spine, small vertebral components of the spine can be distinguished in the dorsocranial section of the fetal body [18].

Three-Dimensional Sonoembryology

On the surface-rendered image of the fetus at 10 weeks, you can clearly distinguish the head, neck, and body. External ears are visible on either side of the fetal head. The arms with elbows and legs with knees

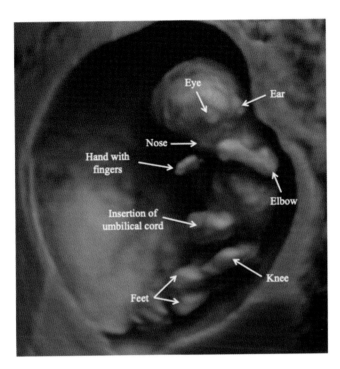

FIGURE 14.18 Surface-rendered three-dimensional image of the fetus at 10 gestational weeks (crown-rump length 33 mm). The fetal face demonstrates human features. It is possible to distinguish fetal nose and eyes and—on either side of the head—the external ears. Both arms and legs with elbows and knees are visible; hands and fingers are also identified. The abdominal insertion of the fetal cord is still wide due to the herniated bowel.

are now visible. Feet can be seen approaching the midline. The dorsal column, the early spine, can be examined in its whole length. Herniation of the midgut is still present [19,22] (Figure 14.18) (Video 14.4).

All structures of the fetal brain are more apparent with 3D imaging. Multiplanar mode is used to demonstrate simultaneously on the screen all three cardinal orthogonal planes together, while TUI (GE Healthcare) or multislice (SAMSUNG) displays several consecutive parallel sections through the sagittal, coronal, or axial plane of the brain (Figure 14.19). Rendered 3D images of the cerebral cavities in inversion mode enable easier study of the brain as they are easier to understand than conventional 2D images [4,19,21,22,31].

VIDEO 14.4
Four-dimensional ultrasound with surface rendering of fetal face and body at 10 gestational weeks (crown-rump length 33 mm). It is possible to distinguish the human features on the face (eyes, nose, and mouth), head (ear), and body (legs and arms with knees and elbows) of the fetus. Fetal movements can be followed. The whole umbilical cord with its tiny placental and thick abdominal insertion (due to bowel herniation) is also visible. (https://youtu.be/ig0OgXEPAvw)

Eleven to Twelve Gestational Weeks

Two-Dimensional Sonoembryology

From the 11th to 12th weeks, the CRL is between 42 and 66 mm [10,14]. Human features of the developing fetus are clearly visible [26]. Development of the head and neck continues. The nose and lips achieve their final stage of development already at 11 weeks. From the 11th week onward, it is possible to analyze in the coronal section the symmetry of the face, which consists of two orbits—the maxilla and the mandible.

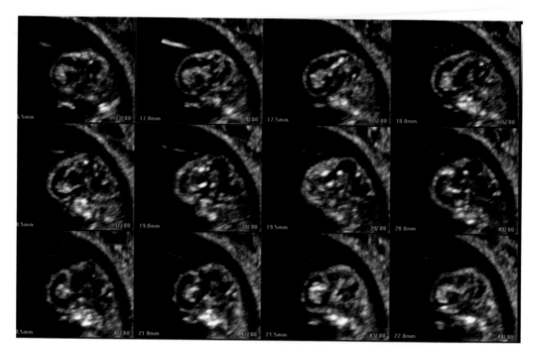

FIGURE 14.19   Three-dimensional image postprocessed in multislice (SAMSUNG ultrasound systems, Korea) displaying several consecutive parallel sections through the sagittal plane of fetal brain at 10 gestational weeks (crown-rump length 33 mm). The exact midline section of fetal brain with several parasagittal sections (lateral ventricles filled with choroid plexuses) can be studied.

The maxilla initially grows faster than the mandible, but by 12 weeks, the mandible reaches the size of the maxilla. The palate forms over a long period of time, from the seventh to the twelfth week, when fusion finally occurs [18]. By 12 weeks, a complete study of the palate, the lips, and the nasal bones can be consistently performed [18,34,35].

Abdominal insertion of the umbilical cord becomes thin as the herniated midgut returns into the abdominal cavity. The stomach and urinary bladder are filled with fluid and are thus clearly visible. Even fetal kidneys can often be identified using a transvaginal transducer. Arms and legs continue developing [3,19,22]. From the beginning of the 11th week, it is possible to image the entire length of the arms and legs, as well as hands and feet [18,34,35]. Long bones can be visualized as hyperechogenic elongated structures inside upper and lower extremities. Fingers and toes are visible [3,19,22].

The fetal cardiac ventricles, atria, septa, valves, veins, and outflow tracts become identifiable [26,35,36]. The heart rate slows to 165 bpm at the end of the 11th week.

The fetal brain in axial and coronal section is clearly divided by falx cerebri into two halves. Lateral ventricles are fully filled by the choroid plexuses, and the diencephalon lies between the hemispheres followed by mesencephalon located in the center of the head. The third ventricle starts narrowing; cerebellar hemispheres seem to meet in the midline. The choroid plexus of the fourth ventricle can always be visualized [26]. In midsagittal plane, it is possible to observe in an anteroposterior direction (together with craniocaudal direction) the diencephalon, midbrain, brainstem, and medulla oblongata. Behind the brainstem, the fourth ventricle can easily be identified, with its choroid plexus creating its posterior border, followed by the cavity of the future cerebellomedullaris [37,38] (Figure 14.20).

At 11–13 weeks (CRL 45–84 mm), it is the best time to screen for fetal aneuploidies [39]. First-trimester combined screening based on maternal age, fetal age, heart rate, and nuchal translucency (NT), and maternal serum markers (free β-hCG and PAPP-A) represent the gold standard of screening for chromosomal abnormalities in most countries. Several studies have demonstrated that for a 5% false-positive rate, the first-trimester combined test identifies about 90% of fetuses with Down syndrome

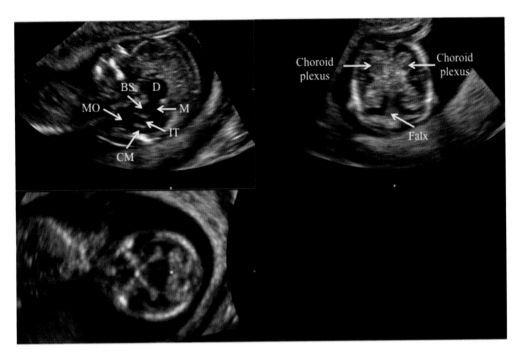

FIGURE 14.20 Three-dimensional image of all three cardinal orthogonal planes of embryonic brain (crown-rump length 63 mm) displayed in multiplanar mode. A-plane (upper left image) displays an exact midsagittal section of fetal brain, showing midline central nervous system structures, respectively, diencephalon (D), midbrain (M), brainstem (BS), and medulla oblongata (MO). The fourth ventricle normally presents as an intracranial translucency (IT) behind the brainstem, between it and cisterna magna (CM). Absence of intracranial translucency represents an important marker of neural tube defects. In the B-plane (upper right image), falx can clearly be distinguished with choroid plexuses filling lateral ventricles.

[33,39–41]. The most important part of first-trimester screening represents ultrasound measurement of fetal NT, which should be performed by an appropriately trained and certified sonographer according to national or international guidelines (https://fetalmedicine.org) [3] (Figure 14.21). Nuchal translucency normally increases with gestation (CRL); however, NT measurement above the 95th percentile can be found in 75%–80% of fetuses with trisomy 21 and other major aneuploidies and only in 5% of chromosomally normal fetuses [33]. Not only is NT measurement useful for detection of aneuploidy, a thickened NT also raises suspicion of a wide range of fetal structural defects (in particular cardiac) and genetic syndromes and generally increases the risk of fetal morbidity and mortality [39,42,43]. Screening for Down syndrome can be further improved by the addition of other markers, including assessment of fetal nasal bone, blood flow through the tricuspid valve in the heart, and in fetal ductus venosus [3,33,39,41]. Absence of the nasal bone, reversed a-wave with increased pulsatility index (PI) in the ductus venosus, and tricuspid regurgitation are observed in only 1%–3% of euploid fetuses but in more than half of fetuses with Down syndrome [33]. The addition of these markers to the routine combined test increases the detection rate for Down syndrome to 98% at the fixed false-positive rate of 5% [33,40]. In screening for other major aneuploidies—trisomy 18 and 13—assessment for the presence of typical associated structural defects (omphalocele, megacystis, and holoprosencephaly) should be included. The combined test including assessment of these typical structural defects allows for the detection of more than 90% of fetuses with trisomy 18, 13, Turner syndrome, and triploidy, and about 50% of fetuses with other chromosomal abnormalities [33,44].

In the last decade, first-trimester screening has evolved from a simple measurement of fetal NT into a complex first-trimester risk assessment that focuses not only on chromosomal abnormalities but also on numerous pregnancy-related complications, such as major structural defects, preeclampsia, and fetal growth restriction [43]. Success of the assessment of fetal anatomy, in particular of the heart, increases with advanced gestation. From a CRL of about 55 mm, all organs apart from the heart can be visualized

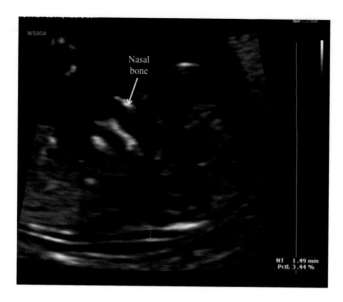

FIGURE 14.21   Nuchal translucency (NT) measurement according to FMF (Fetal Medicine Foundation) protocol. Calipers mark NT. Moreover, a second first-trimester marker of Down syndrome, respectively, nasal bone, can be assessed (present nasal bone) (fetus with crown-rump length of 58 mm).

at a diagnostic quality in more than 90% of pregnancies [35]. Half of all structural malformations can already be diagnosed at 11- to 13-week gestation [43,45,46]. In expert hands, even 90% of major cardiac defects can be detected from 12 weeks onward [36,47].

Three-Dimensional Sonoembryology

Human features of the developing fetus are clearly visible [26]. Striking changes in the development of the head and neck continue. Details of the face such as the nose, orbits, maxilla, and mandible are visible. Herniated midgut returns into the abdominal cavity. Planar mode enables a detailed analysis of the embryonic body with visualization of the stomach and urinary bladder. Kidneys are also often visible. Arms and legs continue with development and can be seen in the whole length. Fingers and toes are visible. The fetus at this stage is moving most of the time (Video 14.5). Detailed 3D analysis of the fetal spine, chest, and limbs is obtainable by using the transparent x-ray–like rendering mode [18,19,22].

VIDEO 14.5
Four-dimensional ultrasound with surface rendering of fetal face and body at 11 weeks and 6 days of gestation (crown-rump length 52 mm); it is possible to distinguish human features of the fetus and observe its prominent movements. (https://youtu.be/YNEH5Heoj3I)

Conclusion

During the first 12 weeks of gestation, rapid development of the human embryo occurs in the first 10 weeks and the fetus in the following weeks. The major development happens during the embryonic period, as after 9 gestational weeks, only fetal face and brain development continues. The other organs only continue to grow, and some of them become functional. Table 14.1 summarizes the gestational age (in postmenstrual weeks) at which embryonic structures are consistently visible using transvaginal sonography. With continuous technical developments and improvement of ultrasound image quality obtained by high-frequency transvaginal and transabdominal transducers, it is possible

TABLE 14.1

Summary of Embryonic Structures and Gestational Age in Postmenstrual Weeks at Which They Become Consistently Visible Using Transvaginal Sonography

Embryonic Structure	Postmenstrual Week										
	4	5	6	7	8	9	10	11	12	13	14
Gestational sac	x	x	x	x	x	x	x	x	x	x	x
Yolk sac	—	x	x	x	x	x	x	x	x	x	x
Fetal heart rate	—	—	x	x	x	x	x	x	x	x	x
Neural tube	—	—	—	x	x	x	x	x	x	x	x
Fetal head	—	—	—	x	x	x	x	x	x	x	x
Single lateral ventricle	—	—	—	x	x	x	—	—	—	—	—
Midgut herniation	—	—	—	—	x	x	x	x	—	—	—
Falx cerebri	—	—	—	—	—	x	x	x	x	x	x
Choroid plexus	—	—	—	—	—	x	x	x	x	x	x
Thalamus	—	—	—	—	—	x	x	x	x	x	x
Anterior and posterior contour	—	—	—	—	—	x	x	x	x	x	x
Humerus and femur	—	—	—	—	—	x	x	x	x	x	x
Finger	—	—	—	—	—	x	x	x	x	x	x
Tibia and radius	—	—	—	—	—	—	x	x	x	x	x
Toes	—	—	—	—	—	—	—	x	x	x	x
Cerebellum	—	—	—	—	—	—	—	x	x	x	x
Face	—	—	—	—	—	—	—	x	x	x	x
Lens	—	—	—	—	—	—	—	—	x	x	x
Palate	—	—	—	—	—	—	—	x	x	x	x
Heart, four chambers	—	—	—	—	—	—	—	x	x	x	x
Stomach	—	—	—	—	—	—	—	—	—	x	x

Source: Modified from Warren WB et al. *Am J Obstet Gynecol.* 1989;161:747–53.

to observe in greater detail the anatomical changes of living embryo and fetus in later gestation. While in the early stages of pregnancy, the major aims of ultrasound examination are confirmation of viability, estimation of the number of fetuses, and dating of pregnancy, around the 12th week, effective screening for chromosomal and structural defects can be performed. Moreover, screening for the most common obstetric complication, namely, preeclampsia and fetal growth restriction, is performed at 11–13 weeks.

REFERENCES

1. Blaas HG. The examination of the embryo and early fetus: How and by whom? *Ultrasound Obstet Gynecol.* 1999;14(3):153–8.
2. O'Rahilly R, and Muller F. Developmental stages in human embryos: Revised and new measurements. *Cells Tissues Organs.* 2010;192(2):73–84.
3. Salomon LJ, Alfirevic Z, Bilardo CM et al. ISUOG practice guidelines: Performance of first-trimester fetal ultrasound scan. *Ultrasound Obstet Gynecol.* 2013;41(1):102–13.
4. Pooh RK, Shiota K, and Kurjak A. Imaging of the human embryo with magnetic resonance imaging microscopy and high-resolution transvaginal 3-dimensional sonography: Human embryology in the 21st century. *Am J Obstet Gynecol.* 2011;204(1):77.e1–16.
5. Mall F. On stages in the development of human embryos from 2 to 25 mm long. *Anat Anz.* 1914(46):78–84.
6. Bagratee JS, Regan L, Khullar V, Connolly C, and Moodley J. Reference intervals of gestational sac, yolk sac and embryo volumes using three-dimensional ultrasound. *Ultrasound Obstet Gynecol.* 2009;34(5):503–9.
7. Papaioannou GI, Syngelaki A, Poon LC, Ross JA, and Nicolaides KH. Normal ranges of embryonic length, embryonic heart rate, gestational sac diameter and yolk sac diameter at 6–10 weeks. *Fetal Diagn Ther.* 2010;28(4):207–19.

8. Hoffman CS, Messer LC, Mendola P, Savitz DA, Herring AH, and Hartmann KE. Comparison of gestational age at birth based on last menstrual period and ultrasound during the first trimester. *Paediatr Perinat Epidemiol.* 2008;22(6):587–96.

9. Khalil A, Rodgers M, Baschat A et al. ISUOG Practice Guidelines: Role of ultrasound in twin pregnancy. *Ultrasound Obstet Gynecol.* 2016;47(2):247–63.

10. Robinson HP. Sonar measurement of fetal crown-rump length as means of assessing maturity in first trimester of pregnancy. *Br Med J.* 1973;4(5883):28–31.

11. Hadlock FP, Shah YP, Kanon DJ, and Lindsey JV. Fetal crown-rump length: Reevaluation of relation to menstrual age (5–18 weeks) with high-resolution real-time US. *Radiology.* 1992;182(2):501–5.

12. Nelson LH. Comparison of methods for determining crown-rump measurement by real-time ultrasound. *J Clin Ultrasound.* 1981;9(2):67–70.

13. Verburg BO, Steegers EA, De Ridder M et al. New charts for ultrasound dating of pregnancy and assessment of fetal growth: Longitudinal data from a population-based cohort study. *Ultrasound Obstet Gynecol.* 2008;31(4):388–96.

14. Robinson HP, and Fleming JE. A critical evaluation of sonar "crown-rump length" measurements. *Br J Obstet Gynaecol.* 1975;82(9):702–10.

15. Smith BR. Visualizing human embryos. *Sci Am.* 1999;280(3):76–81.

16. Yamada S, Uwabe C, Nakatsu-Komatsu T et al. Graphic and movie illustrations of human prenatal development and their application to embryological education based on the human embryo specimens in the Kyoto collection. *Dev Dyn.* 2006;235(2):468–77.

17. Smith BR, Huff DS, and Johnson GA. Magnetic resonance imaging of embryos: An Internet resource for the study of embryonic development. *Comput Med Imaging Graph.* 1999;23(1):33–40.

18. Timor-Tritsch IE, Peisner DB, and Raju S. Sonoembryology: An organ-oriented approach using a high-frequency vaginal probe. *J Clin Ultrasound.* 1990;18(4):286–98.

19. Benoit B, Hafner T, Kurjak A, Kupesic S, Bekavac I, and Bozek T. Three-dimensional sonoembryology. *J Perinat Med.* 2002;30(1):63–73.

20. Timor-Tritsch IE, and Monteagudo A. Three and four-dimensional ultrasound in obstetrics and gynecology. *Curr Opin Obstet Gynecol.* 2007;19(2):157–75.

21. Timor-Tritsch IE, Monteagudo A, and Pilu G. *Ultrasonography of the Prenatal Brain.* 3rd ed. New York, NY: McGraw-Hill Professional; 2012. pp. xiv, 490.

22. Kurjak A, Pooh RK, Merce LT, Carrera JM, Salihagic-Kadic A, and Andonotopo W. Structural and functional early human development assessed by three-dimensional and four-dimensional sonography. *Fertil Steril.* 2005;84(5):1285–99.

23. Pooh RK. Neurosonoembryology by three-dimensional ultrasound. *Semin Fetal Neonatal Med.* 2012;17(5):261–8.

24. Pooh RK, and Kurjak A. 3D/4D sonography moved prenatal diagnosis of fetal anomalies from the second to the first trimester of pregnancy. *J Matern Fetal Neonatal Med.* 2012;25(5):433–55.

25. Pooh RK. Sonoembryology by 3D HDlive silhouette ultrasound—What is added by the "see-through fashion"? *J Perinat Med.* 2016;44(2):139–48.

26. Nicolaides KH. The 11–13 + 6 week scan. Fetal medicine Foundation 2004. https://fetalmedicine.org/education/the-11-13-weeks-scan (accessed April 30, 2019).

27. Borenstein M, Azumendi Perez G, Molina Garcia F, Romero M, and Anderica JR. Gestational sac volume: Comparison between SonoAVC and VOCAL measurements at 11 + 0 to 13 + 6 weeks of gestation. *Ultrasound Obstet Gynecol.* 2009;34(5):510–4.

28. Rolo LC, Nardozza LM, Araujo Junior E, Nowak PM, and Moron AF. Gestational sac volume by 3D-sonography at 7–10 weeks of pregnancy using the VOCAL method. *Arch Gynecol Obstet.* 2009;279(6):821–7.

29. Rolo LC, Nardozza LM, Araujo Junior E, Nowak PM, and Moron AF. Yolk sac volume assessed by three-dimensional ultrasonography using the VOCAL method. *Acta Obstet Gynecol Scand.* 2008;87(5):499–502.

30. Goncalves LF, Lee W, Espinoza J, and Romero R. Three- and 4-dimensional ultrasound in obstetric practice: Does it help? *J Ultrasound Med.* 2005;24(12):1599–624.

31. Kim MS, Jeanty P, Turner C, and Benoit B. Three-dimensional sonographic evaluations of embryonic brain development. *J Ultrasound Med.* 2008;27(1):119–24.

32. Hyett JA, Noble PL, Snijders RJ, Montenegro N, and Nicolaides KH. Fetal heart rate in trisomy 21 and other chromosomal abnormalities at 10–14 weeks of gestation. *Ultrasound Obstet Gynecol.* 1996;7(4):239–44.

33. Nicolaides KH. Screening for fetal aneuploidies at 11 to 13 weeks. *Prenat Diagn.* 2011;31(1):7–15.

34. Timor-Tritsch IE, Fuchs KM, Monteagudo A, and D'Alton ME. Performing a fetal anatomy scan at the time of first-trimester screening. *Obstet Gynecol.* 2009;113(2 Pt 1):402–7.

35. Souka AP, Pilalis A, Kavalakis Y, Kosmas Y, Antsaklis P, and Antsaklis A. Assessment of fetal anatomy at the 11–14-week ultrasound examination. *Ultrasound Obstet Gynecol.* 2004;24(7):730–4.

36. Huggon IC, Ghi T, Cook AC, Zosmer N, Allan LD, and Nicolaides KH. Fetal cardiac abnormalities identified prior to 14 weeks' gestation. *Ultrasound Obstet Gynecol.* 2002;20(1):22–9.

37. Chaoui R, Benoit B, Mitkowska-Wozniak H, Heling KS, and Nicolaides KH. Assessment of intracranial translucency (IT) in the detection of spina bifida at the 11–13-week scan. *Ultrasound Obstet Gynecol.* 2009;34(3):249–52.

38. Chaoui R, and Nicolaides KH. From nuchal translucency to intracranial translucency: Towards the early detection of spina bifida. *Ultrasound Obstet Gynecol.* 2010;35(2):133–8.

39. Sonek J. First trimester ultrasonography in screening and detection of fetal anomalies. *Am J Med Genet C Semin Med Genet.* 2007;145C(1):45–61.

40. Abele H, Wagner P, Sonek J et al. First trimester ultrasound screening for Down syndrome based on maternal age, fetal nuchal translucency and different combinations of the additional markers nasal bone, tricuspid and ductus venosus flow. *Prenat Diagn.* 2015;35(12):1182–6.

41. Santorum M, Wright D, Syngelaki A, Karagioti N, and Nicolaides KH. Accuracy of first-trimester combined test in screening for trisomies 21, 18 and 13. *Ultrasound Obstet Gynecol.* 2017;49(6):714–20.

42. Souka AP, Krampl E, Bakalis S, Heath V, and Nicolaides KH. Outcome of pregnancy in chromosomally normal fetuses with increased nuchal translucency in the first trimester. *Ultrasound Obstet Gynecol.* 2001;18(1):9–17.

43. Kagan KO, Sonek J, Wagner P, and Hoopmann M. Principles of first trimester screening in the age of non-invasive prenatal diagnosis: Screening for other major defects and pregnancy complications. *Arch Gynecol Obstet.* 2017;296(4):635–43.

44. Syngelaki A, Guerra L, Ceccacci I, Efeturk T, and Nicolaides KH. Impact of holoprosencephaly, exomphalos, megacystis and increased nuchal translucency on first-trimester screening for chromosomal abnormalities. *Ultrasound Obstet Gynecol.* 2017;50(1):45–8.

45. Rossi AC, and Prefumo F. Accuracy of ultrasonography at 11–14 weeks of gestation for detection of fetal structural anomalies: A systematic review. *Obstet Gynecol.* 2013;122(6):1160–7.

46. Syngelaki A, Chelemen T, Dagklis T, Allan L, and Nicolaides KH. Challenges in the diagnosis of fetal non-chromosomal abnormalities at 11–13 weeks. *Prenat Diagn.* 2011;31(1):90–102.

47. Persico N, Moratalla J, Lombardi CM, Zidere V, Allan L, and Nicolaides KH. Fetal echocardiography at 11–13 weeks by transabdominal high-frequency ultrasound. *Ultrasound Obstet Gynecol.* 2011;37(3):296–301.

15

Assisted Reproductive Technology and Multiple Pregnancy

Rezan A. Kadir and Zdravka Veleva

Introduction

In industrialized countries, multiple birth rates began to decline in the 1950s, reaching a minimum in the 1970s. While a definitive explanation has not been found, this decline of multiple births has been attributed to the increased use of oral contraceptives and to unidentified environmental pollutants [1]. Starting in the 1970s, the rates of both twin and triplet deliveries have followed the same rising trend until 1998–2000.

There were two main reasons behind this phenomenon: increasing maternal age because of delayed childbearing, as well as the use of ovulation induction and assisted reproductive technologies (ARTs). These treatments have accounted for similar proportions of both twin births (20%–30%) and triplet births (30%–40%) during that time [2]. In the dawn of ART, the transfer of multiple embryos was the only way to compensate for very low implantation rates. However, with improvement in laboratory culture and ovarian stimulation protocols, embryo quality and implantation rates increased, which gave rise to the so-called "multiple birth epidemic" that was observed in the 1990s and early 2000s.

In 2002, the World Collaborative Report on ART that published data from Europe, the United States, Australia and New Zealand, and individual Latin American and Middle Eastern countries [3], showed an overall twin rate of 25.7% and an overall triplet rate of 2.5%. The triplet delivery rate varied markedly, from 0.2% in Finland and Sweden, to greater than 10% in Guatemala and the United Arab Emirates. This meant that slightly less than half of the infants born in 2002 after ART treatment originated in a multiple pregnancy. With up to 246,000 children born in 2002, the high rate of multiple pregnancies was estimated to be a significant problem.

Multiple pregnancy is associated with significant maternal, fetal, and neonatal complications and remains the most common treatment-related adverse outcome of ART. By 2011, the multiple birth epidemic already showed signs of being contained in certain regions of the world. European data revealed a multiple birth rate of 19% after fresh *in vitro* fertilization (IVF) treatment [4]. However, the Centers for Disease Control and Prevention (CDC) data from the United States showed 46% of births following IVF treatment were either twins or higher-order multiples [5].

Elective Single Embryo Transfer

The way to curb the increase in the multiple birth rate after ART was to restrict the number of embryos transferred to the uterus. In the 1990s, the number of embryos transferred decreased in most countries from three to two. This, however, was still associated with about 20%–30% of multiple births. In order to restore the multiple birth rate to a lower level, elective single embryo transfer (eSET) was introduced to clinical practice. In eSET, more than one good-quality embryos are created after oocyte pickup, but only one of them is transferred in the fresh cycle. All other good-quality embryos are cryopreserved for later use in frozen-thawed transfers. The first report of eSET was published in 1999, when the strategy was tested in Finnish women with contraindications for multiple pregnancy [6]. The first randomized controlled trials (RCTs) came from Belgium [7] and Finland [8] and showed similarly good implantation and ongoing pregnancy rates. In view of these encouraging early studies, eSET became the recommended embryo transfer strategy by the European Society of Human Reproduction and Embryology (ESHRE) [9] and the American Society of Reproductive Medicine (ASRM) [10].

However, initial studies were performed in patients with good prognoses, and the strategy became subject to strong criticism. There was widespread suspicion that if eSET was used on a wider scale, it would result in lower live birth rates and increased treatment costs [11]. A multitude of studies examined different scenarios for use with eSET. Most showed that costs of eSET were lower, compared with the costs associated with the transfer of two embryos (double embryo transfer, DET) [12–15]). There was, however, some controversy regarding clinical outcome. RCTs showed lower pregnancy rates with eSET (21.4%–47.9%), compared with DET (36%–74%) [7,8,16–18]). By contrast, retrospective studies observed similar pregnancy rates in eSET (29.7%–49%) and DET (29.4%–54%) [6,19,13,20].

The definitive evidence about the applicability of eSET came from several large retrospective studies, the first of which was from Sweden [21], and showed that despite successive reduction in the number of embryos transferred from 2.7 in 1992 to 1.3 in 2004, live birth rates were maintained at around 26%, while multiple birth rates decreased dramatically, from about 35% to around 5%.

A Finnish study from a single university hospital analyzed data collected between 1995 and 2005 when eSET was gradually introduced into clinical practice [22]. During 1995–1999, eSET was used experimentally in 4.2% of patients, while it was used routinely in almost half (42.6%) of ART cycles during 2000–2005. A comparison of these two periods revealed that the rate of multiple births decreased from 19.6% to 8.9%, with most multiple births initiating in the frozen-thawed cycles. In the same time, the term live birth rate (greater than 37 gestational weeks) increased significantly from 36.6% to 41.7%. A single term live birth in the period with routine use of eSET was 19,889 euros less expensive than in the previous time period. The usefulness of eSET was later confirmed in patients from Quebec [23] and from the United States [24]. Furthermore, a meta-analysis of RCTs observed that even if only one frozen-thawed embryo transfer was performed after an eSET cycle compared to the transfer of two frozen-thawed embryos, the term live birth rate increases dramatically with an odds ratio (OR) of 4.93 (95% confidence interval [CI] 2.98–8.18) [25].

In the United Kingdom, the Human Fertilisation and Embryology Authority (HFEA) introduced a two-embryo policy in 2001. This led to a significant reduction in triplets and higher-order multiple births. However, the contribution of ART continued to rise for twin births. In 2006, one in four IVF pregnancies resulted in the birth of twins, a ten times higher risk than after spontaneous conception [26]. In 2009, HFEA set out a maximum multiple birth rate target for IVF clinics with a target of 24% to be reduced in steps over a period of years to an end goal of no more than 10% of all live births with a policy of eSET. National Institute for Health and Care Excellence (NICE) guidelines published in February 2013 also recommend single embryo transfer (SET) in many cases. This has been a successful program and has led to a reduction of the national multiple birth rate from 24% in 2008 to a current rate of 11%, without reducing birth rates [27].

Risks of Multiple Pregnancy

Early Pregnancy Risks

Multiple pregnancy (Figure 15.1) is associated with an increased risk of vaginal bleeding during the first trimester, with an increased risk of miscarriage in triplets and higher-order multiples. In twin pregnancy, particularly those conceived by ART, there is also an increased incidence of first-trimester bleeding, but it is not associated with increased risk of spontaneous miscarriage, although it increases the risk for low birth weight for at least one twin [28].

Several studies have shown a lower incidence of first-trimester complete pregnancy loss and miscarriage per gestational sac among twins compared to singletons conceived by ART. This has been attributed to a better cohort of embryos and higher placental volume and hormone production from early in the first

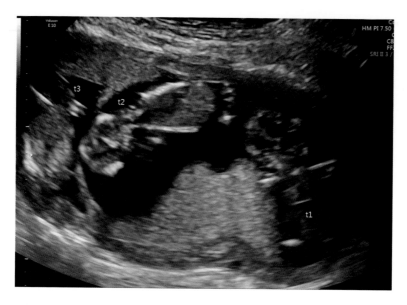

FIGURE 15.1   Triplet pregnancy.

trimester in twin pregnancies [29]. However, multiple pregnancy confers a greater risk of second-trimester loss. In one study, multiple pregnancy accounted for 48% of second-trimester pregnancy loss in women with ongoing second-trimester IVF-conceived pregnancy (defined as ultrasound confirmation of at least one fetus with fetal heart tones at 12 weeks' gestation), with an adjusted OR of 1.93 compared to singleton pregnancies [30].

Vanishing twin syndrome (VTS) (Figure 15.2) is a spontaneous reduction of a fetus *in utero*. It occurs in approximately half and one-third of pregnancies starting as triplets and twins, respectively. It has been reported that VTS is associated with adverse perinatal outcome with an increased risk for congenital anomalies, malformations of cortical development in monochorionic twins, low birth weight, preterm labor, and increased perinatal mortality [31].

The risk of congenital anomaly is increased in multiple pregnancy, especially in monochorionic type (Figure 15.3). The risk of chromosomal abnormality is also higher per pregnancy. Diagnosis and management of these abnormalities often pose a clinical challenge. These include reliability of screening

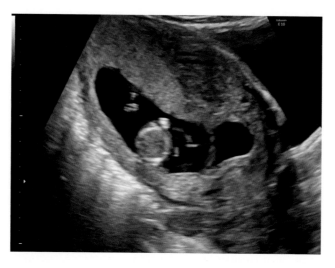

FIGURE 15.2   Vanishing twin syndrome.

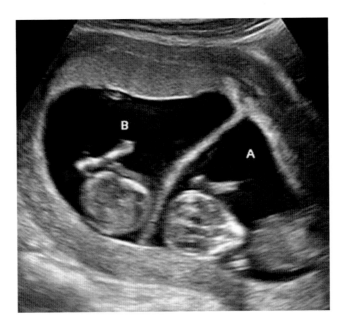

FIGURE 15.3   Monochroinic diamniotic (MCDA) twin pregnancy.

tests and their inability to identify which fetus is affected, higher risk of pregnancy loss with invasive diagnostic tests, as well as potential sampling error. For twins discordant for fetal anomaly or aneuploidy, decision-making in relation to the use of selective feticide is complex because of the potential risks to the healthy co-twin. Conversely, conservative management may also compromise the well-being of the normal twin in some abnormalities, for example, abnormalities associated with polyhydramnios leading to preterm labor.

Fetal and Neonatal Risks

A systematic review of 25 studies [32] looking at perinatal outcome in singleton and twin pregnancy after assisted conception showed preterm birth of 2% and 6.8% for very preterm (less than 32 weeks) and 11.4% and 45.6% for preterm (less than 37 weeks) for singleton and twin pregnancies, respectively. The rate of singleton babies weighing less than 1500 g (very low birth weight [VLBW]) ranged from 1.5% to 3.9% in singleton pregnancies compared to 5%–25% for twin pregnancies. Cesarean section was the mode of delivery in 47% of twins and 26% of singletons. Among the twins, 65% required admission to the neonatal intensive care unit compared to only 17% of the singletons. In the same study, perinatal mortality was 12.4/1000 for singleton pregnancies and 23/1000 for twin pregnancies in 14 matched studies. When compared to naturally conceived pregnancies, singletons from ART are significantly disadvantaged, but the difference is less for twins. In a population-based study in the United States, ART twins were less likely to be very preterm (OR 0.75, 95% CI 0.58–0.97) and VLBW (less than 1500 g) (OR 0.75, CI 0.58–0.95) with less infant death (OR 0.55, CI 0.35–0.88) than non-ART twins [33]. Possible reasons for these attenuated risks for ART twins are enhanced antenatal care and peripartum monitoring and lower frequency of high-risk monozygotic twins. However, ART is strongly associated with twin pregnancies, and twins carry a higher risk for adverse perinatal outcome compared to singletons. In the previous study, 30% of ART deliveries were twins compared to 1.5% of non-ART deliveries. In a subset analysis restricted to a higher sociodemographic group, the singleton rate for preterm, very preterm, low birth weight (LBW; less than 2500 g), and VLBW were 6.6%, 0.8%, 3.6%, and 0.6%, respectively. While for the twins, 50% were preterm, 9% were very preterm, 49.5% were LBW, and 8% were VLBW.

Multiple pregnancies are also associated with a higher risk of stillbirth, neonatal death (death under 28 days). The infant mortality rate is ten times higher for twin deliveries (with at least one infant death) compared to singleton delivery, and each ART twin infant individually has a sixfold higher risk of infant death than a singleton infant [33]. Twins often require long periods of hospitalization at the beginning of life, with a higher risk of child disability and longer-term health and cognitive effects. Twins are also more likely than singletons to suffer from cerebral palsy. All these adverse outcomes seem to be mainly due to prematurity and LBW in multiple pregnancy.

The mechanisms of preterm birth in twins and higher multiples are multifactorial and not well understood. Thus, methods for prediction and prevention of preterm birth are very limited. Cervical cerclage and the use of progesterone are ineffective in preventing preterm birth, and the value of antenatal steroids is not fully established in twin pregnancy [34]. There is also an increased risk of intrauterine growth restriction, in particular, selective intrauterine growth restriction (sIUGR) in twins. Again, management of these cases remains challenging with a high risk of intrauterine demise of the smaller twin and a high rate of preterm delivery less than 32 weeks [35]. Therefore, eSET strategy seems the only viable option of reducing perinatal mortality and morbidity and achieving a successful outcome with ART.

Maternal Risks

Multiple pregnancy is also associated with increased maternal risks and complications during pregnancy, intrapartum and postpartum. These risks are often overlooked and underestimated when counseling women about risks of multiple pregnancy. Mothers carrying twins undergo an exaggerated physiological response to pregnancy. They suffer nausea and vomiting of pregnancy more commonly compared to women with singleton pregnancy, often with severe intensity requiring repeated hospital admissions. They are also more likely to develop hyperemesis gravidarum. There is also an increased risk of ovarian hyperstimulation syndrome after IVF treatment, with more severe symptoms.

There is a higher cardiac output due to both higher stroke volume and heart rate in pregnant women with a twin pregnancy compared to a singleton pregnancy. In one study, an increase in left atrial diameter and left ventricular end-diastolic diameter were reported in association with twin pregnancies [36]. These changes may put women with preexisting cardiovascular conditions at risk of decompensation and serious cardiac complications during pregnancy. Exaggerated hemostatic response to pregnancy with increased coagulation factors and the effect of pressure that the large uterus puts on the pelvic veins puts women with multiple pregnancy at an increased risk of venous thromboembolism during the antenatal and postnatal periods. Multiple pregnancy leads to increased caloric intake and nutrient requirements. Women with twin pregnancy have a two- to fourfold increase in iron deficiency anemia [37].

Women with multiple pregnancies have a higher risk of developing hypertensive disorders. There is a higher incidence of preeclampsia in twin pregnancy compared to singleton pregnancy, with an increasing risk in higher-order multiples. Preeclampsia is more likely to develop earlier and be more severe, with its associated complications, need for hospitalization, and early delivery [38]. There is also an increased risk of antepartum hemorrhage due to a higher rate of placenta previa and placental abruption in multiple pregnancy. Delivery is more likely to be by cesarean section in twin pregnancy due to these complications, and there is a higher rate of malpresentation and fetal growth restriction. Higher-order multiples are always delivered by cesarean section. For twin pregnancies in labor, there is a risk of cord prolapse, fetal distress, abnormal or unstable lie, and placental abruption, especially during the delivery of the second twin. Thus, there is a high rate of instrumental delivery and emergency cesarean section, including a small risk of a combined vaginal-cesarean delivery. In a large study of 61,845 twin births, a 9.5% rate of emergency cesarean section was reported for second twins after vaginal delivery of the first twin [39]. Postpartum hemorrhage (PPH) is more common during twin birth, with more than a twofold increase in PPH (500 mL or greater) and progression to severe PPH (1500 mL or greater) [40]. This is attributed to uterine overdistention and a high rate of uterine atony as well as a higher rate of operative deliveries. Thus, women with multiple pregnancies are more likely to require blood transfusion during the intrapartum and postpartum periods, with associated transfusion risks. A significantly higher rate of blood transfusion has been reported in women with twin pregnancies during primary and repeat cesarean section compared to singleton pregnancies [41].

Multiple pregnancy is associated with excessive weight gain, and coupled with the effect of a large gravid uterus changing the center of gravity, there may be a significant mechanical strain on the musculoskeletal system. Back pain and pelvic joint dysfunction are more likely to occur and be severe with a negative impact on the mother's mobility and sleep and her quality of life.

Due to higher risks of complications, neonatal and maternal morbidity, and fetal loss, a multiple pregnancy has a greater impact on the mother's physical and emotional well-being than a singleton pregnancy. A higher rate of depression has been reported in mothers of twins, with the highest risk in mothers who lost one twin [42]. Having a multiple birth puts strain on the family with financial difficulties and marital problems. Mothers of multiple births are less likely to return to work, reducing the family's income and the need to use up their savings. Families with multiple births are also more likely to report tiredness and lower levels of confidence and competence in looking after their children, and they are more likely to separate or divorce than other families [43].

Data from a recent large nationwide population study from Sweden showed that multiple gestations mediated most of the associations with preeclampsia, preterm birth, and cesarean delivery in pregnancies conceived by ART [44]. In Sweden, a SET policy was implemented in 2003 and led to a reduction of multiple pregnancies from 13% before 2004 to 6% after, with an associated reduction in preeclampsia and preterm births. These findings support the policy of eSET and confirm that interventions to restrict multiple pregnancy can reduce the risk of these pregnancy complications in ART.

Conclusions

Major advances have taken place in ARTs since the birth of the first test tube baby in 1978, and they are increasingly utilized for a wide range of indications in couples with infertility or genetic conditions. With the focus on improving pregnancy rates, there have been some adverse outcomes. Increased risk of multiple pregnancy due to transfer of multiple embryos is one of the most common complications, with serious health risks for the mother and child/children. Over the last three decades, efforts to reduce the number of embryos transferred have helped reduce this risk. Research has shown that the policy of eSET can eliminate the risk of multiple pregnancies associated with ARTs without reducing the pregnancy and live birth rates, with additional cost-saving benefits. Thus, this policy is now the recommended embryo transfer strategy by ESHRE, ASRM, and many national authorities, and should be practiced by all clinicians working in the field to optimize patient safety and experience.

REFERENCES

1. Botting BJ, Davies IM, and Macfarlane AJ. Recent trends in the incidence of multiple births and associated mortality. *Arch Dis Child.* 1987;62(9):941–50.
2. Collins J. Global epidemiology of multiple birth. *Reprod Biomed Online.* 2007;15(Suppl 3):45–52.
3. International Committee for Monitoring Assisted Reproductive Technology; de Mouzon J, Lancaster P, Nygren KG et al. World collaborative report on Assisted Reproductive Technology, 2002. *Hum Reprod.* 2009;24(9):2310-20.
4. Kupka MS, D'Hooghe T, Ferraretti AP et al.; The European IVF-Monitoring Consortium (EIM), for the European Society of Human Reproduction and Embryology (ESHRE). Assisted reproductive technology in Europe, 2011: Results generated from European registers by ESHRE. *Hum Reprod.* 2016;31:233–48.
5. Sunderam S, Kissin DM, Crawford SB, Folger SG, Jamieson DJ, and Barfield WD; Centers for Disease Control and Prevention (CDC). Assisted reproductive technology surveillance—United States, 2011. *MMWR Surveill Summ.* 2014;63:1–28.
6. Vilska S, Tiitinen A, Hydén-Granskog C, and Hovatta O. Elective transfer of one embryo results in an acceptable pregnancy rate and eliminates the risk of multiple birth. *Hum Reprod.* 1999;14:2392–5.
7. Gerris J, De Neubourg D, Mangelschots K, Van Royen E, Van de Meerssche M, and Valkenburg M. Prevention of twin pregnancy after *in-vitro* fertilization or intracytoplasmic sperm injection based on strict embryo criteria: A prospective randomized clinical trial. *Hum Reprod.* 1999;14:2581–7.
8. Martikainen H, Tiitinen A, Tomás C et al. One versus two embryo transfer after IVF and ICSI: A randomized study. *Hum Reprod.* 2001;16:1900–3.
9. ESHRE Campus Course Report. Prevention of twin pregnancies after IVF/ICSI by single embryo transfer. *Hum Reprod.* 2001;16(4):790–800.

10. The Practice Committee of the Society for Assisted Reproductive Technology and the Practice Committee of the American Society for Reproductive Medicine. Guidelines on number of embryos transferred. *Fertil Steril.* 2006;86:S51–2.
11. Gleicher N, and Barad D. The relative myth of elective single embryo transfer. *Hum Reprod.* 2006;21(6):1337–44.
12. Wølner-Hanssen P, and Rydhstroem H. Cost-effectiveness analysis of *in-vitro* fertilization: Estimated costs per successful pregnancy after transfer of one or two embryos. *Hum Reprod.* 1998;13(1):88–94.
13. Gerris J, De Sutter P, De Neubourg D et al. A real-life prospective health economic study of elective single embryo transfer versus two-embryo transfer in first IVF/ICSI cycles. *Hum Reprod.* 2004;19(4):917–23.
14. Fiddelers AA, van Montfoort AP, Dirksen CD et al. Single versus double embryo transfer: Cost-effectiveness analysis alongside a randomized clinical trial. *Hum Reprod.* 2006;21(8):2090–7.
15. Thurin Kjellberg A, Carlsson P, and Bergh C. Randomized single versus double embryo transfer: Obstetric and paediatric outcome and a cost-effectiveness analysis. *Hum Reprod.* 2006;21(1):210–6.
16. Thurin A, Hausken J, Hillensjo T et al. Elective single-embryo transfer versus double-embryo transfer in *in vitro* fertilization. *N Engl J Med.* 2004;351(23):2392–2402.
17. Lukassen HG, Braat DD, Wetzels AM et al. Two cycles with single embryo transfer versus one cycle with double embryo transfer: A randomized controlled trial. *Hum Reprod.* 2005;20(3):702–8.
18. van Montfoort AP, Fiddelers AA, Janssen JM et al. In unselected patients, elective single embryo transfer prevents all multiples, but results in significantly lower pregnancy rates compared with double embryo transfer: A randomized controlled trial. *Hum Reprod.* 2006;21(2):338–43.
19. Tiitinen A, Halttunen M, Harkki P, Vuoristo P, and Hyden-Granskog C. Elective single embryo transfer: The value of cryopreservation. *Hum Reprod.* 2001;16(6):1140–4.
20. van Montfoort AP, Dumoulin JC, Land JA, Coonen E, Derhaag, and Evers JL. Elective single embryo transfer (eSET) policy in the first three IVF/ICSI treatment cycles. *Hum Reprod.* 2005;20(2):433–6.
21. Karlström PO, and Bergh C. Reducing the number of embryos transferred in Sweden—Impact on delivery and multiple birth rates. *Hum Reprod.* 2007;22:2202–7.
22. Veleva Z, Karinen P, Tomás C, Tapanainen JS, and Martikainen H. Elective single embryo transfer with cryopreservation improves the outcome and diminishes the costs of IVF/ICSI. *Hum Reprod.* 2009;24:1632–9.
23. Vélez MP, Connolly MP, Kadoch IJ, Phillips S, and Bissonnette F. Universal coverage of IVF pays off. *Hum Reprod.* 2014;29(6):1313–9.
24. Mancuso AC, Boulet SL, Duran E, Munch E, Kissin DM, and Van Voorhis BJ. Elective single embryo transfer in women less than age 38 years reduces multiple birth rates, but not live birth rates, in United States fertility clinics. *Fertil Steril.* 2016;106:1107–14.
25. McLernon DJ, Harrild K, Bergh C et al. Clinical effectiveness of elective single versus double embryo transfer: Meta-analysis of individual patient data from randomised trials. *BMJ.* 2010;341:c6945.
26. Braude P. *One child at a time. Reducing multiple births after IVF.* Report of the Expert Group on Multiple Births after IVF. HFEA October 2006.
27. Fertility treatment 2014–2016 Trends and figures. HFEA March 2018. https:// www.hfea.gov.uk
28. Eaton JL, XingqiAhang MC, and Kazer RR. First-trimester bleeding and twin pregnancy outcomes after *in vitro* fertilization. *Fertil Steril.* 2016;106:140–3.
29. Póvoa A, Matias A, Xavier P, and Blickstein I. Can early ultrasonography explain the lower miscarriage rates in twin as compared to singleton pregnancies following assisted reproduction? *J Perinat Med.* 2018;46(7):760–3.
30. Bressler HL, Correia KF, Srouii SS, Hornstein MD, and Missmer SA. Factors associated with second-trimester pregnancy loss in women with normal uterine anatomy undergoing *in vitro* fertilization. *Obstet Gynecol.* 2015;125:621–7.
31. Evron E, Sheiner E, Friger M, Sergienko R, and Harlev A. Vanishing twin syndrome: Is it associated with adverse perinatal outcome. *Fertil Steril.* 2015;103:1209–14.
32. Helmerhorst FM, Perquin D, Donker D, and Keirse M. Perinatal outcome of singletons and twins after assisted conception: A systematic review of controlled studies. *BMJ.* 2004;328:261.
33. Boulet S, Schieve L, Nannini A et al. Prenatal outcomes of twin births conceived using assisted reproduction technology: A population-based study. *Hum Reprod.* 2008;23(8):1941–8.
34. Stock S, and Norman J. Preterm and term labour in multiple pregnancies. *Semin Fetal Neonatal Med.* 2010;15:336–41.

35. Kilby M. Multiple pregnancy. *Semin Fetal Neonatal Med.* 2010;15:305.
36. Kametas NA, McAuliffe F, and Krampl E. Maternal cardiac function in twin pregnancy. *Obstet Gynecol.* 2003;102:806–15.
37. Goodnight W, and Newman R. Optimal nutrition for improved twin pregnancy outcome. *Obstet Gyecol.* 2009;114:1121–34.
38. Henry D, McElrath T, and Smith N. Preterm severe preeclampsia in singleton and twin pregnancies. *J Perinatal.* 2013;33:94–7.
39. Wen SW, Fung KF, Oppenheimer L, Demissie K, Yang Q, and Walker M. Occurrence and predictors of cesarean delivery for the second twin after vaginal delivery of the first twin. *Obstet Gynecol.* 2004;103(3):413–9.
40. Briley A, Seed PT, Tydeman G et al. Reporting errors, incidence and risk factors for postpartum haemorrhage and progression to severe PPH: A prospective observational study. *BJOG.* 2014;121:876–88.
41. Rose DJ, MacPherson C, and Laudon M. Blood transfusion and cesarean section. 2006. *Obstet Gynaecol.* 2006;108:891–7.
42. Thorpe K, Golding J, and MacGillivray I. Comparison of prevalence of depression in mothers of twins and mothers of singletons. *BMJ.* 1991:302:875–8.
43. McKay S. The Effects of Twins and Multiple Births on Families and Their Living Standards. Aldershot, UK: Tamba (Twins and Multiple Births Association) [now Twins trust]; 2010. https://twinstrust.org/uploads/assets/f01090b4-013a-4495-97102255a16f89d4/Financial-Report-FINAL.pdf
44. Oberg AS, VanerWeele TJ, Almgvist C, and Hetnandez-Diaz S. Pregnancy complications following fertility treatment-disentangling the role of multiple gestation. *Int J Epidemiol.* 2018;47(4):1333–42.

16

Miscarriage and Gestational Trophoblastic Disease

Rudaina Hassan and Caryl Thomas

Introduction

An early or first-trimester miscarriage occurs at less than or equal to 12 weeks' gestation; a late miscarriage is when a miscarriage occurs between 13 and 24 weeks. It is estimated to occur in 10%–15% of clinically recognized pregnancies with 80% occurring in the first trimester. The frequency of miscarriage increases further with maternal age [1].

Miscarriage can be further classified as missed, incomplete, complete, inevitable, and threatened miscarriage.

Missed Miscarriage

This is defined as a nonviable intrauterine pregnancy retained within the uterine cavity. The diagnosis is usually confirmed on ultrasound with an absent fetal heartbeat. In some cases, there is a gestational sac without a detectable fetal pole, described as "blighted ovum" or "anembryonic pregnancy"; however, these terms are now avoided with the use of set ultrasound criteria to diagnose miscarriage.

Incomplete Miscarriage

This is also often referred to as retained products of conception. It is where there has been passage of some tissue, but there are retained products of conception within the uterine cavity with no identifiable gestational sac. Ultrasound may show that some of the products of conception are still present in the uterus.

Complete Miscarriage

This is where there is usually a history of bleeding and tissue passed, and ultrasound demonstrates an empty uterus where an intrauterine pregnancy has previously been visualized.

Inevitable Miscarriage

This is an early pregnancy where a women presents with vaginal bleeding and dilatation of the cervix but with no pregnancy tissue passed. On ultrasound, the products of conception are located in the lower uterine segment or the cervical canal.

Threatened Miscarriage

This is usually diagnosed in women with a history of vaginal bleeding with a live embryo visualized on ultrasound. About 15% of these will result in a miscarriage [2].

Etiology

The majority of miscarriages in the first trimester are due to chromosomal anomalies [3]. Other etiological factors include thrombophilias, maternal systemic disease or its treatment, uterine anomalies, and environmental factors.

Presentation

The clinical symptoms of miscarriage include pelvic pain, cramps, and vaginal bleeding; however, some women may present with no symptoms.

Ultrasound Diagnosis of Miscarriage

Since the development of transvaginal sonography, ultrasound has become the main modality for diagnosing miscarriage. In the United Kingdom, dedicated early pregnancy assessment units have been established which offer assessment and ultrasound for women with pain and/or bleeding in early pregnancy. The ultrasound scanning is carried out by trained health-care professionals, which may include nurses, midwives, or sonographers trained in early pregnancy scanning. In addition to assessment and management of early pregnancy complications, these services offer support and counseling [4].

In 2013, the Society of Radiologists in Ultrasound published new criteria on using ultrasonography for diagnosing first-trimester miscarriage. The ultrasound criteria have been determined to have 100% specificity with 100% positive predictive value in order to prevent the possibility of potentially terminating a viable pregnancy [5].

Diagnostic criteria for first-trimester miscarriage (transvaginal ultrasound) [5]:

- An embryo with a crown-rump length (CRL) of 7 mm or more and no heartbeat on a transvaginal scan (Figure 16.1)
- A gestational sac with mean sac diameter (MSD) of 25 mm or more and no embryo on a transvaginal scan (Figure 16.2)
- Absence of an embryo with heartbeat 2 weeks or more after a scan that demonstrated a gestational sac without a yolk sac
- Absence of an embryo with heartbeat 11 days or more after a scan that demonstrated a gestational sac with a yolk sac

If these criteria are not met, then a repeat scan at 7 or 14 days should be performed depending on the findings. It is recommended that a second operator confirms the diagnosis of miscarriage. If a second operator is unavailable, a repeat scan on a separate occasion should be done to confirm the diagnosis. If a woman has fetal cardiac activity noted on an initial scan and re-presents, then the absence of cardiac activity on repeat assessment is diagnostic of miscarriage without the need to fulfill the measurement criteria.

There are ultrasound features that may suggest an increased chance of miscarriage, but they are not diagnostic of miscarriage. The presence of one or more of these findings should prompt a further repeat scan in 7 or 14 days depending on the findings.

Findings that are suspicious for, but not diagnostic of, a miscarriage (transvaginal ultrasound) [5]:

- An embryo with a CRL of less than 7 mm and no heartbeat
- A gestational sac with MSD of 16–24 mm and the absence of an embryo

(a)

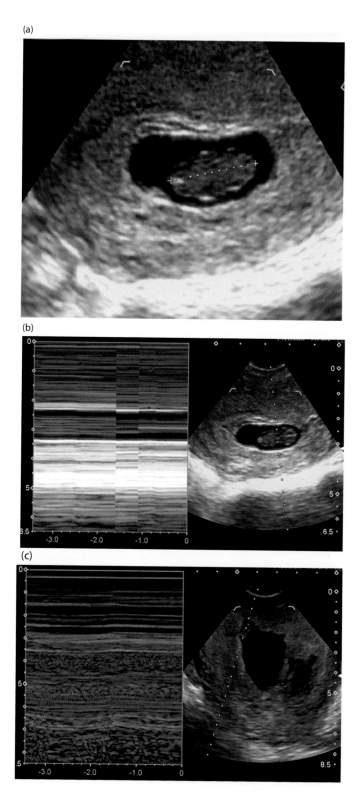

(b)

(c)

FIGURE 16.1   (a,b) Missed miscarriage: embryo with crown-rump length of 15.9 mm with no fetal heart activity, diagnostic of miscarriage. (c) Missed miscarriage: embryo with crown-rump length of 8.6 mm with no fetal heart activity, diagnostic of miscarriage.

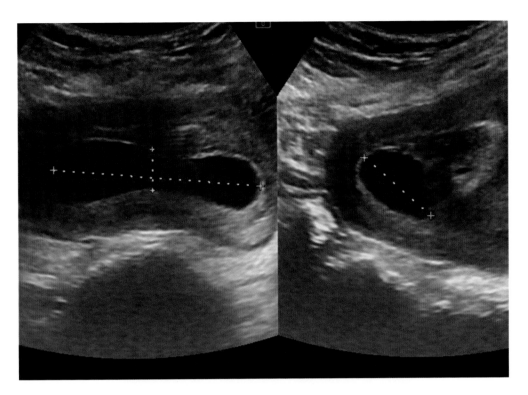

FIGURE 16.2   Missed miscarriage: empty gestation sac with mean sac diameter of 28.6 mm, diagnostic of miscarriage.

- The absence of an embryo with heartbeat 7–13 days following a scan that showed a gestational sac with no yolk sac
- The absence of an embryo with heartbeat 7–10 days following a scan that showed a gestational sac with a yolk sac
- The absence of an embryo 6 weeks or more after the last menstrual period
- An empty amnion seen adjacent to yolk sac, with no visible embryo (empty amnion sign)
- An enlarged yolk sac (greater than 7 mm) (Figure 16.3)
- A small gestational sac in relation to the size of the embryo (less than 5 mm difference between MSD and CRL) (Figure 16.4)
- Large amniotic cavity (expanded amnion sign) (Figure 16.5)

If a transvaginal scan is unacceptable to a woman and a transabdominal scan is performed, the limitations of this type of scan at early gestation should be explained and a repeat scan performed at 14 days to confirm the diagnosis.

Once the diagnosis of miscarriage has been established, the woman can be offered the various options for management of miscarriage, which include expectant, medical or surgical depending on the clinical findings and patient preference. The management options are not covered in this book.

Retained Products of Conception

Retained products of conception (RPOC) or incomplete miscarriage refer to placental or fetal tissue that remains in the uterus following a miscarriage, termination of pregnancy, or delivery.

The clinical symptoms include pelvic pain and vaginal bleeding, and in some cases, women may present with pyrexia and signs of infection.

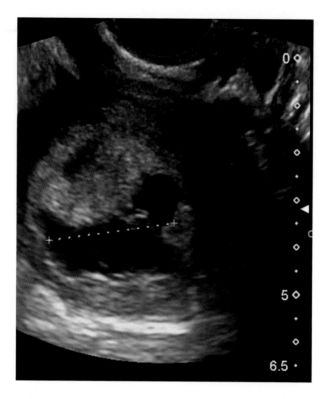

FIGURE 16.3   Irregular gestation sac with enlarged yolk sac, suspicious but not diagnostic of miscarriage.

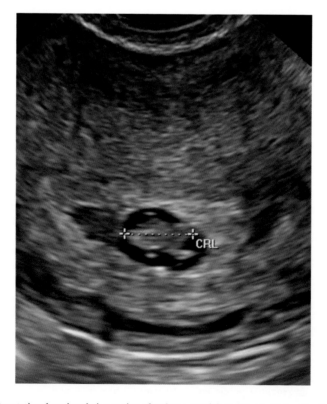

FIGURE 16.4   Small gestational sac in relation to size of embryo, suspicious but not diagnostic of miscarriage.

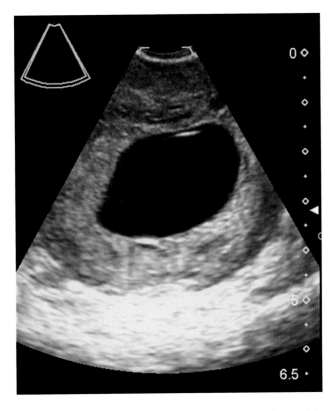

FIGURE 16.5   Expanded amnion sign. Gestation sac with enlarged amniotic cavity, suspicious but not diagnostic of miscarriage.

Ultrasound

- A variable amount of echogenic or heterogeneous material within the endometrial cavity, with an endometrial thickness usually greater than 15 mm (Figure 16.6). There is no consensus in the literature on the endometrial thickness that is diagnostic of RPOC.
- In some instances, this may present like an endometrial or intrauterine mass.

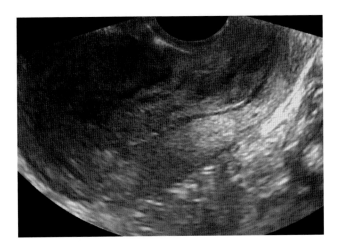

FIGURE 16.6   Retained products of conception or incomplete miscarriage. Heterogenous mixed echogenic material within the endometrial cavity.

- The presence of vascularity within the echogenic material supports the diagnosis, but the absence of color Doppler flow has a low negative predictive value, as retained products of conception may be avascular [6] (Figure 16.7).
- Calcification may be present, especially if diagnosis is delayed (Figure 16.8).

Once the diagnosis is made, women are offered various management options depending on clinical and ultrasound findings. These include expectant management, medical management, and surgical management with dilatation and curettage. The management options are not covered in this book.

(a)

(b)

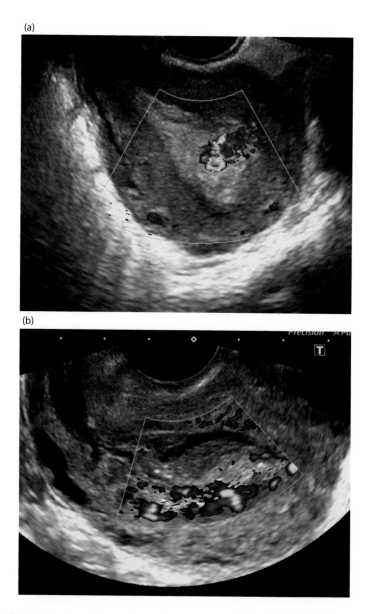

FIGURE 16.7   (a) Retained products of conception or incomplete miscarriage: vascularity within the tissue supports the diagnosis of retained products. (b) Retained products of conception or incomplete miscarriage: area of mixed echogenicity within the endometrial cavity with vascularity within the tissue that supports the diagnosis of retained products.

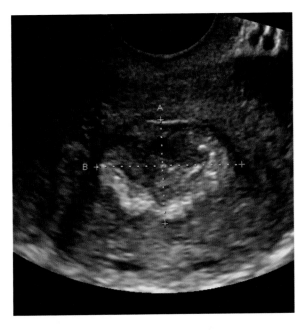

FIGURE 16.8 Retained products of conception or incomplete miscarriage. Area of mixed echogenicity within the endometrial cavity with calcification within the tissue.

Subchorionic Hematoma

Subchorionic hematoma occurs when there is perigestational hemorrhage and blood collects between the uterine wall and the chorionic membrane in pregnancy. It often occurs within the first 20 weeks' gestation. Some women experience vaginal bleeding. When the subchorionic hematomas is large, it is associated with an increased risk of miscarriage [7]. In early pregnancy, the size of the hematoma is a subjective assessment; a subchorionic hematoma is considered small if it is less than 20% of the size of the sac, and large if it is greater than 50%.

Ultrasound

On ultrasound, a subchorionic hematoma appears as a crescent-shaped hypoechoic or anechoic area around part of the gestational sac and outside the chorion (Figure 16.9). With time, the echotexture of the hematoma will vary and may contain internal echoes and debris (Figure 16.10).

In most cases, the hematoma gradually decreases in size on follow-up.

Gestational Trophoblastic Disease

Gestational trophoblastic disease (GTD) encompasses a number of conditions that arise from the abnormal proliferation of trophoblastic tissue. These include the following:

- Hydatidiform mole
  - Complete mole (CHM)
  - Partial mole (PHM)
- Invasive mole, approximately 10%
- Choriocarcinoma (gestational choriocarcinoma) 1%
- Placental site trophoblastic tumor (PSTT)

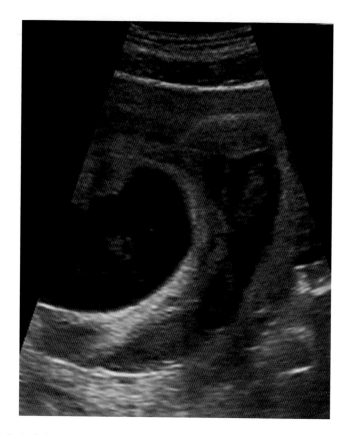

FIGURE 16.9 Subchorionic hematoma. Crescent-shaped hypoechoic area around part of the gestational sac.

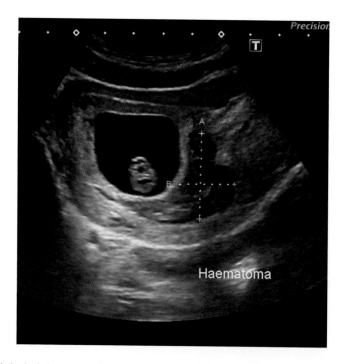

FIGURE 16.10 Subchorionic hematoma. Crescent-shaped hypoechoic area around part of the gestational sac.

Epidemiology

Gestational trophoblastic disease is rare, and studies have reported wide regional variations in the incidence of hydatidiform mole ranging from 0.57–1.1 per 1000 pregnancies in North America, Australia, New Zealand, and Europe, to 2 per 1000 pregnancies in Southeast Asia and Japan [8]. It is more common at the extremes of reproductive age, with women older than 40 years and younger than 20 years at increased risk [9].

In the United Kingdom, there is an effective registration and treatment program at designated centers. The program has been successful and achieved high cure (98%–100%) and low (5%–8%) chemotherapy rates.

Presentation

In the majority of cases, bleeding is the most common presenting symptom. Women may also present with various other symptoms including larger uterus than expected for gestational age, abnormally high serum beta-human chorionic gonadotropin (β-hCG) levels, hyperemesis, hypertension, theca-lutein cysts, and hyperthyroidism. However, as most molar pregnancies are now diagnosed in the first trimester with the advancement of ultrasound, the onset of these signs and symptoms is seen less often.

Hydatidiform Mole

A hydatidiform mole is abnormality characterized by diffuse swelling of villi, trophoblastic hyperplasia, and trophoblastic atypia.

Complete Hydatidiform Mole

Complete mole is the most common type of GTD accounting for 80% of cases. In a complete mole, the chromosomes are usually 46XX, with both sets of chromosomes originating from the father, and absent fetal tissue [10]. Women with complete hydatidiform moles typically present with bleeding during the first trimester. The human chorionic gonadotropin (β-hCG) levels are markedly elevated, and multiple large ovarian cysts ("theca lutein" cysts) may develop. Treatment involves evacuation of products from the uterus with follow-up urinary β-hCG for 6–12 months. Up to 15% of cases may progress to invasive mole and 5% to choriocarcinoma.

A complete hydatidiform mole is characterized on ultrasound by a large complex mass within the endometrial cavity. The mass usually contains multiple small cystic spaces within echogenic tissue (Figure 16.11), and no fetus is present. Prior to high-resolution ultrasonography, the classic appearance using older ultrasound machines was described as a snowstorm pattern representing the hydropic chorionic villi.

Partial Hydatidiform Mole

Partial molar pregnancies are a type of GTD that comprises both fetal tissue and abnormal placental tissue. These are usually triploid, 69 XXX or 69XXY, and occur when two sperm fertilize an ovum. The fetus is severely abnormal and tends to be incompatible with life. The serum β-hCG levels tend to be moderately elevated. The diagnosis is often made pathologically following a miscarriage.

On ultrasound, a partial molar pregnancy is seen as a gestational sac containing a fetus in the uterus and thickened placenta with focal cystic spaces (Figure 16.12). The fetus may be abnormal in appearance, and it is often demised at the time of the sonographic examination. In some cases, the placenta may appear similar to a hydropic placenta following demise of a nontriploid fetus, and the diagnosis is made only after pathological examination. If theca lutein cysts are seen in addition to the above findings, then a partial mole is more likely.

Treatment of hydatidiform moles involves evacuation of the uterus. In the majority of cases, this completely resolves the disease, but in a small number of cases, it recurs (persistent mole) and further treatment is necessary. Persistent moles may progress to invasion into the myometrium (invasive mole) or development into a malignancy (choriocarcinoma) that can metastasize. These complications, particularly persistent mole, occur in approximately 20% of complete moles and much less frequently with partial moles.

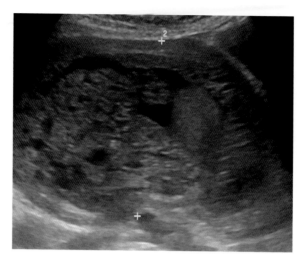

FIGURE 16.11   Complete hydatidiform mole. Large mass within the uterine cavity containing multiple small cystic spaces within echogenic tissue, and no fetus is present.

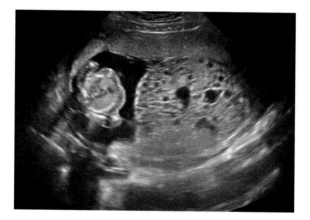

FIGURE 16.12   Partial hydatidiform mole. Gestational sac containing a fetus in the uterus and thickened placenta with focal cystic spaces.

Invasive Mole

An invasive mole is a benign tumor that results from myometrial invasion of a hydatidiform mole. It presents with persistently elevated β-hCG following hydatidiform mole. Up to 15% metastasize to lungs or vagina. Treatment involves chemotherapy, which carries high cure rates.

On ultrasound, the molar tissue is seen extending into the myometrium and distorting the uterine zonal structures. It may also invade parametrial tissue and blood vessels, and color Doppler demonstrates increased vasculature.

Gestational Choriocarcinoma

Choriocarcinoma is a rare malignant disease that arises following known molar pregnancy (50%), miscarriage (30%), or normal pregnancy (20%). Metastasis can occur, mainly to the lungs but can affect other areas including vagina, pelvis, liver, and brain [10,11].

Patients tend to present with significantly elevated β-hCG and may have multiple metastases without an identifiable primary.

On ultrasound, it can appear similar to hydatidiform mole or as a solid component in the uterus.

Placental Site Trophoblastic Tumor

Placental site trophoblastic tumor is a very rare form of GTD that develops at the placental implantation site. It often occurs following a normal pregnancy or miscarriage and produces small amounts of β-hCG. The tumor invades the myometrium, and the diagnosis is made after surgery and pathological examination.

Summary

The development of high-resolution transvaginal sonography has had a significant impact on the management of early pregnancy complications. The accuracy of diagnosis of first-trimester miscarriage allows women to receive treatment options and counseling at earlier gestations. The detection of gestational trophoblastic disease during early pregnancy scanning allows for prompt initiation of treatment and referral to specialist centers.

REFERENCES

1. Nybo Andersen AM, Wohlfahrt J, Christens P, Olsen J, and Melbye M. Maternal age and fetal loss: Population based register linkage study. *BMJ.* 2000;320:1708–12.
2. Sotiriadis A, Papatheodorou S, and Makrydimas G. Threatened miscarriage: Evaluation and treatment. *BMJ.* 2004;329(7458):152–5.
3. Van den Berg MM, van Maarle MC, van Wely M, and Goddijn M. Genetics of early miscarriage. *Biochim Biophys Acta.* 2012;1822:1951–9.
4. National Institute for Health and Care Excellence (NICE). Ectopic pregnancy and miscarriage: Diagnosis and initial management. *NICE Clinical Guidance* 126. 2019.
5. Doubilet P, Benson C, Bourne T, et al. Diagnostic criteria for nonviable pregnancy early in the first trimester. *N Eng J Med.* 2013;369:1443–51.
6. Atri M, Rao A, Boylan C, Rasty G, and Gerber D. Best predictors of grayscale ultrasound combined with color Doppler in the diagnosis of retained products of conception. *J Clin Ultrasound.* 2011;39(3):122–7.
7. Bennett GL, Bromley B, Lieberman E, and Benacerraf BR. Subchorionic hemorrhage in first-trimester pregnancies: Prediction of pregnancy outcome with sonography. *Radiology.* 1996;200(3):803–6.
8. Atrash HK, Hogue CJR, and Grimes DA. Epidemiology of hydatidiform mole during early gestation. *Am J Obstet Gynecol.* 1986;154:906–9.
9. Sebire NJ, Foskett M, Fisher RA, et al. Risk of partial and complete molar pregnancy in relation to maternal age. *Br J Obstet Gynecol.* 2002;109:99–102.
10. Lurain J. Gestational trophoblastic disease I; epidemiology, pathology, clinical presentation and diagnosis of gestational trophoblastic disease, and management of hydatiform mole. *AJOG.* 2010;203:531–9.
11. Royal College of Obstetricians and Gynaecologists. The management of gestational trophoblastic disease. Green-Top Guideline 38. 2010.

17

Ectopic Pregnancy and Pregnancy of Unknown Location

Ghada Salman

Tubal Ectopic Pregnancy

Definition

Tubal ectopic pregnancy is a pregnancy that implants outside the uterine cavity and within the ampullary (73%), isthmic (13%), or fimbrial (12%) portions of the Fallopian tube [1].

Incidence

The three most commonly used denominators to record the incidence of ectopic pregnancies are number of births, number of pregnancies, and number of women of reproductive age (15–44 years) in the population [2]. The incidence of ectopic pregnancy in the developed world has been reported to be 1%–2% of all pregnancies and has remained relatively static in recent years. The incidence is thought to be higher in the developing countries, but specific numbers are not very well known [3–7].

Etiology

Abnormalities of the tubal morphology and/or changes in the tubal microenvironment resulting from damage to the tubal mucosa and/or disturbance to tubal muscular contractility due to tubal inflammation have been implicated in impairing migration of the fertilized ovum and halting it within the fallopian tube, permitting early implantation and leading to delay in embryo transfer and incorrect signaling, resulting in abnormal implantation. It has also been suggested that an altered estrogen/progesterone ratio can cause malfunction of the tubal smooth muscle [8–13]. The etiology behind ectopic pregnancy in the absence of any tubal factors remains unclear. Poor quality of the morula or a chromosomally abnormal pregnancy have been suggested [14]. However, Goddijn et al. showed in his study that the rate of chromosomally abnormal ectopic pregnancies is not higher than intrauterine pregnancies [15]. The effect of the male factor has also been suggested in the pathophysiology behind ectopic pregnancies, but more studies are needed to confirm this.

Prognosis

Despite advances in the diagnosis and management of ectopic pregnancy, it remains one of the most important causes of morbidity and mortality in women of reproductive age worldwide. The estimated maternal mortality is 0.3 per 100,000 maternities or 0.2 per 1000 ectopics. This figure is even higher in developing countries, accounting for as high as 6%–10% of pregnancy-associated mortality [16–19], while the rate of a normal intrauterine pregnancy after ectopic pregnancy is around 60%–66%. The recurrence rate of tubal ectopic pregnancy has been reported to be 5%–20% after one previous ectopic pregnancy and around 32% if greater than one previous ectopic [20–22].

Risk Factors

Most of the risk factors are related to distortion of the Fallopian tube anatomy or to their effect on its microenvironment (Box 17.1) [23–37].

BOX 17.1　SOME OF THE RISK FACTORS FOR ECTOPIC PREGNANCY

- Assisted reproductive techniques (ART) especially *in vitro* fertilization (IVF) and ovulation induction
- Pelvic inflammatory disease (PID), especially *Chlamydia trachomatis*
- Pelvic surgery
- Endometriosis
- Previous ectopic pregnancy
- Some contraception, especially progestogen-only pills and failure of intrauterine contraceptive devices (IUCDs)
- Smoking, significantly higher risk if more than 20 cigarettes per day

---

Clinical Presentation

Traditionally, patients who presented with pain and vaginal bleeding in early pregnancy were suspected to have an ectopic pregnancy. However, these symptoms are not uncommon in the early weeks of gestation and can occur in about one-third of women [38–40]. According to Shwartz and Di Pietro, the classic triad of amenorrhea, abdominal pain, and vaginal bleeding happened in less than 50% of the women with ectopic pregnancy, and in only 10%–15% of the women who had a clinical suspicion of ectopic pregnancy was the diagnosis confirmed. It is also interesting to know that about 9% of women with ectopic pregnancy have no clinical symptoms, and about 30% have no clinical signs of ectopic pregnancy [41]. Women with ruptured ectopic pregnancy usually present with symptoms and signs of shock, including syncope, tachycardia, pallor and collapse, abdominal distension, and severe tenderness that indicates significant intraperitoneal bleed [42–46].

An atypical presentation, such as diarrhea, vomiting, and rectal pressure, has also been reported by women with ectopic pregnancy. Death reports over the years have shown that most deaths from ectopic pregnancy were related to misdiagnosis [16,18,47,48]. Ectopic pregnancy can also mimic other gynecological and nongynecological conditions (Box 17.2) [47,49]. It is therefore of vast importance that clinicians are aware of the atypical clinical presentations of ectopic pregnancy and to have a low threshold for suspecting it in any woman in the reproductive age who presents with abdominal pain and vaginal bleeding.

BOX 17.2　ECTOPIC PREGNANCY CAN MIMIC OTHER CONDITIONS

- Gynecological condition:
  - Ruptured ovarian cysts
  - Ovarian torsion
  - Pelvic inflammatory disease (PID)
  - Miscarriage
- Urinary tract disorders: such as urinary tract infection
- Gastrointestinal disorders: such as gastroenteritis and appendicitis

---

Diagnosis

Early identification and correct diagnosis of women with ectopic pregnancies are crucial for reducing the risk of rupture and allowing a more conservative approach to be used. A combination of ultrasound scanning, serum beta-human chorionic gonadotropin (β-hCG) with or without serum progesterone measurements have been used over the years to diagnose ectopic pregnancies [50–52].

Ultrasound Diagnosis

Although the first ultrasound criteria for the diagnosis of ectopic pregnancy were published in 1969 [53], the introduction of high-definition transvaginal ultrasonography (TVS) has revolutionized the diagnosis of both intrauterine and extrauterine gestations, and it is now considered as the diagnostic method of choice and an acceptable imaging tool for women presenting with early pregnancy complications such as pain or bleeding [54–56]. Using the vaginal probe will also enable the palpation of the pelvic organs under vision. This helps to assess pelvic organ mobility (sliding sign) and to locate the site of tenderness more accurately [57].

The TVS has been shown by several studies to have a high sensitivity (87%–99%), specificity (94%–99.9%), and accuracy (75%–80%) when used to diagnose ectopic gestations [58–60]. However, the accuracy of ultrasound will depend among other factors on the size of the ectopic at the time of presentation. A study looking at the accuracy of diagnosing ectopic pregnancy at first presentation found that women with higher levels of β-hCG and more advanced gestational age or larger size ectopic pregnancy had a better diagnosis on transvaginal scan [61,62].

The benefit of transabdominal sonography (TAS) examination in the diagnosis of early pregnancy is doubtful. A high rate of false negatives and false positives has been reported with its use due to the difficulty in identifying early intrauterine pregnancy or a small size ectopic pregnancy. This would result in uncertainty when excluding ectopic pregnancy. However, the TAS may be useful in women with a large fibroid uterus or in the presence of a large pelvic mass [63]. Abdominal scans should also be considered in women with previous abdominal surgeries, such as multiple cesarean sections due to the likelihood of extensive adhesions between the uterus and anterior abdominal wall [49,64].

Ultrasound Criteria for Diagnosis of Tubal Ectopic Pregnancy

Tubal ectopic pregnancy usually presents as an adnexal mass (within the fallopian tube) adjacent to but separate from the ovary that moves away from it on gentle pressure (sliding sign) and with no evidence of an intrauterine pregnancy. It is important to note that around 70% to 80% of ectopic pregnancies will be on the same side as the corpus luteum. This is useful when localizing the site of the ectopic pregnancy [43,65].

In a meta-analysis of 2216 women, the presence of an adnexal mass separate to the ovary had a sensitivity of 84.4% and a specificity of 98.9% when diagnosing ectopic pregnancy [66].

The adnexal mass will have one of the following sonographic features (Box 17.3) [58,61,65–69] (Figures 17.1–17.5).

BOX 17.3   TUBAL ECTOPIC PREGNANCY

- An adnexal (tubal) mass that moves separate to the ovary—it can have one of the following criteria:
  - An inhomogeneous or solid echogenic mass (50%–60%)
  - An empty gestational sac surrounded by a hyperechoic ring (bagel sign) (20%–40%)
  - A gestational sac surrounded by a hyperechoic ring and containing a yolk sac or a yolk sac and an embryo with or without cardiac activity (15%–20%)
- Color Doppler sonography demonstrate increased vascularity at the adnexal mass
- Pulsed Doppler sonography demonstrate a high-velocity, low-resistance blood flow pattern in the adnexal mass; this reflects the trophoblastic blood flow

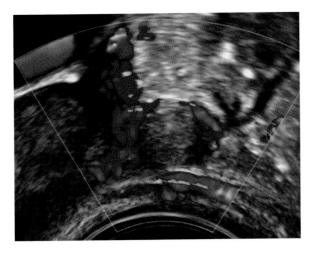

FIGURE 17.1   Tubal ectopic: Tubal pregnancy presenting as an inhomogeneous or solid echogenic tubal mass.

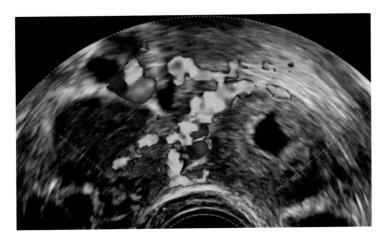

FIGURE 17.2   Tubal ectopic: An empty gestational sac surrounded by a hyperechoic ring (bagel sign). Color Doppler sonography demonstrating trophoblastic blood flow.

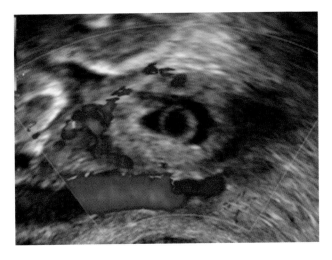

FIGURE 17.3   Tubal ectopic: A gestational sac surrounded by a hyperechoic ring with a yolk sac.

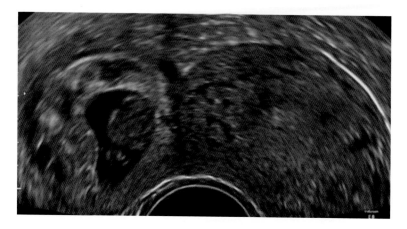

FIGURE 17.4   Tubal ectopic: A gestational sac surrounded by a hyperechoic ring with a yolk sac and an embryo.

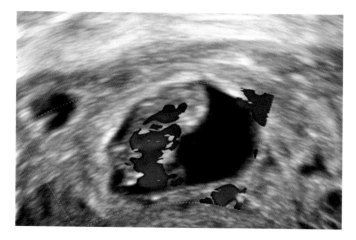

FIGURE 17.5   Tubal ectopic: A gestational sac surrounded by a hyperechoic ring containing an embryo with cardiac activity. This is diagnostic of ectopic pregnancy.

Other suspicious but inconclusive sonographic features that can coexist with ectopic pregnancy include the following:

Hemoperitoneum: Blood within the pouch of Douglas or around the uterus that occurs with ruptured ectopic. This is different from the small amount of free fluid (transudate) that is commonly seen in the pouch of Douglas of women with early pregnancy due to increased vascular permeability [70]. (Figure 17.6).

Pseudosac: An area of fluid collected within the endometrial cavity due to the hormonal changes associated with pregnancy, resulting from a localized breakdown of the decidualized endometrium. It is reported to be seen in 8% of all ectopic pregnancies. An experienced ultrasound operator should be able to differentiate a pseudosac from an early intrauterine gestational sac (Box 17.4) [71,72] (Figure 17.7).

Empty uterus and endometrial thickness: The measurement of endometrial thickness in patients with an empty uterus and a β-hCG level below the discriminatory zone (less than 1500 mIU/mL) has been suggested to aid in the diagnoses of ectopic pregnancy. A high sensitivity (100%) with an endometrial thickness of less than 6 mm and a high specificity (100%) with an endometrial thickness greater than 13 mm was reported by some studies [73,74]. However, other studies suggested little value in measuring endometrial thickness [75,76] (Figure 17.8).

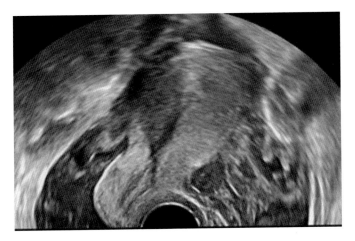

FIGURE 17.6   Hemoperitoneum: Blood visualized within the pouch of Douglas or around the uterus can occur with a ruptured ectopic pregnancy. When blood is noted anterior to the uterus, it indicates significant bleed.

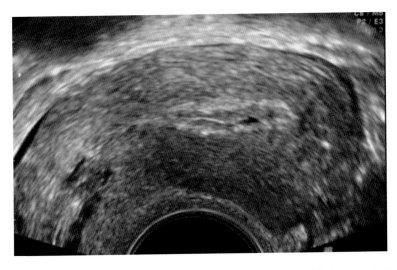

FIGURE 17.7   Pseudosac: Central location within the endometrial cavity and absence of the hyperechoic decidual reaction.

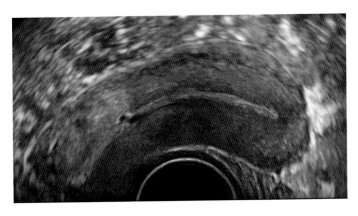

FIGURE 17.8   Endometrial thickness: The association between thin endometrium and diagnosis of ectopic pregnancy has been reported.

In a recent systematic review and meta-analysis, a low sensitivity (32.4%) but a high specificity (93.3%) for predicting ectopic pregnancy were demonstrated when an empty uterus was found on ultrasound examination. Similarly, the pseudosac had a very low sensitivity (3.3%) and a high specificity (95%). The presence of adnexal mass and free fluid showed a sensitivity of 66.2% and 41.2% and a specificity of 91.3% and 90.6%, respectively. The conclusion was that in the absence of an extrauterine viable pregnancy, the ultrasound had a good specificity but a poor sensitivity for identifying tubal ectopic pregnancy [77].

BOX 17.4   PSEUDO-SAC

This is differentiated from a true gestational sac by the following:

- Its central location within the endometrial cavity, unlike a true early gestation sac that is typically eccentrically placed
- Transient, and changes position during the examination
- Absence of the hyperechoic decidual reaction (double ring sign)

Magnetic Resonance Imaging

Magnetic resonance imaging (MRI) can be useful when the ultrasound scan is inconclusive, especially in cases where a precise and early diagnosis of ectopic pregnancy is essential, such as with a damaged contralateral fallopian tube or in cases of persistent pregnancy of unknown location (PUL). The MRI can diagnose ectopic pregnancy by visualizing tubal wall enhancements and fresh tubal hematoma [78,79].

Nontubal Ectopic Pregnancy

Ectopic pregnancy can occur in other locations within the pelvis or abdomen other than the fallopian tubes. Despite the fact that these types of ectopic pregnancies are less common (less than 10% of all ectopic pregnancies), they are usually associated with more adverse outcomes and a higher maternal morbidity and mortality rate when compared with tubal ectopic pregnancies [1,16]. This is mainly due to their tendency to remain symptom free in early gestation until they rupture in the later stages of the first trimester or in the second trimester, causing severe hemorrhage and acute clinical symptoms and signs. In addition, clinicians are often less familiar with these types of gestations, which can lead to delay in the correct diagnosis and initiation of the appropriate treatment [80,81]. The use of three-dimensional (3D) ultrasound scan and in selected cases the use of other imaging modalities such as MRI have helped provide more precise information on the location of the pregnancy and thus facilitated an early and more accurate diagnosis of these nontubal ectopic pregnancies [78,79,82,83].

Cesarean Scar Ectopic Pregnancy

Definition

Cesarean scar ectopic pregnancy (CSP) is a form of ectopic pregnancy in which the implantation occurs in the scar of a previous cesarean section (CS) delivery. The gestational sac is located outside the endometrial cavity and is completely surrounded by the myometrium and fibrous tissue of the scar [84,85].

Incidence

The reported incidence ranges between 1 in 1800 and 1 in 2500 pregnancies or approximately 1 in 2000 pregnancies and this incidence is believed to be increasing in parallel with the increase in cesarean section rate world-wide [86,87].

Etiology

Invasion of the myometrium through a microtubular tract between the CS scar and the endometrium as a result of the damage created by the previous CS. A similar tract can also develop from the trauma of other uterine surgery, such as uterine curettage and endometrial sampling [84–88].

Risk Factors

The relationship between multiple cesarean deliveries, increase in scar surface area, and the size of anterior uterine wall defect have been described by many studies [89,90]. Evidence from a recent cohort study is that the risk of CSP increases progressively with the number of previous cesarean deliveries. Compared with one CS, the odds ratio (OR) is 3.1 (95% confidence interval [CI] 1.6–5.9) for women with two previous CS, 4.9 (95% CI 1.7–14.4) for three previous CS, and 7.8 (95% CI 1.4–18.6) with four or more previous CS [91].

Prognosis

A high percentage of CSP will end up with a miscarriage. In one study, 44% of CSPs ended in spontaneous first-trimester miscarriage [92]. If CSP is developing and left untreated, it can progress into an abnormally invasive placenta, which can result in uterine rupture and life-threatening hemorrhage [93,94].

The rate of recurrence of CSP has been reported by different studies to be 5%–15.6%, while the rate of successful pregnancy post CSP is 60%–65% [92,95–97].

Diagnosis

The clinical presentation of CSP can range widely from an incidental finding in a completely asymptomatic women to severe abdominal pain and profuse bleeding with rupture. However, the more common presentation is a painless first-trimester vaginal bleeding. Other presentations include vaginal bleeding with mild abdominal pain or abdominal pain without bleeding [98–101]. The first case of scar ectopic pregnancy was reported in 1990 by Rempen and Albert and coincided with the introduction of transvaginal ultrasound that allowed more accurate diagnosis of early pregnancies [102].

Two types of CSP have been described in the literature depending on the site of trophoblast implantation. These were first described 18 years ago by Vial et al. The first type (type I, endogenic type) refers to implantation in the scar with the progression of the pregnancy into the uterine cavity. This can allow the pregnancy to reach an advanced stage and viable birth, but with the increased risks of abnormal placental adherence (30%–40%) and massive bleeding from the placental site at delivery. The second type (type II, exogenic type) is more serious, and it involves deep implantation and invasion of the trophoblast tissue into the uterine myometrium with progression toward the bladder and abdominal cavity. This type usually results in uterine rupture and life-threatening hemorrhage in the first trimester of pregnancy [103]. Hwang et al. categorized CSPs slightly differently into intramural and nonintramural [104], while Zhang et al. classified them into risky type and stable type. The risky type is further divided into type 1 (1a, 1b, 1c), type 2, and type 3 [105]. More recently, Lin and colleagues classified CSP into four grades based on their ultrasound criteria, including the depth of implantation of the gestational sac into the anterior uterine wall and the thickness of the overlying myometrium [106]. All of these classifications were suggested with the intention to develop a better management strategy for CSP.

An early and accurate diagnosis of CSP needs a great awareness from the examining physician, a detailed history taking, and a highly experienced ultrasound operator. It is also essential that pregnant women with a history of cesarean delivery are screened early in the first trimester of pregnancy to rule out scar implantation. Using TVS, CSP can be diagnosed with a high accuracy (96%) and a good sensitivity (86%). The sonographic features are shown in Box 17.5 [65,107–112] (Figures 17.9–17.13).

BOX 17.5   CESAREAN SCAR ECTOPIC

- Empty uterine cavity.
- Discontinuity in the anterior uterine wall.
- A pregnancy mass or a gestational sac ± a yolk sac ± a fetal pole ± heartbeat activity is seen embedded in the anterior uterine wall in the cesarean/hysterotomy scar, usually at the level of the internal os.
- A thin (less than 5 mm) or absent myometrial layer between the pregnancy sac and the urinary bladder.
- Empty endocervical canal.
- Doppler sonography typically shows (prominent) high-velocity, low-impedance peritrophoblastic flow vascularity and is useful for assessing the proximity to or the possible invasion of the bladder wall.
- Negative sliding sign. By applying gentle pressure during a transvaginal ultrasound scan, the gestational sac will not move or change position. A miscarriage on the other hand will be easily displaced.
- Three-dimensional ultrasound can be used to enhance the diagnostic accuracy. Surface-rendered images help identify subtle anatomical details of the trophoblastic ring around the gestational sac.

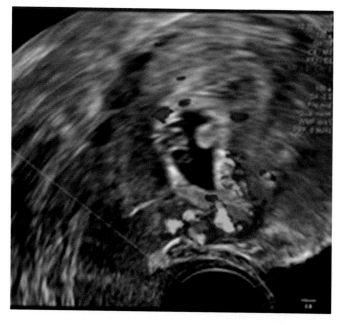

FIGURE 17.9   Type 1 or endogenic cesarean scar ectopic: An implantation on the cesarean scar with progression toward the uterine cavity.

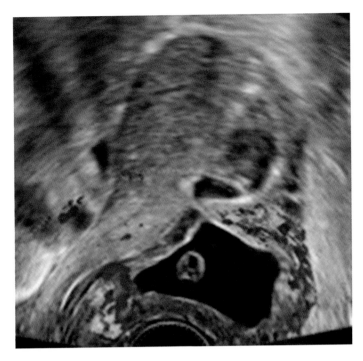

FIGURE 17.10 Type 2 or exogenic cesarean scar ectopic: A deep implantation into the cesarean scar defect and the surrounding myometrium growing toward the bladder and abdominal cavity.

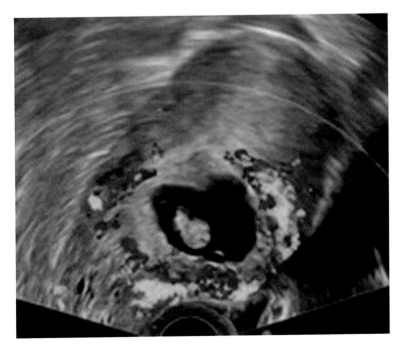

FIGURE 17.11 Cesarean scar ectopic: Color flow Doppler shows a distinct peritrophoblastic perfusion surrounding the gestation sac which can add to the diagnostic efficacy.

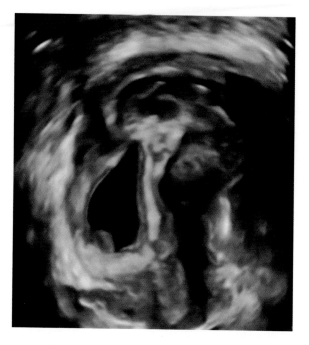

FIGURE 17.12   Cesarean scar ectopic: Three-dimensional imaging can be used to enhance the diagnostic accuracy.

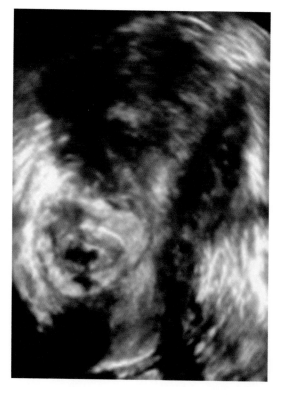

FIGURE 17.13   Cesarean scar ectopic—three-dimensional image: The surface-rendered image helps identify subtle anatomical details of the trophoblastic ring and its position.

Cervical Pregnancy

Definition

Cervical pregnancy is the implantation of the pregnancy in the wall of the endocervical canal below the level of the internal os [113,114].

Incidence

The incidence is about 1 in 2500 to 1 in 18,000 pregnancies or less than 1% of all ectopic pregnancies [114,115].

Risk Factors

Few risk factors have been linked to cervical ectopic pregnancy including intrauterine adhesions, fibroids, previous instrumentation of the cervix, intrauterine device, and ART, which has contributed to a higher incidence of cervical pregnancy (1 in 1000 *in vitro* fertilization [IVF] pregnancies) [114,116,117].

Etiology

Although the exact etiology remains unclear, damage to the cervical/endometrial lining during uterine procedures or a fast travel of the fertilized egg toward the cervical canal before its implantation in the endometrial cavity are thought to be the main causes [114,115,116].

Clinical Presentation

The typical presentation is usually first-trimester painless vaginal bleeding; however, the bleeding can be major and life threatening due to penetration of the trophoblast into the uterine vasculature [118–120].

Diagnosis

Historically, cervical ectopics were suspected at the time of uterine curettage due to heavy intraoperative bleeding. With time, the diagnosis and management of cervical ectopic have changed [121,122]. Using ultrasound, the first reported cervical ectopic pregnancy was diagnosed in 1978 [123]. As with other types of ectopic pregnancies, early and accurate diagnosis is essential to prevent morbidity and mortality. It is also very important to consider the differential diagnosis of cervical ectopic pregnancy, especially an early low implanted intrauterine pregnancy and a miscarriage with a gestational sac passing through the cervical canal [124–126]. The sonographic features are shown in Box 17.6 [65,113,118,126,127] (Figures 17.14 and 17.15).

BOX 17.6   CERVICAL ECTOPIC

- Empty uterine cavity
- A ballooned cervical canal
- An hourglass (barrel-shaped) uterine shape
- Evidence of trophoblast tissue invading the cervical wall substance
- A gestational sac seen below the level of the internal cervical os
- Closed internal os
- Negative sliding sign, when the gestational sac does not change its shape or location with gentle pressure with the vaginal probe
- Doppler sonography—demonstrate trophoblastic blood flow

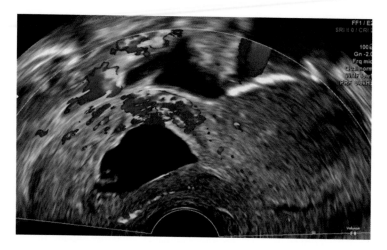

FIGURE 17.14 Cervical ectopic: Empty uterine cavity and a ballooned cervical canal. Evidence of trophoblast tissue invading the cervical wall substance.

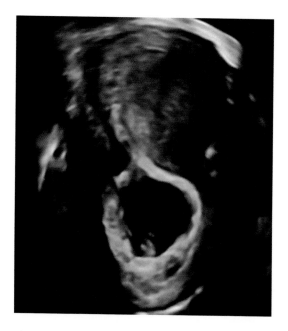

FIGURE 17.15 Cervical ectopic—three-dimensional image: A ballooned cervical canal and an hourglass uterine shape.

Heterotopic Pregnancy

Definition

A heterotopic pregnancy is a combination of an intrauterine pregnancy and an ectopic pregnancy of any kind occurring simultaneously [1,128].

Incidence

The reported incidence is 1 in 2600–30,000 pregnancies. The incidence is higher (1–3 in 100 pregnancies) in women undergoing ART with the risk increasing with more embryos transferred, reaching as high as 1 in 45 if more than four embryos are returned [129,130].

Risk Factors

In addition to the general risk factors, congenital or acquired uterine cavity abnormalities have been linked to this type of pregnancy [131–133].

Diagnosis

The clinical presentations are slightly different from other types of ectopics in the fact that vaginal bleeding is not common due to the presence of a normal intrauterine gestation. Other more frequent presentations include abdominal pain due to peritoneal irritation, or acute abdomen with signs of shock if the ectopic pregnancy has ruptured [134,135].

The diagnosis of heterotopic pregnancy is considered as one of the most challenging conditions due to the presence of the intrauterine pregnancy, which can give the clinician a false reassurance of a normally located pregnancy. In one study, 50% of heterotopic pregnancies were missed by ultrasound [136,137]. Early diagnosis is crucial for optimal management; thus, caution should always be taken when examining women who have clinical symptoms and/or signs of ectopic pregnancy, even if a normal intrauterine pregnancy is visualized and this is even more important if the pregnancy is through an IVF [128,134,138]. The diagnosis should also be considered in the presence of more than one corpus luteum on scan. The sonographic features of heterotopic pregnancy are essentially similar to those of an intrauterine pregnancy in addition to ectopic pregnancy. Although in most of the cases the ectopic component is tubal, other types of ectopic pregnancies have been reported [136,139,140–142] (Figures 17.16–17.22).

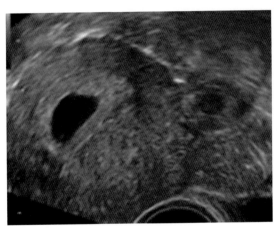

FIGURE 17.16 Heterotopic pregnancy: A normally positioned intrauterine pregnancy is seen in combination with a tubal ectopic pregnancy.

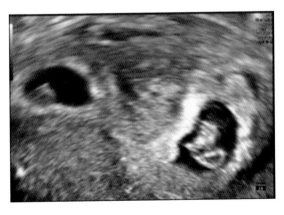

FIGURE 17.17 Heterotopic pregnancy: A gestational sac seen inside the uterine cavity and another sac seen separate and lateral; connected to the endometrial cavity by an echogenic line.

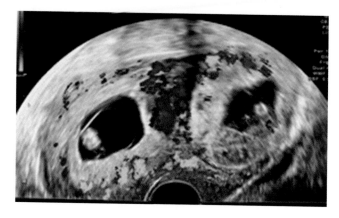

FIGURE 17.18 Heterotopic pregnancy: A normally positioned intrauterine pregnancy is seen alongside a cesarean scar ectopic pregnancy.

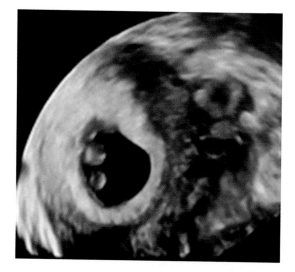

FIGURE 17.19 Heterotopic pregnancy—three-dimensional image: An intrauterine pregnancy is seen in addition to a tubal ectopic pregnancy.

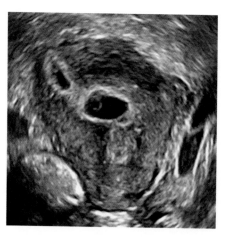

FIGURE 17.20 Heterotopic pregnancy: Three-dimensional ultrasound can facilitate diagnosis. Accurate position of the interstitial ectopic pregnancy is demonstrated.

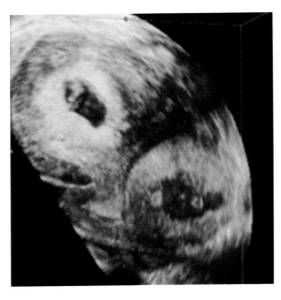

FIGURE 17.21 Heterotopic pregnancy—three-dimensional image: An intrauterine pregnancy is seen in addition to a caesarean scar ectopic.

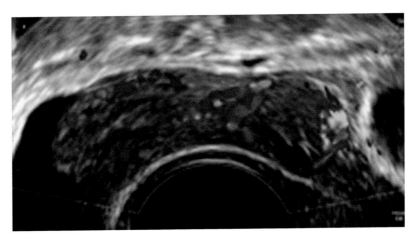

FIGURE 17.22 The diagnosis of heterotopic pregnancy should be considered in the presence of more than one corpus luteum on scan.

Abdominal Pregnancy

Definition

An abdominal pregnancy occurs if there is implantation of the ectopic pregnancy in the peritoneal cavity outside the fallopian tubes and the ovaries [143].

Incidence

The incidence is one in 2200–10,200 of all pregnancies or less than 1% of all ectopic gestations. However, this incidence is reported to be higher in developing countries [143,144].

Risk Factors

The risk factors are similar to those described for other ectopic pregnancies, especially pelvic inflammatory disease. However, the use of cocaine has been reported to be exclusively associated with abdominal pregnancy [143–145].

Prognosis

Despite its rarity, abdominal pregnancy can be a life-threatening condition if not diagnosed and treated early, with a maternal mortality rate of 0.5%–20% and a perinatal mortality rate of 40%–95% [146–148].

Etiology

Two types of abdominal pregnancies have been described in the literature, a primary and a secondary. The primary type is rare, and it results from direct peritoneal implantation of the fertilized egg. The secondary type is more common, and it occurs from reimplantation of an ectopic pregnancy in the peritoneal cavity after dislodging from its original position, most commonly after it ruptures or miscarry from the fallopian tube. Another classification for abdominal pregnancies is early (less than 20 weeks) and advanced (more than 20 weeks) [1,143,144,149].

Diagnosis

The most common presentation is lower abdominal pain. The pain can be generalized or localized to the site of implantation, such as the pouch of Douglas, bowel, or bladder. Distant locations such as the liver, spleen, or diaphragm have also been described. In advanced gestations, the diagnosis can be suspected on examination when the fetal parts are easily palpated through the abdominal wall and/or when there is an abnormal lie of the fetus [150–152].

Although ultrasound is the main diagnostic method, it remains challenging with greater than 50% of cases missed antenatally [153,154]. MRI can be used to confirm the diagnosis and delineate the degree of peritoneal involvement for the preoperative management plan [155].

The sonographic features are shown in Box 17.7 [65,156–159] (Figure 17.23).

BOX 17.7   ABDOMINAL ECTOPIC

- Empty uterus.
- Pregnancy is outside uterus, tubes, and ovaries.
- Absence of a myometrium around the pregnancy/fetus.

In advanced pregnancy:

- Abnormal fetal lie, and relative oligohydramnios.
- Fetal parts close to maternal abdominal wall.
- Poorly visualized placenta that is located outside the uterus.
- Magnetic resonance imaging (MRI) is useful to confirm the diagnosis and identify placental implantation over vital structures, such as the bowel or major blood vessels to prevent major intraoperative complications.

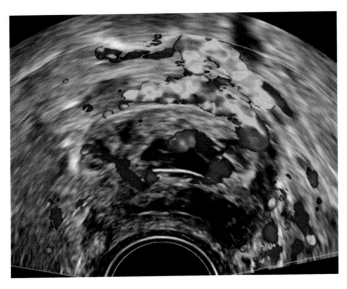

FIGURE 17.23 Abdominal ectopic: Absence of a myometrium around the pregnancy. Pregnancy located outside the uterus, tubes and ovaries seen at the left side of the pelvis.

Ovarian Pregnancy

Definition

An ovarian pregnancy is an ectopic pregnancy that is implanted in the ovary [160].

Incidence

The incidence can vary from 1 in 7000 to 1 in 40,000 deliveries. It is one of the most common types of nontubal ectopic pregnancy and accounts for 0.5%–3% of all ectopic gestations [161,162].

Etiology

Ovarian pregnancy is classified into primary and secondary types. The primary type is one of the rarest types of ectopic pregnancy, and it happens when the fertilization takes place within the ovary due to lack of release of the ovum from the ruptured follicle. The secondary type occurs due to tubal miscarriage, resulting in implantation of the pregnancy in the ovarian stroma [163–166].

Risk Factors

Although primary ovarian ectopic pregnancy may occur without the presence of any risk factors, intrauterine device use, history of tubal sterilization, and use of assisted reproductive technique, especially ovulation induction, have been linked to ovarian ectopic pregnancy [167–170]. Razeiel et al. reported in his study that 90% of ovarian pregnancy occurred in women who have an intrauterine contraceptive device [159], while Grimes et al. reported infertility factors to be the risk factor in more than 50% of women [171].

Prognosis

Ovarian ectopic pregnancy will usually (91%) result in rupture in the first weeks of gestation. Progression beyond early stages is rare. However, there have been cases of ovarian ectopic pregnancies progressing into the second or third trimester before rupture. There have been no reported cases of recurrent ovarian ectopic pregnancies [172–177].

Diagnosis

The first case of ovarian pregnancy was reported in 1876 [175]. Women with ovarian pregnancy most commonly present with pelvic pain with or without vaginal bleeding early in gestation due to ovarian tissue invasion by the trophoblastic tissue, while a ruptured ovarian pregnancy can present with severe lower abdominal pain and signs of acute abdomen. These signs and symptoms are similar to tubal ectopic gestation or ruptured hemorrhagic corpus luteum cyst. In one study, two-thirds of ovarian ectopics were diagnosed clinically as hemorrhagic corpus luteum [178–181]. Sonographic features are shown in Box 17.8 [65,139,182–185] (Figures 17.24–17.26).

> **BOX 17.8   OVARIAN ECTOPIC**
>
> - Empty uterus
> - Complex ovarian mass
> - An enlarged ovary containing a gestational sac–like (cystic) structure with or without yolk sac or embryo surrounded by a thick echogenic ring
> - The presence of an ovarian tissue around the pregnancy sac/mass
> - Negative sliding sign—not possible to separate the cystic structure from the ovary on gentle pressure with the vaginal probe
> - The corpus luteum can be on the same or contralateral side
> - Doppler sonography detection of a trophoblast implantation and/or fetal heart pulsation within the ovary

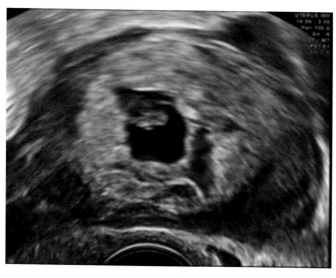

FIGURE 17.24   Ovarian ectopic: An enlarged ovary containing a gestational sac–like (cystic) structure surrounded by a thick echogenic ring. The presence of an ovarian tissue around the pregnancy sac.

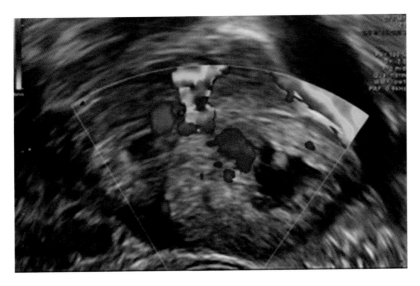

FIGURE 17.25 Ovarian ectopic: The corpus luteum can be on the same side. Doppler flow helps to detect trophoblast implantation within the ovary.

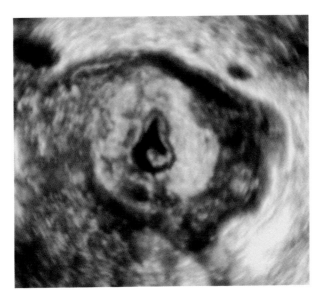

FIGURE 17.26 Ovarian ectopic—three-dimensional image: Thick echogenic ring surrounding the gestational sac within the ovary.

Interstitial Ectopic Pregnancy

Definition

An interstitial ectopic pregnancy develops in the uterine (interstitial) portion of the fallopian tube, implanting in the myometrium and growing either medially or bulging laterally [1,186].

Incidence

The incidence is 2%–7% of all ectopic pregnancies or 1 in 2500–5000 live birth [186,187].

Etiology

The etiology is abnormal transfer of the fertilized ovum within the fallopian tube. This can occur secondary to a damaged tube or due to hormonal imbalances causing a change in the transport mechanism of the tube [187–189].

Risk Factors

Risk factors include partial salpingectomy in addition to others [187–189].

Prognosis

Interstitial ectopic pregnancy is associated with a high incidence of complications. The maternal mortality rate is high at 2%–2.5% or 1 per 1000 interstitial pregnancies, which is twice the reported mortality rate from tubal ectopic pregnancies [188–190]. This is attributable to the fact that the muscular component of the interstitial part can provide distensibility and support, allowing the pregnancy to grow much further (12–14 weeks) than if it was implanted in other parts of the fallopian tube. In addition, the high vascularity means its rupture is usually associated with significant bleeding. Rupture of an interstitial ectopic pregnancy has been reported at all gestational ages, including advanced pregnancy [188,190,191].

Diagnosis

The common clinical symptoms of tubal ectopic pregnancy can be found in only one-quarter of women with interstitial ectopics. However, the use of 3D ultrasound, which provides superior images of the fundal aspect of the uterus and the interstitial section of the Fallopian tubes, has helped improve the diagnosis of this form of ectopics. The sonographic features are shown in Box 17.9 [65,192–196] (Figures 17.27–17.30).

BOX 17.9   INTERSTITIAL ECTOPIC

- An empty uterine cavity.
- A gestational sac/pregnancy mass located laterally, in the interstitial (intramural part) portion of the fallopian tube.
- An incomplete ring of thin uterine myometrium (less than 5 mm) surrounding the chorionic sac.
- The interstitial line sign—An echogenic line is seen connecting the endometrial cavity to the medial edge of the pregnancy mass (80% sensitivity, 98% specificity).
- Color Doppler sonography demonstrates a circular peritrophoblastic perfusion surrounding the gestational sac.
- Three-dimensional ultrasound is useful in most cases to show the position of the interstitial pregnancy.

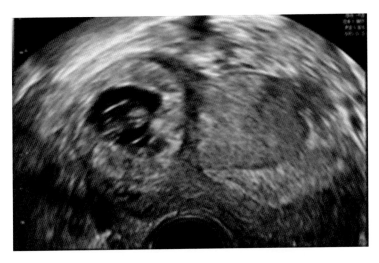

FIGURE 17.27 Interstitial ectopic: An empty uterine cavity with a gestational sac noted separate and lateral to the corner of the uterine cavity. A line is seen connecting the endometrial cavity to the medial edge of the pregnancy sac (the interstitial line sign).

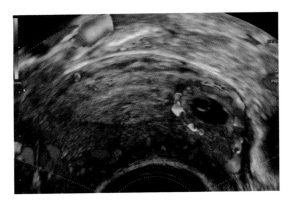

FIGURE 17.28 Interstitial ectopic: Color Doppler sonography demonstrating trophoblastic blood flow surrounding the gestation sac.

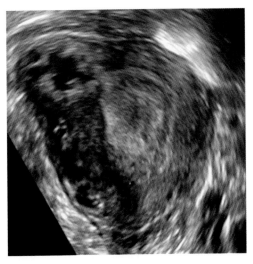

FIGURE 17.29 Interstitial ectopic: Three-dimensional imaging can show accurately the position of the ectopic gestational sac.

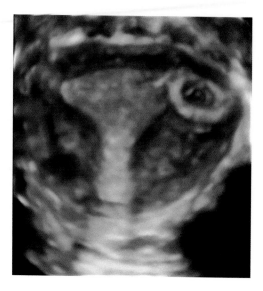

FIGURE 17.30   Interstitial ectopic: Three-dimensional imaging can demonstrate accurate details of the trophoblastic ring and the interstitial line.

Cornual Pregnancy

Definition

The terms *interstitial, cornual,* and *angular pregnancy* have been used as synonymous by some authors; however, a true cornual pregnancy is a pregnancy that develops in a rudimentary, noncommunicating horn of a unicornuate uterus [82,197–200].

Risk Factors

Congenital uterine anomaly [202,203].

Incidence

The incidence is 1/76,000 of all pregnancies [1,65,197].

Diagnosis

Similar to interstitial pregnancy, in around 50% of cases, the pregnancy can remain symptom free in the early weeks of gestation until it ruptures in the second trimester with major internal bleeding. The sonographic features are shown in Box 17.10 [65,200–207] (Figures 17.31–17.33).

BOX 17.10   CORNUAL ECTOPIC

- A unicornuate uterus with a single interstitial portion of fallopian tube.
- The gestational sac or products of conception separate from the main uterine body and completely surrounded by myometrium.
- A thick vascular pedicle adjoining the pregnancy to the main uterine body.

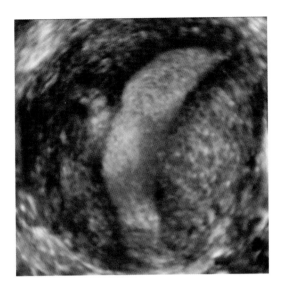

FIGURE 17.31   A unicornuate uterus with a single interstitial portion of fallopian tube.

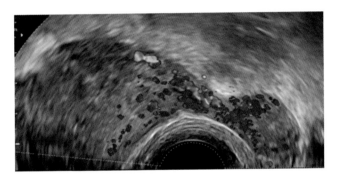

FIGURE 17.32   A thick vascular pedicle adjoining the horn to the main uterine body.

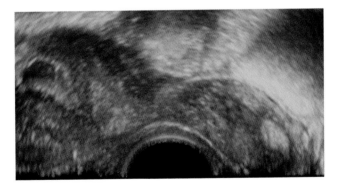

FIGURE 17.33   Three-dimensional imaging can demonstrate accurate details of the congenital uterine anomaly.

Pregnancy of Unknown Location

PUL is a descriptive term used to classify the diagnosis of the ultrasound scan when the pregnancy is not identified inside or outside the uterine cavity in women with a positive pregnancy test [208]. Despite the advances in imaging, it is estimated that the initial ultrasound examination fails to confirm the diagnosis in 8%–31% of women with early pregnancy complications [59,209]. This will depend on the quality of ultrasound scanning, including the skills of the ultrasound operator, the route of the ultrasound examination (transvaginal or transabdominal), and the quality of the ultrasound equipment used as well as the patient's body habitus and/or the presence of large pelvic masses [211,212]. A consensus statement published by the International Society of Ultrasound in Obstetrics and Gynecology suggested that modern early pregnancy units should try to sustain a PUL rate of 15% [209,213].

Many women present nowadays early in gestation before a pregnancy can be identified on ultrasound due to very sensitive urine pregnancy tests and easy access to the early pregnancy units. The majority of these women will either have a normal intrauterine pregnancy that is too small to be visualized on ultrasound scan or have a failed pregnancy [214–217].

Several markers have been used to predict the outcome of PULs, including β-hCG and serum progesterone [218–221]. Both the β-hCG discriminatory level (which indicates the level of serum β-hCG when a pregnancy can be visualized on ultrasound scan (1000–1500 IU/L for TVS and 6500 IU/L for TAS) [222–227] and the serial changes in the serum β-hCG level over 2 days have been described [228,229]. In general, a decreasing β-hCG value on serial measurements and/or a low serum progesterone level can help recognize women in whom pregnancy is failing, regardless of its location [230,231]. It is important to note that many ectopic pregnancies can be seen with β-hCG levels well below the discriminatory zone [221,229,232]. Thus, an ultrasound scan assessment should be offered to all symptomatic women and not be delayed until the β-hCG level is above this zone. In 7%–20%, ectopic pregnancy will be eventually diagnosed, and a small minority (2%) will have a persistent PUL, a term used in cases were β-hCG levels are either static or slowly increasing or decreasing in the absence of a visible pregnancy on ultrasound scan [201,210,224].

Mortality secondary to ruptured ectopic pregnancy diagnosed initially as PUL had been reported. It is therefore essential that all women with the diagnosis of PUL are followed up until the final location or outcome of the pregnancy is known [18].

REFERENCES

1. Bouyer J. Sites of ectopic pregnancy: A 10 year population-based study of 1800 cases. *Hum Reprod.* 2002;17(12):3224–30.
2. Salman G, and Irvine L. Ectopic pregnancy, the need for standardisation of rate. *J Obstet Gynaecol.* 2008;28(1):32–5.
3. Coste J, Job-Spira N, Aublet-Cuvelier B, Germain E, Glowaczower E, Fernandez H, and Pouly JL Incidence of ectopic pregnancy. First results of a population-based register in France. *Hum Reprod.* 1994;9(4):742–5.
4. Centers for Disease Control and Prevention. Ectopic pregnancy in the United States 1990–1992. *Morb Mortal Wkly Rep.* 1995;44(3):46–8.
5. Leke R, Goyaux N, Matsuda T, and Thonneau P. Ectopic pregnancy in Africa: A population-based study. *Obstet Gynecol.* 2004;103(4):692–7.
6. Boufous S, Quartararo M, Mohsin M, and Parker J. Trends in the incidence of ectopic pregnancy in New South Wales between 1990–1998. *Aust N Z J Obstet Gynaecol.* 2001;41(4):436–8.
7. Hoover KW, Tao G, and Kent CK. Trends in the diagnosis and treatment of ectopic pregnancy in the United States. *Obstet Gynecol.* 2010;115:495–502.
8. Shaw JL, Dey SK, Cricthley HOD, and Horne AW. Current knowledge of the aetiology of human tubal ectopic pregnancy. *Hum Reprod Update.* 2010;16(4):432–44.
9. Horne AW, and Critchley HO. Mechanisms of disease: The endocrinology of ectopic pregnancy. *Expert Rev Mol Med.* 2012;14:e7.
10. Shaw JL, Oliver E, Lee KF, Entrican G, Jabbour HN, Critchley HO, and Horne AW. Cotinine exposure increases fallopian tube PROKR1 expression via nicotinic AChRα-7. *Am J Pathol.* 2010;177(5):2509–15.
11. Parazzini F. Increasing rates of ectopic pregnancy: Oestrogens and progesterone concentrations and risk of ectopic pregnancy: An epidemiological point of view. *Hum Reprod.* 1996;11(2):236–8.
12. Shaw J, Wills G, Lee K et al. *Chlamydia trachomatis* infection increases fallopian tube PROKR2 via TLR2 and NFKB activation resulting in a microenvironment predisposed to ectopic pregnancy. *Am J Pathol.* 2011;178(1):253–60.

13. Bouyer J. Epidemiology of ectopic pregnancy: Incidence, risk factors and out- comes. *J Gynecol Obstet Biol Reprod (Paris)*. 2003;32:S8–17.
14. Coste J, Fernandez H, Joyé N, Benifla J, Girard S, Marpeau L, and Job-Spira N. Role of chromosome abnormalities in ectopic pregnancy. *Fertil Steril*. 2000;74(6):1259–60.
15. Goddijn M, van der Veen F, Schuring-Blom G, Ankum W, and Leschot N. Pregnancy: Cytogenetic characteristics of ectopic pregnancy. *Hum Reprod*. 1996;11(12):2769–71.
16. Lewis G. *The Confidential Enquiry into Maternal and Child Health (CEMACH). Saving Mothers' Lives: Reviewing Maternal Deaths to Make Motherhood Safer 2003–2005*. London, UK: RCOG Press; 2007.
17. Khan KS, Wojdyla D, Say L, Gülmezoglu AM, and van Look PF. WHO analysis of causes of maternal death: A systematic review. *Lancet*. 2006;367:1066–74.
18. Centre for Maternal and Child Enquiries (CMACE). Saving Mothers' Lives: Reviewing maternal deaths to make motherhood safer: 2006–08. The Eighth Report on Confidential Enquiries into Maternal Deaths in the United Kingdom. *BJOG*. 2011;118(Suppl. 1):1–203.
19. Job-Spira N, Bouyer J, Pouly JL, Germain E, Coste J, Aublet-Cuvelier B, and Fernandez H. Fertility after ectopic pregnancy: First results of a population-based cohort study in France. *Hum Reprod*. 1996;11(1):99–104.
20. Bhattacharya S, McLernon DJ, Lee AJ, and Bhattacharya S. Reproductive outcomes following ectopic pregnancy: Register-based retrospective cohort study. *PLOS MED*. 2012;9(6):e1001243.
21. Akande V, Turner C, Horner P, Horne A, and Pacey A. Impact of *Chlamydia trachomatis* in the reproductive setting: British Fertility Society Guidelines for practice. *Hum Fertil*. 2010;13(3):115–25.
22. Hillis SD, Owens LM, Marchbanks PA, Amsterdam LF, and MacKenzie WR. Recurrent chlamydial infections increase the risks of hospitalisation for ectopic pregnancy and pelvic inflammatory disease. *Am J Obstet Gynecol*. 1997;176:103–7.
23. Ankum WM, Mol BW, van Der Veen F, and Bossuyt PM. Risk factors for ectopic pregnancy: A meta-analysis. *Fertil Steril*. 1996;65:1093–9.
24. Marchbanks PA, Annegers JF, Coulam CB, Strathy JH, and Kurland LT. Risk factors for ectopic pregnancy. A population-based study. *JAMA*. 1988;259:1823–7.
25. Westrom L, Bengtsson LPH, and Mardh P-A. Incidence, trends and risks of ectopic pregnancy in a population of women. *BMJ*. 1981;282:15–8.
26. Karaer A, Avsar FA, and Batioglu S. Risk factors for ectopic pregnancy: A case-control study. *Aust N Z J Obstet Gynaecol*. 2006;46:521–7.
27. Marion LL, and Meeks GR. Ectopic pregnancy: History, incidence, epidemiology, and risk factors. *Clin Obstet Gynecol*. 2012;55:376–86.
28. Clayton H, Schieve L, Peterson H, Jamieson D, Reynolds M, and Wright V. Ectopic pregnancy risk with assisted reproductive technology procedures. *Obstet Gynecol*. 2006;107(3):595–604.
29. Strandell A, Thorburn J, and Hamberger L. Risk factors for ectopic pregnancy in assisted reproduction. *Fertil Steril*. 1999;71:282–6.
30. Steptoe PC, and Edwards RG. Reimplantation of a human embryo with subsequent tubal pregnancy. *Lancet*. 1976;1:880–2.
31. Mol BW, Ankum WM, Bossuyt PM, and Van der Veen F. Contraception and the risk of ectopic pregnancy: A meta-analysis. *Contraception*. 1995;52:337–41.
32. Benagiano G, Gabelnick H, and Farris M. Contraceptive devices: Intravaginal and intrauterine delivery systems. *Expert Rev Med Devices*. 2008;5:639–54.
33. Furlong LA. Ectopic pregnancy risk when contraception fails. A review. *J Reprod Med*. 2002;47:881–5.
34. Butts S, Sammel M, Hummel A, Chittams J, and Barnhart K. Risk factors and clinical features of recurrent ectopic pregnancy: A case control study. *Fertil Steril*. 2003;80(6):1340–4.
35. Bouyer J. Risk factors for ectopic pregnancy: A comprehensive analysis based on a large case-control, population-based study in France. *Am J Epidemiol*. 2003;157(3):185–94.
36. de Mouzon J, Spira A, and Schwartz D. A prospective study of the relation between smoking and fertility. *Int J Epidemiol*. 1988;17:378–84.
37. Talbot P, and Riveles K. Smoking and reproduction: The oviduct as a target of cigarette smoke. *Reprod Biol Endocrinol*. 2005;3:52.
38. Ramakrishnan K, and Scheid DC. Ectopic pregnancy: Forget the "classic presentation" if you want to catch it sooner. *J Fam Pract*. 2006;55(5):388–95.

39. Patel M, Chavda D, and Prajapati S. A retrospective study of 100 cases of ectopic pregnancy: Clinical presentation, site of ectopic and diagnosis evaluation. *Int J Reprod Contracept Obstet Gynecol.* 2016;5(12):4313–6.
40. Hassan N, Zaheen Z, and Jatoi N. Risk factors, clinical presentation and management of 62 cases of ectopic pregnancy at tertiary care centre. *JLUMHS.* 2009;8(3):238–41.
41. Schwartz RO, and Di Pietro DL. β-hCG as a diagnostic aid for suspected ectopic pregnancy. *Obstet Gynecol.* 1980;56(2):197–203.
42. Stovall TG, Kellerman AL, and Ling FW. Emergency department diagnosis of ectopic pregnancy. *Ann Emerg Med.* 1990;19:1098–103.
43. Sivalingam V, Duncan W, Kirk E, Shephard L, and Horne A. Diagnosis and management of ectopic pregnancy. *J Fam Plann Reprod Health Care.* 2011;37(4):231–40.
44. Murray H. Diagnosis and treatment of ectopic pregnancy. *CMAJ.* 2005;173(8):905–12.
45. Farquhar CM. Ectopic pregnancy. *Lancet.* 2005;366:583–91.
46. Nama V, and Manyonda I. Tubal ectopic pregnancy: Diagnosis and management. *Arch Gynecol Obstet.* 2009;279:443–53.
47. National Institute for Health and Care Excellence (NICE). Ectopic pregnancy and miscarriage: Diagnosis and initial management. *NICE guideline (NG126)*; April 17, 2019. https://www.nice.org.uk/guidance/ng126
48. Confidential Enquiry into Maternal and Child Health (CEMACH). Saving mothers' lives: Reviewing maternal deaths to make motherhood safer—2006-2008. The eighth report of the Confidential Enquiries into Maternal Deaths in the United Kingdom. *BJOG.* 2011;118:1–203.
49. Jurkovic D, and Wilkinson H. Diagnosis and management of ectopic pregnancy? *BMJ.* 2011;342:d3397.
50. Lozeau AM, and Potter B. Diagnosis and management of ectopic pregnancy. *Am Fam Physician.* 2005;72:1707–14.
51. Weckstein LN, Boucher, Tucker H, Gibson D, and Rettenmaier MA. Accurate diagnosis of early ectopic pregnancy. *Obstet Gynecol.* 1985;65(3):393–7.
52. Horne AW, Duncan WC, and Critchley HO. The need for serum biomarker development for diagnosing and excluding tubal ectopic pregnancy. *Acta Obstet Gynecol Scand.* 2010;89:299–301.
53. Kobayashi M, Hellman LM, and Fillisti LP. Ultrasound: An aid in the diagnosis of ectopic pregnancy. *Am J Obstet Gynecol.* 1969;103:1131–40.
54. Basama FM, Crosfill F, and Price A. Women's perception of transvaginal sonography in the first trimester; in an early pregnancy assessment unit. *Arch Gynecol Obstet.* 2004;269:117–20.
55. Atri M, Valenti D, Bret P, and Gillett P. Effect of transvaginal sonography on the use of invasive procedures for evaluating patients with a clinical diagnosis of ectopic pregnancy. *J Clin Ultrasound.* 2002;31(1):1–8.
56. Dutta RL, and Economides DL. Patient acceptance of transvaginal sonography in the early pregnancy unit setting. *Ultrasound Obstet Gynecol.* 2003;22:503–7.
57. Athey PA, Lamki N, Matyas MA, and Watson AB Jr. Comparison of transvaginal and transabdominal ultrasonography in ectopic pregnancy. *Can Assoc Radiol J.* 1991;42(5):349–52.
58. Condous G, Okaro E, Khalid A, Lu C, Van Huffel S, Timmerman D, and Bourne T. The accuracy of transvaginal ultrasonography for the diagnosis of ectopic pregnancy prior to surgery. *Hum Reprod.* 2005;20(5):1404–9.
59. Kirk E, Papageorghiou A, Condous G, Tan L, Bora S, and Bourne T. The diagnostic effectiveness of an initial transvaginal scan in detecting ectopic pregnancy. *Hum Reprod.* 2007;22(11):2824–8.
60. Stein JC, Wang R, Adler N, Boscardin J, Jacoby VL, Won G, Goldstein R, and Kohn MA. Emergency physician ultrasonography for evaluating patients at risk for ectopic pregnancy: A meta-analysis. *Ann Emerg Med.* 2010;56(6):674–83.
61. Kirk E, Daemen A, Papageorghiou AT, Bottomley C, Condous G, De Moor B, Timmerman D, and Bourne T. Why are some ectopic pregnancies characterized as pregnancies of unknown location at the initial transvaginal ultrasound examination?. *Obstet Gynecol Surv.* 2009;64(3):162–3.
62. Cacciatore B, Stenman UH, and Ylostalo P. Diagnosis of ectopic pregnancy by vaginal ultrasonography in combination with a discriminatory serum hCG level of 1000 IU/L. *BJOG.* 1990;97:904–8.
63. Cacciatore B, Stenman UH, and Ylostalo P. Comparison of abdominal and vaginal sonography in suspected ectopic pregnancy. *Obstet Gynecol.* 1989;73:770–4.
64. Moro F, Mavrelos D, Pateman K, Holland T, Hoo W, and Jurkovic D. Prevalence of pelvic adhesions on ultrasound examination in women with a history of Cesarean section. *Ultrasound Obstet Gynecol.* 2014;45(2):223–8.

65. Elson CJ, Salim R, Potdar N, Chetty M, Ross JA, and Kirk EJ on behalf of the Royal College of Obstetricians and Gynaecologists. Diagnosis and management of ectopic pregnancy. *BJOG*. 2016;123:e15–55.
66. Brown DL, and Doubilet PM. Transvaginal sonography for diagnosing ectopic pregnancy. *J Ultrasound Med*. 1994;13:259–66.
67. Kirk E, and Bourne T. Diagnosis of ectopic pregnancy with ultrasound. *Best Pract Res Clin Obstet Gynaecol*. 2009;23(4):501–8.
68. De Crespigny LC. Demonstration of ectopic pregnancy by transvaginal ultrasound. *Br J Obstet Gynaecol*. 1988;95(12):1253–6.
69. Fleischer A. Transvaginal sonography of ectopic pregnancy. *Contemp Diagn Radiol*. 1990;13(12):1–7.
70. Nyberg D, Hughes M, Mack L, and Wang K. Extrauterine findings of ectopic pregnancy of transvaginal US: Importance of echogenic fluid. *Radiology*. 1991;178(3):823–6.
71. Ahmed AA, Tom BD, and Calabrese P. Ectopic pregnancy diagnosis and the pseudo-sac. *Fertil Steril*. 2004;81:1225–8.
72. Perriera L, and Reeves MF. Ultrasound criteria for diagnosis of early pregnancy failure and ectopic pregnancy 2008. *Semin Reprod Med*. 26:373–82.
73. Spandorfer SD, and Barnhart KT. Endometrial stripe thickness as a predictor of ectopic pregnancy. *Fertil Steril*. 1996;66:474–7.
74. Hammoud A, Hammoud I, Bujold E, Gonik B, Diamond M, and Johnson S. The role of sonographic endometrial patterns and endometrial thickness in the differential diagnosis of ectopic pregnancy. *Am J Obstet Gynecol*. 2005;192(5):1370–5.
75. Wachsburg RH, and Karimi S. Sonographic endometrial three-layer pattern in symptomatic first-trimester pregnancy: Not diagnostic of ectopic pregnancy. *JCU*. 1998;26(4):199–201.
76. Mol BW, Hajenius PJ, Engelsbel S, Ankum WM, van der Veen F, Hemrika DJ, and Bossuyt PM. Are gestational age and endometrial thickness alternatives for serum human chorionic gonadotropin as criteria for the diagnosis of ectopic pregnancy? *Fertil Steril*. 1999;72(4):643–5.
77. Richardson A, Gallos I, Dobson S, Campbell B, Coomarasamy A, and Raine-Fenning N. Accuracy of first-trimester ultrasound in diagnosis of tubal ectopic pregnancy in the absence of an obvious extrauterine embryo: Systematic review and meta-analysis. *Ultrasound Obstet Gynecol*. 2015;47(1):28–37.
78. Kataoka M, Togashi K, Kobayashi H, Inoue T, Fujii S, and Konishi J. Evaluation of ectopic pregnancy by magnetic resonance imaging. *Hum Reprod*. 1999;14(10):2644–50.
79. Kao LY, Scheinfeld MH, and Chernyak V. Beyond ultrasound: CT and MRI of ectopic pregnancy. *AJR*. 2014;202:904–11.
80. Panelli D, Phillips C, and Brady P. Incidence, diagnosis and management of tubal and nontubal ectopic pregnancies: A review. *Fertil Res Pract*. 2015;1:15.
81. Lin E, Shweta Bhatt S, and Dogra V. Diagnostic clues to ectopic pregnancy. *Radiographics*. 2008;28:1661–71.
82. Singh N, Tripathi R, Mala Y, and Batra A. Diagnostic dilemma in cornual pregnancy—3D ultrasonography may aid! *J Clin Diagn Res*. 2015;9(1):QD12–3.
83. Lawrence A, and Jurkovic D. Three-dimensional ultrasound diagnosis of interstitial pregnancy. *Ultrasound Obstet Gynecol*. 1999;14(4):292–3.
84. Godin PA, Bassil S, and Donnez J. An ectopic pregnancy developing in a previous caesarean section scar. *Fertil Steril*. 1997;67:398–400.
85. Rotas MA, Haberman S, and Levgur M. Caesarean scar ectopic pregnancies: Aetiology, diagnosis, and management. *Obstet Gynecol*. 2006;107:1373–81.
86. Majangara R, Madziyire MG, Verenga C, and Manase M. Cesarean section scar ectopic pregnancy—a management conundrum: A case report. *Journal of Medical Case Reports*. 2019;13:137.
87. Jurkovic D, Knez J, Appiah A, Farahani L, Mavrelos D, and Ross J. Surgical treatment of Cesarean scar ectopic pregnancy: Efficacy and safety of ultrasound-guided suction curettage. *Ultrasound Obstet Gynecol*. 2016;47(4):511–7.
88. Maymon R, Halperin R, Mendlovic S, Schneider D, and Herman A. Ectopic pregnancies in a Caesarean scar: Review of the medical approach to an iatrogenic complication. *Hum Reprod Update*. 2004;10(6):515–23.
89. Shi M, Zhang H, Qi SS, Liu WH, Liu M, Zhao XB, and Mu YL. Identifying risk factors for cesarean scar pregnancy: A retrospective study of 79 cases. *Ginekol Pol*. 2018;89(4):196–200.

90. Ofili-Yebovi D, Ben-Nagi J, Sawyer E, Yazbek J, Lee C, Gonzalez J, and Jurkovic D. Deficient lower-segment Cesarean section scars: Prevalence and risk factors. *Ultrasound Obstet Gynecol.* 2007;31(1):72–7.

91. Harb HM, Knight M, Bottomley C et al. Caesarean scar pregnancy in the UK: A national cohort study. *BJOG.* 2018;125(13):1663–70.

92. Jurkovic D, Hillaby K, Woelfer B, Lawrence A, Salim R, and Elson C. First-trimester diagnosis and management of pregnancies implanted into the lower uterine segment Cesarean section scar. *Ultrasound Obstet Gynecol.* 2003;21(3):220–7.

93. Timor-Tritsch IE, Monteagudo A, Cali G, Vintzileos A, Viscarello R, Al-Khan A, Zamudio S, Mayberry P, Cordoba MM, and Dar P. Cesarean. Cesarean scar pregnancy is a precursor of morbidly adherent placenta. *Ultrasound Obstet Gynecol.* 2014;44(3):346–53.

94. Timor-Tritsch IE, and Monteagudo A. Unforeseen consequences of the increasing rate of Caesarean deliveries: Early placenta accreta and Caesarean scar pregnancy. A review. *Am J Obstet Gynecol.* 2012;207:14–29.

95. Wang Q, Peng H-L, He L, and Zhao X. Reproductive outcomes after previous cesarean scar pregnancy: Follow up of 189 women. *Taiwan J Obstet Gynecol.* 2015;54:551–3.

96. Gao L, Huang Z, Zhang X, Zhou N, Huang X, and Wang X. Reproductive outcomes following cesarean scar pregnancy—A case series and review of the literature. *Eur J Obstet Gynecol Reprod Biol.* 2016;200:102–7.

97. Ben Nagi J, Helmy S, Ofili-Yebovi D, Yazbek J, Sawyer E, and Jurkovic D. Reproductive outcomes of women with a previous history of Caesarean scar ectopic pregnancies. *Hum Reprod.* 2007;22(7):2012–5.

98. Zhang Y, Gu Y, Wang J, and Li Y. Analysis of cases with cesarean scar pregnancy. *J Obstet Gynaecol Res.* 2012;39(1):195–202.

99. Timor-Tritsch IE, Monteagudo A, Santos R, Tsymbal T, Pineda G, and Arslan AA. The diagnosis, treatment, and follow-up of cesarean scar pregnancy. *Am J Obstet Gynecol.* 2012;207:44.e1–13.

100. Gonzalez N, and Tulandi T. Cesarean scar pregnancy: A systematic review. *J Minim Invasive Gynecol.* 2017;24(5):731–8.

101. Pedraszewski P, Wlaźlak E, Panek W, and Surkont G. Cesarean scar pregnancy—A new challenge for obstetricians. *J Ultrason* 2018;18:56–62.

102. Rempen A, and Albert P. Diagnosis and therapy of an in the cesarean section scar implanted early pregnancy. *Z. Geburtshilfe Perinatol.* 1990;194(1):46–8.

103. Vial Y, Petignat P, and Hohlfeld P. Pregnancy in a cesarean scar. *Ultrasound Obstet Gynecol.* 2000;16:592–3.

104. Wang HY, Zhang J, Li YN, Wei W, Zhang DW, Lu YQ, and Zhang HF. Laparoscopic management or laparoscopy combined with transvaginal management of type II caesarean scar pregnancy. *JSLS.* 2013;17(2):263–72.

105. Hwang JH, Lee JK, Oh MJ, Lee NW, Hur JY, and Lee KW. Classification and management of cervical ectopic pregnancies: Experience at a single institution. *J Reprod Med.* 2010;55(11–12):469–76.

106. Lin SY, Hsieh CJ, Tu YA, Li YP, Lee CN, Hsu WW, and Shih JC. New ultrasound grading system for cesarean scar pregnancy and its implications for management strategies: An observational cohort study. *PLOS ONE.* 2018;13(8):e0202020.

107. Timor-Tritsch I, El-Refaey H, and Monteagudo A. Proposal for easy and reliable sonographic diagnosis of the first trimester Caesarean scar pregnancy. *Ultrasound Obstet Gynecol.* 2015;46:154.

108. Zhang H, Huang J, Wu X, Fan H, Li H, and Gao T. Clinical classification and treatment of cesarean scar pregnancy. *J Obstet Gynaecol Res.* 2017;43(4):653–61.

109. Timor-Tritsch IE, Khatib N, Monteagudo A, Ramos J, Berg R, and Kovacs S. Cesarean scar pregnancies: Experience of 60 cases. *J Ultrasound Med.* 2015;34(4):601–10.

110. Seow KM, Hwang JL, and Tsai YL. Ultrasound diagnosis of a pregnancy in a Cesarean section scar. *Ultrasound Obstet Gynecol.* 2001;18:547–9.

111. Seow K, Huang L, Lin Y, Yan-Sheng Lin M, Tsai Y, and Hwang J. Cesarean scar pregnancy: Issues in management. *Ultrasound Obstet Gynecol.* 2004;23(3):247–53.

112. Osborn DA, Williams TR, and Craig BM. Caesarean scar pregnancy: Sonographic and magnetic resonance imaging findings, complications, and treatment. *J Ultrasound Med.* 2012;31:1449–56.

113. Jurkovic D, Hacket E, and Campbell S. Diagnosis and treatment of early cervical pregnancy: A review and a report of two cases treated conservatively. *Ultrasound Obstet Gynecol.* 1996;8:373–80.

114. Singh S. Diagnosis and management of cervical ectopic pregnancy. *J Hum Reprod Sci.* 2013;6(4):273–6.

115. Uludag S, Kutuk M, Aygen E, and Sahin Y. Conservative management of cervical ectopic pregnancy: Single-center experience. *J Obstet Gynaecol Res.* 2017;43(8):1299–304.

116. Karande VC, Flood JT, Heard N, Veeck L, and Muasher SJ. Analysis of ectopic pregnancies resulting from *in-vitro* fertilization and embryo transfer. *Hum Reprod.* 1991;6:446–9.

117. Ginsburg ES, Frates MC, Rein MS, Fox JH, Hornstein MD, and Friedman AJ. Early diagnosis and treatment of cervical pregnancy in an *in vitro* fertilization program. *Fertil Steril.* 1994;61:966–9.

118. Vela G, and Tulandi T. Cervical pregnancy: The importance of early diagnosis and treatment. *J Minim Invasive Gynecol.* 2007;14:1–4.

119. Verma U, and Goharkhay N. Conservative management of cervical ectopic pregnancy. *Fertil Steril.* 2009;91:671–4.

120. Benson CB, and Doubilet PM. Strategies for conservative treatment of cervical ectopic pregnancy. *Ultrasound Obstet Gynecol.* 1996;8:371–2.

121. Kirk E, Condous G, Haider Z, Syed A, Ojha K, and Bourne T. The conservative management of cervical ectopic pregnancies. *Ultrasound Obstet Gynecol.* 2006;27:430–7.

122. Murji A, Garbedian K, and Thomas J. Conservative management of cervical ectopic pregnancy. *J Obstet Gynaecol Can.* 2015;37(11):1016–20.

123. Raskin M. Diagnosis of cervical pregnancy by ultrasound: A case report. *Am J Obstet Gynecol.* 1978;130:234–5.

124. Kung FT, Lin H, Hsu TY, Chang CY, Huang HW, Huang LY, Chou YJ, Huang KH. Differential diagnosis of suspected cervical pregnancy and conservative treatment with the combination of laparoscopy-assisted uterine artery ligation and hysteroscopic endocervical resection. *Fertil Steril.* 2004;81(6):1642–9.

125. Saha E, and Paul A. Cervical ectopic pregnancy mimicking missed abortion. *Bangladesh Med J Khulna.* 2012;44:28–30.

126. Vas W, Suresh PL, Tang-Barton P, Salimi Z, and Carlin B. Ultrasonographic differentiation of cervical abortion from cervical pregnancy. *J Clin Ultrasound.* 1984;12:553–7.

127. Leeman LM, and Wendland CL. Cervical ectopic pregnancy: Diagnosis with endovaginal ultrasound examination and successful treatment with methotrexate. *Arch Fam Med.* 2000;9:72–7.

128. Li-Ping H, Hui-Min Z, Jun-Bi G, Chao-Yue T, and Xiao-Xiao H. Management and outcome of heterotopic pregnancy. *Ann Clin Lab Res.* 2018;6(1):228.

129. Richards SR, Stempel LE, and Carlton BD. Heterotopic pregnancy: Reappraisal of incidence. *Am J Obstet Gynecol.* 1982;142:928–30.

130. Tal J, Haddad S, Gordon N, and Timor-Tritsch L. Heterotopic pregnancy after ovulation induction and assisted reproduction technologies: A literature review from 1971 to 1993. *Fertil Steril.* 1996;66:1–2.

131. Rizk, B., Tan, S. L., Morcos, S., Riddle, A., Brinsden, P., Mason, B. A., and Edwards, R. G. Heterotopic pregnancies after *in vitro* fertilization and embryo transfer. *Am J Obstet Gynecol.* 1991;164(1):161–4.

132. Govindarajan MJ, and Rajan R. Heterotopic pregnancy in natural conception. *J Hum Reprod Sci.* 2008;1:37–8.

133. Raziel A, Friedler S, Herman A, Strassburger D, Maymon R, and Ron-El R. Recurrent heterotopic pregnancy after repeated *in-vitro* fertilization treatment. *Hum Reprod.* 1997;12(8):1810–2.

134. Yu Y, Xu W, Xie Z, Huang Q, and Li S. Management and outcome of 25 heterotopic pregnancies in Zhejiang, China. *Eur J Obstet Gynecol Reprod Biol.* 2014;80:157–61.

135. Lee JS, Cha H, Han AR, Lee SG, and Seong WJ. Heterotopic pregnancy after a single embryo transfer. *Obstet Gynecol Sci.* 2016;59:316–8.

136. Beyer D, and Dumesic D. Heterotopic pregnancy: An emerging diagnostic challenge. *OBG Management.* 2002;14:36–46.

137. Jerrad D, Tso E, Salik R, and Barish RA. Unsuspected heterotopic pregnancy in a woman without risk factors. *Am J Emerg Med.* 1992;10:58–60.

138. Zhaoxia L, Honglang Q, and Danqing C. Ruptured heterotopic pregnancy after assisted reproduction in a patient who underwent bilateral salpingectomy. *J Obstet Gynaecol.* 2013;33(2):209–10.

139. Ghaneie A, Grajo J, Derr C, and Kumm T. Unusual ectopic pregnancies. *Sonographic Findings Implications Manage.* 2015;34(6):951–62.

140. Li XH, Ouyang Y, and Lu GX. Value of transvaginal sonography in diagnosing heterotopic pregnancy after *in-vitro* fertilization with embryo transfer. *Ultrasound Obstet Gynecol.* 2013;41(5):563–9.

141. Habana A, Dokras A, Giraldo JL, and Jones EE. Cornual heterotopic pregnancy: Contemporary management options. *Am J Obstet Gynecol.* 2000;182:1264–70.

142. Peleg, D., Bar-Hava, I., Neuman-Levin, M., Ashkenazi, J., and Ben-Rafael, Z Early diagnosis and successful non-surgical treatment of viable combined intrauterine and cervical pregnancy. *Fertil Steril.* 1994;62:405–8.

143. Attapattu J, and Menon S. Abdominal pregnancy. *Int J Gynecol Obstet.* 1993;43:51–5.

144. Alto WA. Abdominal pregnancy. *Am Fam Physician.* 1990;41:209–14.

145. Audain L, Brown WE, Smith DM, and Clark JF. Cocaine use as a risk factor for abdominal pregnancy. *J Natl Med Assoc.* 1998;90:277–83.

146. Martin JN Jr, Sessums JK, Martin RW, Pryor JA, and Morrison JC et al. Abdominal pregnancy: Current concepts of management. *Obstet Gynecol.* 1988;71:549–57.

147. Atrash H, Friede A, and Hogue C. Abdominal pregnancy in the United States: Frequency and maternal mortality. *Obstet Gynecol.* 1987;69:333–7.

148. Worley KC, Hnat MD, and Cunningham FG. Advanced extrauterine pregnancy: Diagnostic and therapeutic challenges. *Am J Obstet Gynecol.* 2008;198:297.e1–297.e7.

149. Studdiford WE. Primary peritoneal pregnancy. *Am J Obstet Gynecol.* 1942;44:5.

150. Nkusu Nunyalulendho D, and Einterz EM. Advanced abdominal pregnancy: Case report and review of 163 cases reported since 1946. *Rural Remote Health.* 2008;8:1087.

151. Ombelet W, Vandermerwe JV, and Van Assche FA. Advanced extrauterine pregnancy: Description of 38 cases with literature survey. *Obstet Gynecol Surv.* 1988;43:386–97.

152. Kun KY, Wong PY, Ho MW, Tai CM, and Ng TK. Abdominal pregnancy presenting as a missed abortion at 16 weeks' gestation. *Hong Kong Med J.* 2000;6:425–7.

153. Dahab AA, Aburass R, Shawkat W, Babgi R, Essa O, and Mujallid RH. Full-term extrauterine abdominal pregnancy: A case report. *J Med Case Rep* 2011;5:531.

154. Ludwig M, Kaisi M, Bauer O, and Diedrich K. The forgotten child: A case of heterotopic, intra-abdominal and intrauterine pregnancy carried to term. *Hum Reprod.* 1999;14:1372–4.

155. Malian V, and Lee JH. MR imaging and MR angiography of an abdominal pregnancy with placental infarction. *AJR Am J Roentgenol.* 2001;177:1305–6.

156. Bertrand G, Le Ray C, Simard-Emond L, Dubois J, and Leduc L. Imaging in the management of abdominal pregnancy: A case report and review of the literature. *J Obstet Gynaecol Can.* 2009;31:57–62.

157. Graham D, Johnson TR Jr, and Sanders RC. Sonographic findings in abdominal pregnancy. *J Ultrasound Med.* 1982;1:71–4.

158. Angtuaco TL, Shah HR, Neal MR, and Quirk JG. Ultrasound evaluation of abdominal pregnancy. *Crit Rev Diagn Imaging* 1994;35:1–59.

159. Gerli S, Rossetti D, Baiocchi G, Clerici G, Unfer V, and Di Renzo GC. Early ultrasonographic diagnosis and laparoscopic treatment of abdominal pregnancy. *Eur J Obstet Gynecol Reprod Biol.* 2004;113:103–5.

160. Raziel A, Schachter M, Mordechai E, Friedler S, Panski M, and Ron-El R. Ovarian pregnancy: A 12-year experience of 19 cases in one institution. *Eur J Obstet Gynecol Reprod Biol.* 2004;114:92–6.

161. Gaudoin M, Coulter K, Robin A, Verghese A and Hanretty K. Is the incidence of ovarian ectopic pregnancy increasing? *Eur J Obstet Gynecol Reprod Biol.* 1996;70:141–3.

162. Riethmuller D, Sautiere JL, Benoit S, Roth P, Schaal JP, and Maillet R. Ultrasonic diagnosis and laparoscopic treatment of an ovarian pregnancy: A case report and review of the literature [in French]. *J Gynecol Obstet Biol Reprod (Paris).* 1995;25:378–83.

163. Joseph RJ, and Irvine LM. Ovarian ectopic pregnancy: Aetiology, diagnosis, and challenges in surgical management. *J Obstet Gynaecol.* 2012;32:472–4.

164. Choi HJ, Im KS, Jung HJ, Lim KT, Mok JE, and Kwon YS. Clinical analysis of ovarian pregnancy: A report of 49 cases. *Eur J Obstet Gynecol Reprod Biol.* 2011;158:87–9.

165. Hallatt JG. Primary ovarian pregnancy: A report of twenty-five cases. *Am J Obstet Gynecol.* 1982;143:55–60.

166. Mehmood SA, and Thomas JA. Primary ectopic ovarian pregnancy (report of three cases). *J Postgrad Med.* 1985;31:219–22.

167. Priya S, Kamala S, and Gunjan S. Two interesting cases of ovarian pregnancy after *in vitro* fertilization-embryo transfer and its successful laparoscopic management. *Fertil Steril.* 2009;92:394.e17–394.e19.

168. Dhorepatil B, and Rapol A. A rare case of unruptured viable secondary ovarian pregnancy after IVF/ICSI treated by conservative laparoscopic surgery. *J Hum Reprod Sci.* 2012;5:61–3.

169. Das S, Kalyani R, Lakshmi V, and Harendra Kumar ML. Ovarian pregnancy. *Indian J Pathol Microbiol.* 2008;51:37–8.

170. Tantuway B, Sachdeva P, Triapthi R, and Mala YM. Primary ovarian ectopic pregnancy. *J Case Rep.* 2017;7:130–2. doi:10.17659/01.2017.0036

171. Grimes HG, Nosal RA, and Gallagher JC. Ovarian pregnancy: A series of 24 cases. *Obstet Gynecol.* 1983;61(2):174–80.

172. Prabhala S, Erukkambattu J, Dogiparthi A, Kumar P, and Tanikella R. Ruptured ovarian pregnancy in a primigravida. *Int J Appl Basic Med Res.* 2015;5(2):151.

173. Koo YJ, Choi HJ, Im KS, Jung HJ, and Kwon YS. Pregnancy outcomes after surgical treatment of ovarian pregnancy. *Int J Gynaecol Obstet.* 2011;114:97–100.

174. De Seta, F., Baraggino, E., Strazzanti, C., De Santo, D., Tracanzan, G., and Guaschino, S. Ovarian pregnancy: A case report. *Acta Obstet Gynecol Scand.* 2001; 80(7), 661–2.

175. Gerin-Lajoie L. Ovarian pregnancy. *Am J Obstet Gynecol.* 1951;62:920–9.

176. Shahabuddin AK, and Chowdhury S. Primary term ovarian pregnancy superimposed by intrauterine pregnancy: A case report. *J Obstet Gynaecol Res.* 1998;24:109–14.

177. Meşeci E, Güzel Y, Zemheri E, Eser SK, Özkanlı S, and Kumru P. A 34-week ovarian pregnancy: Case report and review of the literature. *J Turkish-German Gynecol Assoc.* 2013;14:246–9.

178. Begum J. Diagnostic dilemma in ovarian pregnancy: A case series. *J Clin Diagn Res.* 2015;9(4):1–3.

179. Nwanodi O, and Khulpateea N. The preoperative diagnosis of primary ovarian pregnancy. *J Natl Med Assoc.* 2006;98(5):796–8.

180. Nisenblat V, Leibovitz Z, Tal J, Barak S, Shapiro I, Degani S, and Ohel G. Primary ovarian ectopic pregnancy misdiagnosed as first-trimester missed abortion. *J Ultrasound Med.* 2005;24(4):539–45.

181. Hertzberg BS, Kliewer MA, and Paulson EK. Ovarian cyst rupture causing hemoperitoneum: Imaging features and the potential for misdiagnosis. *Abdom Imaging.* 1999;24:304–8.

182. Gupta N, Gupta A, Onyema G, Pantofel Y, Ying SC, Garon JE, Lampley C, and Blankstein J. Accurate preoperative diagnosis of ovarian pregnancy with transvaginal scan. *Case Rep Obstet Gynecol.* 2012;2012:934571.

183. Comstock C, Huston K, and Lee W. The ultrasonographic appearance of ovarian ectopic pregnancies. *Obstet Gynecol.* 2005;105:42–5.

184. Stein MW, Ricci ZJ, Novak L, Roberts JH, and Koenigsberg M. Sonographic comparison of the tubal ring of ectopic pregnancy with the corpus luteum. *J Ultrasound Med.* 2004;23:57–62.

185. Chang FW, Chen CH, and Liu JY. Early diagnosis of ovarian pregnancy by ultrasound. *Int J Gynaecol Obstet.* 2004;85:186–7.

186. Brincat M, Bryant-Smith A, and Holland TK. The diagnosis and management of interstitial ectopic pregnancies: A review. Gynecological Surgery. 2019;16:2.

187. Chen J, Huang D, Shi L, and Zhang S. Prevention, diagnosis, and management of interstitial pregnancy: A review of the literature. Laparoscopic, Endoscopic and Robotic Surgery. 2019;2:12–7.

188. Lau S, and Tulandi T. Conservative medical and surgical management of interstitial ectopic pregnancy. *Fertil Steril.* 1999;72(2):207–15.

189. Poon L, Emmanuel E, Ross J, and Johns J. How feasible is expectant management of interstitial ectopic pregnancy? *Ultrasound Obstet Gynecol.* 2014;43(3):317–21.

190. Eddy CA, and Pauerstein CJ. Anatomy and physiology of the fallopian tube. *Clin Obstet Gynecol.* 1980;23:1177–93.

191. Moore KL, Dalley AF, and Agur AM. *Clinically Oriented Anatomy.* 6th ed. Baltimore, MD: Lippincott Williams & Wilkins; 2010.

192. Honemeyer U, Plavsic SK, and Kurjak A. Interstitial ectopic pregnancy: The essential role of ultrasound diagnosis. *Donald School J Ultrasound Obstet Gynecol* 2010;4:321–5.

193. Ackerman TE, Levi CS, Dashefsky SM, Holt SC, and Lindsay DJ. Interstitial line: Sonographic finding in interstitial (cornual) ectopic pregnancy. *Radiology.* 1993;189:83–7.

194. Araujo Júnior, E., Zanforlin Filho, S. M., Pires, C. R., Guimarães Filho, H. A., Massaguer, A. A., Nardozza, L. M., and Moron, A. F. Three-dimensional transvaginal sonographic diagnosis of early and asymptomatic interstitial pregnancy. *Arch Gynecol Obstet.* 2007;275:207–10.

195. Rastogi R, Meena GL, Rastogi N, and Rastogi V. Interstitial ectopic pregnancy: A rare and difficult clinicosonographic diagnosis. *J Hum Reprod Sci* 2008;1:81–2.

196. de Boer C, van Dongen P, Willemsen W, and Klapwijk C. Ultrasound diagnosis of interstitial pregnancy. *Eur J Obstet Gynecol Reprod Biol.* 1992;47:164–6.

197. Nahum GG. Rudimentary uterine horn pregnancy. The 20th-century worldwide experience of 588 cases. *J Reprod Med.* 2002;47:151–63.

198. Kun WM, and Tung WK. On the lookout for a rarity: Interstitial/cornual pregnancy. *Eur J Emerg Med.* 2001;8:147–50.

199. Johnston LW, and Moir JC. A case of angular pregnancy complicated by gas-gangrene infection of the uterus. *J Obstet Gynaecol Br EMP.* 1952;59:85–7.

200. Malinowski A, and Bates SK. Semantics and pitfalls in the diagnosis of cornual/interstitial pregnancy. *Fertil Steril.* 2006;86:1764.e11–1764.e14.

201. Kirk E, Condous G, Van Calster B, Van Huffel S, Timmerman D, and Bourne T. Rationalizing the follow-up of pregnancies of unknown location. *Hum Reprod.* 2007;22(6):1744–50.

202. Terzi, H., Yavuz, A., Demirtaş, Ö., and Kale, A. Rudimentary horn pregnancy in the first trimester; importance of ultrasound and clinical suspicion in early diagnosis: A case report. *J Turkish Soc Obstet Gynecol.* 2014;11(3):189–92.

203. Jayasinghe Y, Rane A, Stalewski H, and Grover S. The presentation and early diagnosis of the rudimentary uterine horn. *Obstet Gynecol.* 2005;105(6):1456–67.

204. Wangdi T, and Deka D. Rupture of non-communicating rudimentary horn ectopic pregnancy of a unicornuate uterus in first trimester. *Int J Reprod Contracept Obstet Gynecol.* 2015;4(4):1211–3.

205. Timor-Tritsch IE, Monteagudo A, Matera C, and Veit CR. Sonographic evolution of cornual pregnancies treated without surgery. *Obstet Gynecol.* 1992;79:1044–9.

206. Maher PJ, and Grimwade JC. Cornual pregnancy…diagnosis before rupture a report of 2 cases. *Aust N Z J Obstet Gynaecol.* 1982;22:172–4.

207. Mavrelos D, Sawyer E, Helmy S, Holland TK, Ben-Nagi J, and Jurkovic D. Ultrasound diagnosis of ectopic pregnancy in the non-communicating horn of a unicornuate uterus (cornual pregnancy). *Ultrasound Obstet Gynecol.* 2007;30:765–70.

208. Kirk E, Condous G, and Bourne T. Pregnancies of unknown location. *Best Pract Res Clin Obstet Gynaecol.* 2009;23:493–9.

209. Barnhart K, van Mello N, Bourne T et al. Pregnancy of unknown location: A consensus statement of nomenclature, definitions, and outcome. *Fertil Steril.* 2011;95(3):857–66.

210. Cordina M, Schramm-Gajraj K, Ross J, Lautman K, and Jurkovic D. Introduction of a single visit protocol in the management of selected patients with pregnancy of unknown location: A prospective study. *BJOG.* 2011;118(6):693–7.

211. Bottomley, C., Van Belle, V., Mukri, F., Kirk, E., Van Huffel, S., Timmerman, D., and Bourne, T. The optimal timing of an ultrasound scan to assess the location and viability of an early pregnancy. *Hum Reprod.* 2009;24(8):1811–7.

212. van Mello, N. M., Mol, F., Opmeer, B. C., Ankum, W. M., Barnhart, K., Coomarasamy, A., Mol, B. W., van der Veen, F., and Hajenius, P. J. Diagnostic value of serum hCG on the outcome of pregnancy of unknown location: A systematic review and meta-analysis. *Hum Reprod Update.* 2012;18(6):603–17.

213. Condous G, Timmerman D, Goldstein S, Valentin L, Jurkovic D, and Bourne T. Pregnancies of unknown location: Consensus statement. *Ultrasound Obstet Gynecol.* 2006;28(2):121–2.

214. Bobdiwala S, Saso S, Verbakel J, Al-Memar M, Timmerman D, and Bourne T. Diagnostic protocols for the management of pregnancy of unknown location (PUL): A systematic review and meta-analysis. *Ultrasound Obstet Gynecol.* 2017;50:82–2.

215. Condous, G., Van Calster, B., Kirk, E., Haider, Z., Timmerman, D., Van Huffel, S., and Bourne, T. Prediction of ectopic pregnancy in women with a pregnancy of unknown location. *Ultrasound Obstet Gynecol.* 2007;29(6):680–7.

216. Hahlin M, Thorburn J, and Bryman I. The expectant management of early pregnancies of uncertain site. *Hum Reprod.* 1995;10:1223–7.

217. Kirk E, Bottomley C, and Bourne T. Diagnosing ectopic pregnancy and current concepts in the management of pregnancy of unknown location. *Hum Reprod Update.* 2014;20:250–61.

218. Bignardi T, Condous G, Alhamdan D et al. The hCG ratio can predict the ultimate viability of the intrauterine pregnancies of uncertain viability in the pregnancy of unknown location population. *Hum Reprod.* 2008;23(9):1964–7.

219. Condous G, Lu C, Van Huffel S, Timmerman D, and Bourne T. Human chorionic gonadotrophin and progesterone levels in pregnancies of unknown location. *Int J Gynecol Obstet.* 2004;86(3):351–7.
220. Mol BW, Lijmer JG, Ankum W, Van der Veen F, and Bossuyt PM. The accuracy of single serum progesterone measurement in the diagnosis of ectopic pregnancy: A meta-analysis. *Hum Reprod.* 1998;13:3220–7.
221. Seeber B, Sammel M, Guo W, Zhou L, Hummel A, and Barnhart K. Application of redefined human chorionic gonadotropin curves for the diagnosis of women at risk for ectopic pregnancy. *Fertil Steril.* 2006;86(2):454–9.
222. Barnhart KT, Simhan H, and Kamelle. Diagnostic accuracy of ultrasound above and below the β-hCG discriminatory zone. *Obstet Gynecol.* 1999;94(4):583–7.
223. Condous, G., Kirk, E., Lu, C., Van Huffel, S., Gevaert, O., De Moor, B., De Smet, F., Timmerman, D., and Bourne, T. Diagnostic accuracy of varying discriminatory zones for the prediction of ectopic pregnancy in women with a pregnancy of unknown location. *Ultrasound Obstet Gynecol.* 2005;26:770–5.
224. Condous, G., Okaro, E., Khalid, A., Lu, C., Van Huffel, S., Timmerman, D. and Bourne, T. A prospective evaluation of a single-visit strategy to manage pregnancies of unknown location. *Hum Reprod.* 2005;20(5):1398–403.
225. Kadar N, and Romero R. HCG assays and ectopic pregnancy. *Lancet.* 1981;1:1205–6.
226. Kadar N, DeVore G, and Romero R. Discriminatory hCG zone: Its use in the sonographic evaluation for ectopic pregnancy. *Obstet Gynecol.* 1981;58(2):156–61.
227. Romero, R., Kadar, N., Jeanty, P., Copel, J. A., Chervenak, F. A., DeCherney, A., and Hobbins, J. C. Diagnosis of ectopic pregnancy: Value of the discriminatory human chorionic gonadotropin zone. *Obstet Gynecol.* 1985;66:357–60.
228. Dart RG, Mitterando J, and Dart LM. Rate of change of serial β-human chorionic gonadotropin values as a predictor of ectopic pregnancy in patients with indeterminate transvaginal ultrasound findings. *Ann Emerg Med.* 1999;34:703–10.
229. Mol, B. W., Hajenius, P. J., Engelsbel, S., Ankum, W. M., Van der Veen, F., Hemrika, D. J., and Bossuyt, P. Serum human chorionic gonadotropin measurement in the diagnosis of ectopic pregnancy when transvaginal sonography is inconclusive. *Fertil Steril.* 1998;5:972–81.
230. Butts S, Guo W, Cary M, Chung K, Takacs P, Sammel M and Barnhart K. Predicting the decline in human chorionic gonadotropin in a resolving pregnancy of unknown location. *Obstet Gynecol.* 2013;122(2):337–43.
231. Condous G, Kirk E, Van Calster B, Van Huffel S, Timmerman D, and Bourne T. General obstetrics: Failing pregnancies of unknown location: A prospective evaluation of the human chorionic gonadotrophin ratio. *BJOG.* 2006;113(5):521–7.
232. Silva C, Sammel M, Zhou L, Gracia C, Hummel A, and Barnhart K. Human chorionic gonadotropin profile for women with ectopic pregnancy. *Obstet Gynecol Surv.* 2006;61(7):446–7.

18

Quality Aspects of Ultrasound

Ilaria Soave and Roberto Marci

Context

Health-care providers undertaking ultrasound examination in a center for reproductive medicine will often face a working environment that is far from the traditional radiology-based ultrasound service. However, in order to ensure a high-quality service and to safeguard patients, the same principles of governance and quality standards must also apply in *in vitro* fertilization (IVF) units. Generally, the aim of a quality assurance program of an imaging department is to assess and monitor technical and diagnostic quality of medical images (including ultrasound) over time. However, ultrasound (US) differs consistently from other imaging modalities. Indeed, unlike X-rays and other cross-sectional imaging modalities (e.g., computed tomography, magnetic resonance imaging) that display tissue volumes and have measures in place to monitor the quality of the imaging, US displays an operator-dependent, two-dimensional section of a tissue. It has to be recognized that the ability of the sonographer to evaluate and recognize normal and pathological patterns in real time and in different planes plays a pivotal role in the quality of US. Well-validated standards of US practice and a scoring system of US image quality exist. However, diagnostic US often includes many images, taken in several nonconventional planes and angles, making their standardization difficult and impractical. While admitting the inherent difficulties in assessing image quality in US, this remains an important aspect in service quality in all departments using US as a fundamental tool in the daily practice, including in IVF units. To promote best practice, clinicians are strongly encouraged to visit the websites of different organizations and leaders in the field of US imaging (e.g., the British Medical Ultrasound Society, the Society of Radiographers, the Royal College of Radiologists, the Royal College of Obstetrics and Gynaecology) [1–4] and export and apply these organizations' recommendations in their daily routine care.

Standard Operating Procedures

Every center for reproductive medicine should have and follow standard operating procedures (SOPs) that clearly explain what is expected at every step of the patients' journey. SOPs are fundamental tools that help clinicians carry out routine procedures efficiently and ensure quality output and uniformity of performance. In this regard, there should be a clear operational policy for the patient pathway, including when the scan should be performed and how it should be recorded. In some cases, the service could opt for either very detailed guidelines or a vague approach, allowing some flexibility and professional autonomy in their application. However, SOPs should be evidence-based, regularly updated, and known to all staff.

Key Performance Indicators

Key performance indicators (KPIs) are defined by the Joint Commission (formerly the Joint Commission on Accreditation of Healthcare Organizations [JCAHO]) as measurement tools "used to monitor and evaluate the quality of important governance, management, clinical, and support functions" [5]. KPIs were developed to assess and improve the overall quality of health care. An optimal quality of care is based on accurate information, proper and quick problem recognition, rigorous analysis, and the ability to measure and remeasure the performance. The possibility of measuring in quantitative terms the quality of a service is fundamental to determine if a particular intervention has led to an improvement of care. Therefore, KPIs' final target is to evaluate the health of an organization and to measure progress toward specific goals in quantitative terms. Over the past decade, the increasing use of imaging has brought the quality of imaging services to the attention of the public, health-care providers, and policymakers. However, its measure is inherently difficult, and scientific standardized metrics are lacking. For this reason, KPIs have been introduced [6–10]. They are particularly helpful for measuring difficult-to-measure processes. Generally, KPIs reflect an organization's strategy for success, and once they are defined, they are rarely changed (unless there is a change in the organization's goal). The definition of specific KPIs in a center for reproductive medicine should result from a collaborative effort between physicians and quality managers. Usually quality managers are more familiar with institutional vision and values, and the success of the center results from the alignment of its KPIs with the institutional strategy. KPIs should be based on core principles shared by the whole team that should include patient safety, quality of care, stakeholder management, operation management, and financial management. Data collection and analysis should be done regularly.

Quality of Interventional Procedures

Ultrasound Safety

US has been used for more than 40 years and so far, no significant biological effects (mechanically or thermally induced) causing harm to patients or sonographers have been reported. However, despite the huge body of literature on the topic, there are few limitations in assessing low-level effects that should be carefully considered. First, a problem in detecting low-level effects is the inability to prove a negative outcome. Indeed, a null finding could be either the result of no existing effects or it may be related to the insufficient sensitivity of the chosen assay to recognize it. The second explanation is more likely to be the case of early literature, where the assay tools used were less advanced than the modern ones. In addition, many studies conducted *in vitro* used cells either maintained in suspension culture or grown as monolayers. These types of studies are useful to evaluate US effects on cell membranes and organelles (nonthermal effects), but they do not provide any information regarding the interaction with other cells in intact tissues. In addition, these models are not suitable to study thermal mechanisms (which in case of *in vivo* exposure become more important than mechanical ones) and do not take into account the body's normal physiological responses to the increased temperature. Animal models have helped to overcome this limitation but have highlighted other concerns. Investigations in pregnant mice using a clinical diagnostic beam expose the whole fetus to the beam with a certain degree of attenuation. In humans, only a small part of the fetal body is exposed, and the attenuation of the beam by the overlying tissues is considerably higher. Considering all these limitations, the duty of US operators it to obtain optimum quality images while exposing patients to the minimum US "dose." Ideally, sonographers should guarantee that they are using US properly and in accordance with published guidelines. Therefore, when performing a US scan, some key principles should be kept in mind:

- Avoid unnecessary US scans by accurately examining all previous medical records.
- Limit the scan time in order to keep the "dose" to a minimum and optimize the scanner setup in order to keep the dose "as low as reasonably achievable" (ALARA principle).
- Avoid the use of Doppler in early pregnancy.

Equipment

In order to ensure an optimum US quality service, it is mandatory that the equipment is "fit for purpose." US transducers commonly used in reproductive medicine include a curved linear transducer

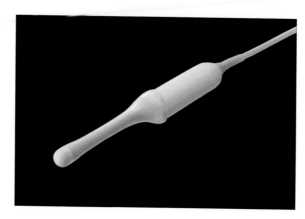

FIGURE 18.1   Transvaginal probe.

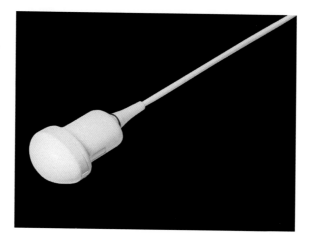

FIGURE 18.2   Transabdominal probe.

for transabdominal scanning and a transvaginal probe for intracavity imaging (Figures 18.1 and 18.2). Additionally, the scanner should be linked to an image management and archiving system.

Maintenance of the equipment is mandatory to ensure optimum performance. The American Institute of Ultrasound in Medicine (AIUM) outlined a quality assurance program that involves sonographers, physicians, medical physicists, and biomedical engineers and includes routine and annual checks that evaluate safety and performance of the US equipment in order to guarantee that the obtained images are accurate and that the equipment is safe [11]. Clinical US personnel are responsible for routine tasks, including cleanliness and safety of the scanning equipment and checks on image display. Routine maintenance recommendations are as follows:

- Machine control panels should be cleaned after each exam (with immediate cleaning if there is a spill of hazardous fluids).
- Transvaginal transducers should be cleaned of gel and disinfected after each exam. Abdominal transducers have lower risks of cross infection as they do not normally come into contact with body fluids. See Chapter 19 for more details.
- Transducer cables and monitors should be checked for damage and cracks daily.
- Power cords and communication systems should be inspected for cracks daily.
- Switches and knobs should be checked daily, and burned-out indicator lights should be identified.
- Brightness, contrast controls, and calibration should be checked daily, as well as gray levels on image hard copy and/or on display workstation.

- The presence of vertical shadows and streaks should be examined daily.
- Machine console air filter should be cleaned for dust weekly.
- Thorough cleaning of the equipment should be done at least monthly.

The AIUM suggests also to carry out detailed performance testing (in order to check cables, housing and transmitting surfaces, transducer uniformity, maximum depth of visualization, target detection, and distance measurement accuracy) on an annual basis. These procedures are generally performed by medical physicists or biomedical engineers who should work closely with sonographers. To organize and efficiently maintain the quality assurance program, it is advisable to designate an individual to be responsible for it.

In an IVF unit, the scanning environment is usually either a common consultation room or an operating room, equipped with a scanner as an additional tool. Consequently, the scanning condition may not be optimal, as expected in a dedicated US service. However, where possible, some small adjustments should be put in place to fulfill the ideal standards. First, the room size should be large enough to enable staff/patients/attendants to have movement with no stumbling hazards. The position of the scanning equipment (seating, console, transducers, display monitor) and of the examination table in the room should allow both patient privacy and dignity and US operator safety. Indeed, there have been reports of work-related musculoskeletal injury disorders in sonographers related to poor posture, repetitive movements, transducer pressure, workload, stress, and limited support [12]. An optimal body mechanic and a neutral posture represent important measures to prevent repetitive strain injuries associated with the profession. An ergonomic workstation, with good postural alignment and equipment position, plays a major role in mitigating these injuries but is only as good as the sonographer's willingness to use it. Some other general rules may help in preventing musculoskeletal injury disorders:

- Alternate between sitting and standing during an examination.
- Readjust the examination table and the monitor whenever necessary.
- Take a few moments to relax the upper extremities during/between the examination/s.
- Choose seating that allows subtle movements.

In addition, US machines generate heat, and without air conditioning, the room temperature can become excessive. Last, low ambient lighting could help and improve visual acuity of the operator.

Recently, increasing attention has been paid to the risk of cross infections following medical procedure using both endocavitary and nonendocavitary US probes. The latter increases the risk only when in contact with broken skin [13,14]. A recent publication reported that US transducers have a significantly higher bacterial contamination than toilets seats or bus poles [15]. Ultrasound gel has also been reported to be another potential source of contamination: a number of pathogens, including *Pseudomonas aeruginosa*, *Escherichia coli*, and *Klebsiella oxytoca*, have been isolated on US probes [15] (Figure 18.3). For this reason, departments should have an evidence-based infection control policy in place to prevent/control infections [15].

Training and Updating

US imaging represents an integral part in reproductive medicine. As previously stated, US is, more than any other imaging modality (e.g., computed tomography, magnetic resonance imaging), highly operator dependent. The sonographer is required to have adequate technical skills (including understanding of the US physics and familiarity with the machine control panel) along with an excellent knowledge of the female pelvic anatomy. However, recent technical improvements in US equipment have increased the potential for diagnostic errors. In some cases, the increasing sophistication of the most advanced scanners may be the cause of image misinterpretation by the operators, who are not properly trained [16].

In a center for reproductive medicine, US plays a pivotal role in clinical decision-making, and ideally, all operators should be "properly trained." The definition of what constitutes appropriate training is, however, complex. In addition, given the increasing educational demands and the recent changes in

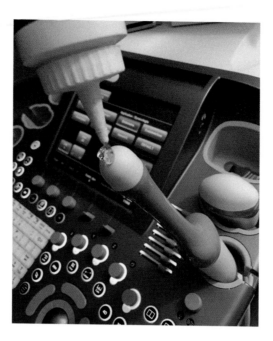

FIGURE 18.3 Ultrasound probes and gel are potential sources of contamination and may increase the risk of cross infections.

residency programs (e.g., work-hours restrictions), less and less time is spent on training and achieving competence in US [16]. Data from the Accreditation Council for Graduate Medical Education on ultrasound performance in obstetrics and gynecology residency programs pinpoint how the average number of US procedures completed during residency does not reach the minimum threshold required for physician qualification as defined by the AIUM [10,11]. Given the clinical importance of US, it is then advisable that all those performing US, especially new operators, should have a mentor. A qualified colleague with expertise in the field could provide advice and give guidance and support on clinical cases. New users should also undergo a period of preceptorship (around 4–6 months) to further develop their practice. It is also recommended to designate a leader in the service who takes on the responsibility for the quality and efficacy of the US service provision. A well-organized and operative framework should include audit on performance and outcome, including adverse event reporting, with time specifically allocated. Conversely, it is everyone's responsibility to keep updated. US operators have the professional responsibility to guarantee that their knowledge and skills evolve constantly as the US evidence base changes. In addition, a critical evaluation of one's own work is a paramount skill that should be engendered in all staff members. To recognize personal limitations and to refer the patient to a more experienced imaging colleague when necessary should also be encouraged.

Diagnostic Sonographic Documentation

Valid Consent and Chaperoning

Pelvic US is considered an intimate procedure, and patient privacy and dignity should be ensured during such a sensitive examination. Valid (verbal or written) consent should be obtained before every gynecological examination, and in case of transvaginal US, the patient should be informed of the need for the movement of the probe during the procedure [1,17]. The policy in the presence of a chaperone varies from one country or institution to another. In some countries, patients may request the presence of a chaperone during the exam, and this demand should be fulfilled whenever possible. In others, the presence of a chaperone is mandatory in all circumstances. Name and designation of the chaperone must be recorded in the medical report.

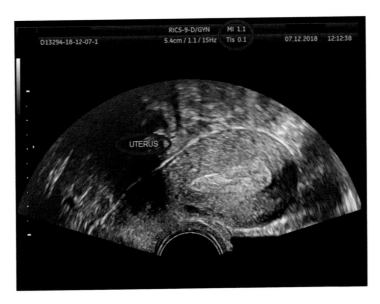

FIGURE 18.4 Example of safety indexes and basic annotations.

Image Labeling and Archiving

Appropriate image labeling and archiving are the operator's responsibility. Before starting the examination, patient data and identification number (when present) should be entered correctly. Besides patient demographics, all images should include date and time of the examination, service identification, system setting (e.g., gain, frame rate), and safety indexes (e.g., mechanical and thermal indexes). Ideally, images should also include a pictogram describing patient and probe position and an annotation stating which organ is scanned along with the anatomical section. However, it is widely recognized that this would extend the exam time and is particularly cumbersome in a busy appointment schedule. Still, basic annotations should be present in order to enable a second observer to interpret the scan (Figure 18.4).

For every US examination, all significant images should be archived in a proper and well-organized manner, and the operator should be able to retrieve them easily. Beyond being precious adjunctive tools to the final report, archived images could also be used for audit purposes [1–3]. Stored images should be of high quality and representative of the examination. Ideally, archiving should be to PACS (Picture Archiving and Communication System). However, some concerns have been raised regarding patient privacy and confidentiality. Some patients may not want their appointment within an IVF unit to be accessible to other health services and providers. In such a case, images could be stored in an external hard drive. However, not every facility is properly equipped for digital archiving, and in this case thermal printing is the only option. Since thermal prints' longevity is poor, it is mandatory to obtain high-quality images on the US system screen. The printer should be checked regularly and set up carefully, in order to ensure that the prints are a good reproduction of the image on the screen.

Reporting the Outcome

A report is defined by the Royal College of Radiologists as "a specialist interpretation of images relating to the findings, both anticipated and unexpected, to the patient's current clinical symptoms and signs in order to diagnose or contribute to the understanding of their medical condition or clinical state" [16]. It represents a primary means of communication between the sonographer and the referring clinician, and it also has medicolegal importance. There is no single "correct" way to report US results, but there are some elements considered necessary for a satisfactory report. Generally, a good report should be accurate, clear, concise, and logically structured. It should address and, where possible, answer the clinical question and, where appropriate, should give suggestions for further investigations and/or management. The sonographer should write it as soon as possible after the examination, and it should be considered as an integral part of the whole examination. The person undertaking the US is responsible for its accuracy. Redundant and long descriptions and technical terminology should be avoided. The adoption of report proforma/worksheet is useful because it is time-saving and also helps in standardizing the procedure and in minimizing errors. The use of a standard template could be particularly helpful when patients undergo multiple scans (e.g., during follicle growth monitoring), which could be performed by different sonographers. The report proforma, when used, should follow the center's scheme of work. The ideal report depends on the variable needs of the patient and on the service providing the scan. A practitioner's personal preference also plays a part, and it is not necessarily appropriate to limit his or her options to communicate as he or she sees fit. Some suggestions on how a report should be structured and what it should contain are set out in Box 18.1.

BOX 18.1   SUGGESTIONS ON WHAT A GOOD REPORT SHOULD INCLUDE

WHAT?	HOW?
Patient identification	• Name and identification number (when present) should be correctly entered • Statement that consent for intimate procedure was obtained should be reported
Staff identification	• Demographics and role of all personnel present during the examination should be reported (US practitioner, trainee, chaperone, etc.)
Date and time	• Must align with the images archived
Clinical indication and nature of the examination	• The reason for performing the scan must be clear • The type of probe used should be mentioned (transvaginal US only, transabdominal US only, transabdominal US progressing to transvaginal US)
Menstrual/reproductive/ hormonal status	• Late menstrual period • Gravida and parity status • Ongoing hormonal treatment
Description of findings	• Note SSOTM (size, shape, outline, texture, relevant measurement) of all analyzed structures • When "normal," it is advisable to record that rather than provide long descriptions • Acoustic terminology (e.g., anechoic, transonic, hypo-/hyperechogenic) should be avoided
Abnormal findings	• SSOTM should also be applied to abnormal findings • Anatomical variants should be noted and, when possible, classified (e.g., congenital uterine malformations)
Technical limitations	• Details should be recorded (e.g., high body mass index, excess bowel gas)
Conclusion	• Conclusion must be clear • Include differential(s) when appropriate • Referral for further investigations, when necessary, should be reported • Report should be signed by the appropriate qualified person

REFERENCES

1. *Guidelines for Professional Ultrasound Standards. Society of Radiographers and British Medical Ultrasound Society.* December 2015. https://www.sor.org/sites/default/files/document-versions/2018.1.5_scor_bmus_guidelines_final.pdf

2. Standards for the provision of an Ultrasound Service. Society and College of Radiographers and the Royal College of Radiologists. December 2014. https://www.rcr.ac.uk/system/files/publication/field_publication_files/BFCR%2814%2917_Standards_ultrasound.pdf

3. *Ultrasound Training Recommendations for Medical and Surgical Specialties.* 2nd ed. Ref No. BFCR(12)17 the Royal College of Radiologists. December 2012. https://www.rcr.ac.uk/system/files/publication/field_publication_files/bfcr173_ultrasound_training_med_surg.pdf

4. *Focused Ultrasound Training Standards.* Ref No. BFCR(12)18. The Royal College of Radiologists. December 2012. https://www.rcr.ac.uk/system/files/publication/field_publication_files/BFCR%2812%2918_focused_training.pdf

5. The Joint Commission (formerly the Joint Commission on Accreditation of Healthcare Organizations). *Primer on Indicator Development and Application.* Oakbrook Terrace, IL: Joint Commission; 1990.

6. Salvesen KA, Lees C, and Tutschek B. Basic European ultrasound training in obstetrics and gynecology: Where are we and where do we go from here? *Ultrasound Obstet Gynecol.* 2010;36(5):525–9.

7. Abuhamad A, Minton KK, Benson CB et al. Obstetric and gynecologic ultrasound curriculum and competency assessment in residency training programs: Consensus report. *Ultrasound Obstet Gynecol.* 2018;51(1):150–5.

8. Baker JP, and Coffin CT. The importance of an ergonomic workstation to practicing sonographers. *J Ultrasound Med.* 2013;32(8):1363–75.

9. Accreditation Council for Graduate Medical Education (ACGME). Obstetrics and Gynecology Case Logs: National Data Report. https://www.acgme.org/Portals/0/PDFs/220_National_Report_Program_Version_2015-2016.pdf

10. *AIUM Ultrasound Practice Accreditation.* American Institute of Ultrasound in Medicine. http://www.aium.org/accreditation/accreditation.aspx

11. *Routine Quality Assurance for Diagnostic Ultrasound Equipment.* American Institute of Ultrasound in Medicine. http://aium.s3.amazonaws.com/resourceLibrary/rqa.pdf

12. Harrison G, and Harris A. Work-related musculoskeletal disorders in ultrasound: Can you reduce risk? *Ultrasound.* 2015;23(4):224–30.

13. Merz E. Is transducer hygiene sufficient when vaginal probes are used in the clinical routine? *Ultraschall Med.* 2016;37(2):137–9.

14. Scott D, Fletcher E, Kane H et al. Risk of infection following semi-invasive ultrasound procedures in Scotland, 2010 to 2016: A retrospective cohort study using linked national datasets. *Ultrasound.* 2018;26(3):168–77.

15. Sartoretti T, Sartoretti E, Bucher C et al. Bacterial contamination of ultrasound probes in different radiological institutions before and after specific hygiene training: Do we have a general hygienical problem? *Eur Radiol.* 2017;27(10):4181–7.

16. Standards for the Reporting and Interpreting of Imaging Investigations BFCR(06)1 RCR Updated. September 2015. https://www.rcr.ac.uk/publication/standardsreporting-and-interpretation-imaging-investigations

17. Obtaining Valid Consent (Clinical Governance Advice No. 6). Royal College of Obstetricians and Gynecologists. London: 2015. https://www.rcr.ac.uk/sites/default/files/bfcr061_standardsforreporting.pdf/

19

Safety Aspects of Ultrasound Scanning

Kelly Tilleman

Brief History on the Covering and Cleaning of the Endovaginal Probe

In the mid-1990s, the American Institute of Ultrasound in Medicine invoked a multidisciplinary task force to tackle the reprocessing of vaginal ultrasound probes between patients. Although very few scientific data existed on the microbial contamination of the probes at that time, it was quite obvious that cleaning the probe with detergent/water should be the cornerstone of the disinfection, since the probes could not be autoclaved as vaginal specula could. The use of chemical disinfection could provide an additional margin of safety and would help in the further reduction in microbial load; however, there were at that time concerns on the toxicity of the chemicals used to both the patient and the sonographers [1]. Ultrasound covers were already routinely used at that time; however, the effectiveness of this barrier in daily clinical practice was not well known. Although these covers sometimes showed small ruptures or breaks after the clinical investigation, a true estimate of the failure rate was unknown. An early study by Rooks et al. [2] demonstrated an 8.3% perforation rate in probe covers and a 1.7% perforation rate in latex condoms by performing a standard leak test by filling the covers or condoms with water. This study already showed the superior quality of condoms, which were a cheaper alternative than the commercially available probe covers. A large study by Milki and Fisch [3] tested more than 800 nonlubricated latex condoms that were used as ultrasound covers and demonstrated a perforation rate of 2%. Although these data were known at that time, apparently not all practitioners routinely disinfected the probes after use because they did not observe any obvious blood or vaginal secretions on the probe, and so it was concluded that the use of a cover was sufficient.

Because of the perforation rate of covers and condoms, both the study of Milki and Fisch [3] and Rooks et al. [2] clearly underlined the use of a germicidal spray or the use of a soaked cloth for disinfection after removal of the cover, since the possibility of microscopic bacterial contamination could not be excluded.

Endovaginal Probe as Semicritical Device

Semicritical devices come directly in contact with mucous membranes or nonintact skin, and these devices should be free from all microorganisms; however, small numbers of bacterial spores are permissible. Since the use of probe covers in transvaginal (TV) ultrasounds made it possible to keep the probe from directly contacting the patient, the ultrasound probe was actually first categorized as a noncritical device. When probe covers were introduced in routine ultrasound practices and changed between every patient, it was considered that a low-level disinfection (LLD) would be sufficient. Since several studies clearly demonstrated that the probe covers were prone to perforation, the guideline for disinfection from the Centers for Disease Control and Prevention (CDC) recommended that even if probe covers were used, the ultrasound probe was to be defined as a semicritical device; thus, the probe had to be first cleaned and subsequently a high-level disinfection (HLD) had to be performed (recommendation 10a; [4]) to ensure the removal of all microorganisms.

Bacterial Contamination of Endovaginal Ultrasound Probe

Results in the literature determine that HLD disinfection is necessary to make sure that ultrasound probes are free of contaminated bacterial flora. Almost all TV probes show bacterial growth when

252

sampled after removal of the probe cover and before disinfection or even after LLD [5]. The microbial testing reveals mostly environmental contaminants, microorganisms originating from vaginal or skin flora. Even after manual disinfection, nosocomial pathogens like *Staphylococcus aureus*, *Klebsiella pneumonia*, *Pseudomonas* spp., or *Escherichia coli* can be identified on ultrasound probes [5–7]. Ngu et al. [6] identified a large portion of isolates containing *S. aureus*, and one of these isolates was found to be methicillin-resistant *S. aureus* (MRSA). Additionally, causative agents of urinary tract infections like *S. aureus*, *S. haemolyticus*, *S. saprophyticus*, and *E. faecium* can be found on TV transducers after manual LLD [6]. Likewise, Westerway et al. [8] showed remaining species derived from normal skin flora of environmental organisms after LLD. When ultrasound probes in this study were subsequently subjected to manual HDL, no bacterial contamination could be found. The authors of these studies already discussed the variability in the residual contamination after manual disinfection, related to the sonographer's compliance with disinfecting procedure. Studies that have included automated disinfection illustrate this to be superior to manual HLD disinfection. The risk for bacterial contamination after manual disinfection was 2.9-fold higher than the risk after automated disinfection using a Trophon EPR automated system in the study of Buescher et al. [5]. Similarly, the use of a disinfection apparatus using ultraviolet-C (UVC) light (Antigermix device) resulted in TV probes where neither bacterial nor viral flora could be detected [9]. Not only can pathogenic microorganisms reside on ultrasound transducers, reports on the presence of human papillomavirus (HPV) gained interest in more recent literature.

Human Papillomavirus Contamination of Endovaginal Ultrasound Probe

The gynecological environment can become contaminated by HPV from health-care workers' hands and gloves. There is, however, conflicting evidence for HPV transmission, and while skin-to-skin and mucosa-to-mucosa contact, predominantly by sexual intercourse, is the most frequent route of transmission, other routes might be involved [10]. HPV can persist in the environment and on medical equipment even after disinfection. The close contact between the transvaginal probe and the cervix uteri or vaginal wall can be a potential risk for transmission of sexually transmitted infections, such as HPV [11].

HPV persists on the probe after disinfection with LLD despite the covering of the probe; thus, LLD is clearly inadequate for preventing contamination of the ultrasound probe [11]. This study found 3.5% HPV DNA positive samples of which 6% were positive for HPV 53, 16, 58, and 31. When the results were analyzed in a successive mode, it was shown that HPV 58 was detected in three out of four subsequent samples suggesting a persistent probe contamination despite each disinfection round. In the second study period, 2.8% were HPV DNA positive, and again, high-risk HPV 53 was detected in the positive samples. Similarly, the study from Ma et al. [12] observed that 7.5% of the TV ultrasound transducers were positive for HPV after disinfection using T-Spray, a quaternary ammonia-based spray.

Not only are ultrasound transducers or handles prone to contamination risk, but the vast majority of gynecological equipment is apparently contaminated with HPV [10].

And even when chemicals are used that are categorized as HLD, they seem to be ineffective against HPV [13,14]. This means that the current guidelines for HLD might not be sufficient in eradicating HPV from TV probes. Although HPV DNA detection does not mean HPV virulence, and consequently, no infectivity of HPV is shown in any of the previously mentioned cross-sectional studies, it is clear that HPV is quite difficult to eliminate.

Recent data show two validation studies using an automated disinfection machine for the complete removal of microorganisms and HPV: one apparatus uses UVC (Antigermix device) [13], and one uses sonicated hydrogen peroxide (Trophon EPR) [14]. These reports present preclinical efficacy for removal of HPV by using a hard surface carrier test in comparison to using chemicals that have been classified as HLD by the CDC (recommendation 10a; [4]). The results of the studies undoubtedly show the possibility for these two automated devices to completely remove and inactivate HPV, as these are the only studies including an HPV infectivity assay [13,14]. See further Table 19.1.

TABLE 19.1

Overview of Cross-Sectional Studies Cited on the Risk of Probe Contamination Following Endovaginal Ultrasound from the Bacterial or Viral Perspective

Study Details	Setting, Population, and Load Tested	Covers Used	Disinfection Used	Method of Sampling	Results	Remarks and Conclusions
Ngu et al. [6]	Single center, prospective study, cross-sectional study, 77 samples GDHO. 75 GDHH • Bacterial contamination	Type of transducers used: not specified, covers used: not specified	The probe: first cleaned with detergent and water, dried with paper towel, then soaking 2.4% GD (GDHO) or automated disinfection using Trophon EPR (using hydrogen peroxide) where both handle and probe are disinfected (GDHH)	Cotton swab dipped in tryptone soya broth, identification by VITEK device (bioMérieux)	80.5% of GDHO versus 5.3 of GDHH showed contamination, most of them associated with health-care infections (*Staphylococcus aureus* and one MRSA)	Ultrasound transducer handles might become contaminated if they are not disinfected if they are not disinfected if HLD methods should include disinfecting the entire transducer. Automated disinfection is more effective than manual disinfection
Buescher et al. [5]	Prospective randomized controlled clinical study, 120 samples pre- and postdisinfection using manual disinfection, 120 samples after Trophon EPR disinfection • Bacterial contamination	TV: transducer covers: not specified	Manual (Mikrozid-sensitive wipes containing quaternary ammonium compounds), Trophon EPR (using hydrogen peroxide)	Polywipe premoistened sponge swabs incubated overnight at 36°C applied to blood-and MacConkey-Agar overnight incubated, next MALDI-TOF analysis for identification	95.4% of the samples before disinfection were positive. After automatic disinfection: 8.6% contaminated, after manual disinfection: 21.2% contaminated	Disinfection reduces bacterial contamination, and automated disinfection shows advantages over manual disinfection
Westerway et al. [8]	Prospective blinded single center study (two ultrasound units), 171 samples were taken before disinfection and after LLD and after LLD and HLD Sampling was also done on the ultrasound unit and on coupling gel • Bacterial contamination	TV: latex condom TA: vinyl cover	Manual LLD using an alcohol-based wipe or HLD by immersion in 2.4% GD	Culture swabs were plated on nutrient agar and incubated at 37°C overnight. CFU were counted and subsequently identified by MALDI-TOF or by PCR	60% TA and 14% TV were positive after removal of the cover. After LLD, 3% (TA) and 4% (TV) were positive. No contamination detected in TV after LLD and HLD	HLD is more effective than LLD. The ultrasound apparatus (keyboard, cord) needs disinfection. Gels are a source of bacterial contamination

(Continued)

TABLE 19.1 (Continued)

Overview of Cross-Sectional Studies Cited on the Risk of Probe Contamination Following Endovaginal Ultrasound from the Bacterial or Viral Perspective

Study Details	Setting, Population, and Load Tested	Covers Used	Disinfection Used	Method of Sampling	Results	Remarks and Conclusions
Casalegno et al. [11]	Single center, prospective study, two study periods; period 1: 200 samples, period 2: 217 samples • Viral (HPV) contamination	TV: disposable probe cover (93/42/EEC CE mark)	Disinfection wipes (sani-cloth active) (containing quaternary ammonium compounds)	Sampling by dry swab, subsequently submerged in EMEM transport medium; DNA extraction (NucliSens easyMAG), genotyping via microarrays (Genomica SAU)	Period 1: 3.5% HV DNA positive Period 2: 2.5% HPV DNA positive	LLD is not sufficient for complete disinfection. HPV DNA detection ≠ HPV virulence. Dry swabbing could result in sensitivity loss for HPV detection
Ma et al. [12]	Two-part cross-sectional study: 2 periods: part 1 (surveillance): 120 samples; part 2: 14 samples originating from TV ultrasound probes used in known HPV+ females • Viral (HPV) contamination	Latex condom	Disinfection with T-spray containing quaternary ammonia	Cotton wool swabs, DNA extraction (QIAamp DNA mini kit), PCR (PGMY09–11)	Part 1: 7.5% HPV positive; Part 2: 21.4% HPV positive	Most positive HPV samples were in the first 20 days of the study. Possibly a more thorough disinfection was performed when staff were aware of the study
Gallay et al. [10]	Cross-sectional study in two centers (public hospital and private setting), 179 samples on gynecological equipment and surfaces • Viral (HPV) contamination	No data	HLD, no further specification	Sampling by flocked swabs submerged in 1 mL PBS saline DNA extraction and identification using real-time PCR (Anyplex II HPV28 test)	18% of samples were HPV DNA positive	Detection of HPV more frequent in samples from private center. Lamp, glove box, specula, and gel tubes were positive for HPV DNA

Abbreviations: CFU, colony-forming units; EMEM, Eagle's minimum essential medium; GD, glutaraldehyde; GDHH, glutaraldehyde disinfection head and handle; GDHO, glutaraldehyde disinfection head only; HLD, high-level disinfection; LLD, low-level disinfection; MRSA, methicillin-resistant *Staphylococcus aureus*; MALDI-TOF, matrix-assisted laser desorption ionization-time of flight; TA, transabdominal; TV, transvaginal.

Clinical Practice in Endovaginal Ultrasound Disinfection

Disinfectants Used

When looking at the literature, a wide variety of chemicals are used for disinfecting ultrasound probes: solutions containing glutaraldehyde, quaternary ammonium salts, peracetic acid, and hydrogen peroxide. All these solutions have to bear a disinfecting activity and be compatible with the functionality of the transducer. Some chemicals can shorten the lifespan of the probe, and insufficient rinsing after using these chemicals can result in a higher risk for irritation to the patient due to damage of the mucosa. HLD chemicals are tested for the removal of bacterial species; however, some studies have shown that glutaraldehyde and orthophthalaldehyde do not have virucidal activity against certain HPV types [13,14]. Nonchemical alternatives, like UVC (Antigermix device) or treatments with H_2O_2 nanodroplets (Trophon EPR automated system) have therefore gained interest and have been shown to be effective in completely disinfecting the probe and removing all bacterial and viral contamination [5,9].

Many hospitals have an infection control department in charge of procedures concerning the overall cleanliness in the hospital, sanitization, and sterilization. It is important to contact this department for information on the disinfectants to be used on semicritical devices such as TV ultrasound probes. On an individual basis, a sonographer could also contact the manufacturer of the disinfectants and the ultrasound machines to get information about utilization of the disinfecting agents and kits.

The Sonographers' Performance

The limited amount of studies on the effectiveness of manual disinfection of TV transducers clearly shows that there is an operator link to the quality of the disinfection. In most studies, the staff was aware of the study, and this aids the compliance to the standard operating procedure (SOP) for disinfection of the probe. Although the cleaning and disinfection of an ultrasound probe might seem futile in the broader package of sonographers' tasks, there is a risk that the disinfection fails simply due to lack of education and training. Knowledge of the disinfecting agents used, compliance to disinfection SOP, especially considering the contact exposure time of the disinfecting chemicals on the probe, and a short literature overview of the possible remaining bacterial and viral load on the probes after disinfecting will reduce the risk of contamination and support the patient safety in ultrasound practice. The study of Ngu et al. [6] clearly showed the importance of the disinfection of the ultrasound handle alongside of the disinfection of the probe. Likewise, data from Buescher et al. [5] showed that disinfection of the handle and the probe (e.g., during automated disinfection) resulted in a 91.4% success rate of disinfection, where manual disinfection had a 78.8% success rate. Finally, Westerway et al. [8] demonstrated high levels of bacterial contamination on the ultrasound unit (keyboards, probe wire) and ultrasound gel. Although most contamination originated from human commensals and environmental species, there was evidence of potential pathogenic species on the keyboard of the ultrasound machine.

Step-by-Step Manual Disinfection Procedure

After the scan has been performed, use new gloves to perform the disinfection procedure and remove the probe cover. First clean the probe by removing any visible remaining residues by using a paper towel or an impregnated cloth (Figure 19.1a). A simple paper towel can already remove 40%–45% of the bacterial load. The use of physiological saline solution reduces the microorganisms further to 76%, and water-soap can eliminate up to 96% of the bacteria [15]. When a soaked cloth has been used, the probe has to be carefully rubbed dry using a paper towel. Next, disinfect the probe by immersing the probe in an HLD agent (Figure 19.1b). If immersing is not possible, then gently rubbing the probe with an impregnated cloth is necessary. It is important to check the desired contact time of the chemical used in order to sufficiently decontaminate the surface (Figure 19.1c). Finally, leave the probe to dry. Next, use new gloves to disinfect the handle of the ultrasound probe. Additionally, disinfect the ultrasound apparatus (keyboard and wire) in

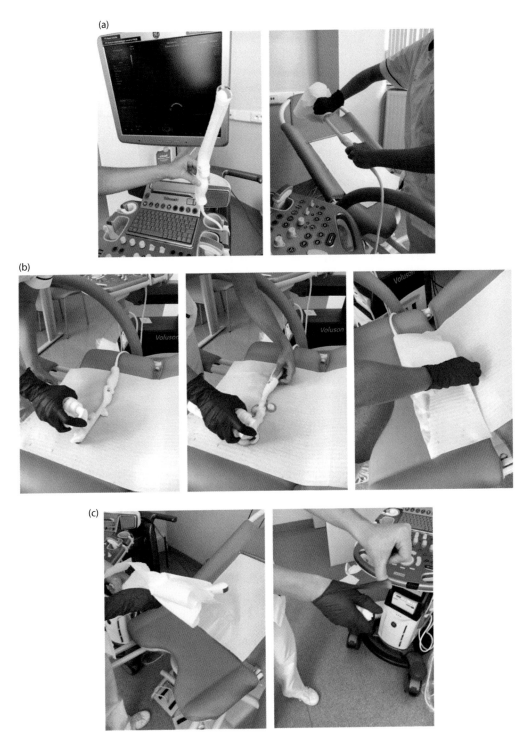

FIGURE 19.1 A step-by-step example of a disinfection protocol: (a) Remove the probe cover and first clean the probe by removing any visible remaining residues by using a paper towel or an impregnated cloth. (b) Disinfect the probe by immersing or covering the probe in a high-level disinfection agent and respect the contact time or gently rub the probe with an impregnated cloth according to the manufacturer's guidelines. (c) If necessary when soaking or covering has been executed, remove the disinfectant with a paper cloth and leave the probe to dry. After disinfecting the probe, new gloves should be used to manually disinfect the handle, the cord, and/or the keyboard.

between patients and, if possible, use single-dose coupling gels. Endorse a vigorous hand hygiene protocol while performing the ultrasound procedure, and take care that during or after the disinfection procedure the transducer, the handle, or the ultrasound unit are not recontaminated.

Conclusion and Published Guidelines

Although there is a limited number of studies in the literature on the disinfection of ultrasound probes, it is clear that recently this subject has gained interest. It is clear that TV probes require HDL disinfection, whereas abdominal probes could still be considered noncritical devices, as abdominal probes do not come directly in contact with mucous membranes or nonintact skin. For the latter, an LLD is sufficient [4].

In order to find out if your disinfection protocol is effective and your staff is adhering to the protocol, a simple practical audit can be carried out. A disinfection exercise was carried out in our fertility department where a total of 71 samples of TV ultrasound probes were analyzed. The samples were taken during a daily practice ultrasound program for controlled ovarian stimulation in fertility patients. After removal of the cover and HLD disinfection, ultrasound probes were sampled by pressing down and rolling the head of the transducer onto a RODAC (replicate organism detection and counting) dish. After 48 hours, mass spectrometry analysis was used for identification of the bacterial residual load. Results showed that the majority of the probes (60.5% [43/71]) were negative, and an average 1.9 colony forming units (CFUs) (min: 0; max: 42) were detected. The majority of the bacterial contaminants originated from skin flora or from environmental contamination, being coagulase-negative staphylococci, micrococci, and *Corynebacterium* sp. (unpublished data from Ghent University Hospital). It was clear that although our protocol consisted of a validated HLD method, the performance of the disinfection procedure among the staff was quite different. A dedicated periodic training in manual disinfection was recommended to aid the consistency of the procedure and to contribute to patient safety. Moreover, an automatic disinfection omits the operator variability of the manual disinfection procedure, additionally reducing the risk for the subsequent use of contaminated ultrasound probes.

Since national guidelines and legislation regulating disinfection procedures vary throughout Europe, the European Society of Radiology Ultrasound Working Group recently published best recommendations on infection prevention and control in ultrasound [16]. The paper is a coherent overview of the transmission risk of infection through ultrasound procedures and describes the normal skin microbial flora and potential pathogens varying from site to site in the human body. There are extensive definitions of the decontamination procedures, and recommendations on disinfection are unambiguously listed. Likewise, the World Federation for Ultrasound in Medicine and Biology (WFUMB) published their guidelines for cleaning transvaginal ultrasound transducers between patients [17]. This document cites relevant disinfecting chemicals and explains how they are effective in eradicating certain bacterial and viral species and spores. Precautions while using these chemicals are mentioned alongside recommendations on the practicalities of disinfection, and automatic disinfection systems (UVC) (Antigermix device) or Trophon EPR are explained [17]. As ultrasound practitioners do not always know which patients carry transmissible pathogens or who may be susceptible to acquiring infections, implementation of clear disinfection recommendations will reassure patients and contribute to their quality of care [16]. Additionally, it is advisable to keep information in the medical file of the disinfection products used and the sonographer or nurse performing the disinfection. These data should be part of traceability and general record keeping.

REFERENCES

1. Goldstein SR. Reprocessing of the vaginal probe between patients. *Ultrasound Obstet Gynecol.* 1996;7:92–3.
2. Rooks VJ, Yancey MK, Elg SA, and Brueske L. Comparison of probe sheaths for endovaginal sonography. *Obstet Gynecol.* 1996;87:27–9.
3. Milki AA, and Fisch JD. Vaginal ultrasound probe cover leakage: Implications for patient care. *Fertil Steril.* 1998;69(3):409–11.

4. Rutala WA, and Weber DJ, HICPAC. *Guideline for Disinfection and Sterilization in Healthcare Facilities.* Washington, DC: Centers for Disease Control and Prevention; 2017.
5. Buescher DL, Möllers M, Falkenberg MK et al. Disinfection of transvaginal ultrasound probes in a clinical setting: Comparative performance of automated and manual reprocessing methods. *Ultrasound Obstet Gynecol.* 2016;47(5):646–51.
6. Ngu A, McNally G, Patel D, Gorgis V, Leroy S, and Burdach J. Reducing transmission risk through high-level disinfection of transvaginal ultrasound transducer handles. *Infect Control Hosp Epidemiol.* 2015;36(5):581–4.
7. Westerway SC, and Basseal JM. The role of infection control within the ultrasound unit. *Ultraschall der Medizin.* 2017;38(6):672–4.
8. Westerway SC, Basseal JM, Brockway A, Hyett JA, and Carter DA. Potential infection control risks associated with ultrasound equipment—A bacterial perspective. *Ultrasound Med Biol.* 2017;43(2):421–6.
9. Kac G, Podglajen I, Si-Mohamed A, Rodi A, Grataloup C, and Meyer G. Evaluation of ultraviolet C for disinfection of endocavitary ultrasound transducers persistently contaminated despite probe covers. *Infect Control Hosp Epidemiol.* 2010;31:165–70.
10. Gallay C, Miranda E, Schaefer S et al. Human papillomavirus (HPV) contamination of gynaecological equipment. *Sex Transm Infect.* 2016;92(1):19–23.
11. Casalegno JS, Le Bail Carval K, Eibach D et al. High risk HPV contamination of endocavity vaginal ultrasound probes: An underestimated route of nosocomial infection? *PLOS ONE.* 2012;7(10):8–11.
12. Ma STC, Yeung AC, Chan PKS, and Graham CA. Transvaginal ultrasound probe contamination by the human papillomavirus in the emergency department. *Emerg Med J.* 2013;30:472–5.
13. Meyers C, Milici J, and Robison R. UVC radiation as an effective disinfectant method to inactivate human papillomaviruses. *PLOS ONE.* 2017;12(10):1–9.
14. Ryndock E, Robison R, and Meyers C. Susceptibility of HPV16 and 18 to high level disinfectants indicated for semi-critical ultrasound probes. *J Med Virol.* 2016;88:1076–80.
15. Miyague AH, Mauad FM, de Paula Martins W, Benedetti ACG, Ferreira AEG, and Mauad-Filho F. Ultrasound scan as a potential source of nosocomial and cross-infection: A literature review. *Radiol Bras.* 2015;48(5):319–23.
16. Nyhsen CM, Humphreys H, Koerner RJ et al. Infection prevention and control in ultrasound—Best practice recommendations from the European Society of Radiology Ultrasound Working Group. *Insights Imaging.* 2017;8(6):523–35.
17. Abramowicz JS, Evans DH, Fowlkes JB, Maršal K, and terHaar G. Guidelines for cleaning transvaginal ultrasound transducers between patients. *Ultrasound Med Biol.* 2017;43(5):1076–9.

20

Ultrasound Training in Assisted Reproduction and Early Pregnancy

Martin G. Tolsgaard, Karin Sundberg, and Henriette Svarre Nielsen

Introduction

The quality of ultrasound examinations depends on the skills of the person performing the ultrasound scan. Ultrasound skills are associated with long learning curves, and the international ultrasound societies have recommended extensive periods of supervision before commencing independent practice [1,2] (training guidelines). This begs the question: are we training new trainees as effectively as we should be? What evidence supports the development of ultrasound skills, and how do we determine when trainees are fit for independent practice? In this chapter, we provide insights into the development of ultrasound skills, methods for training ultrasound skills in the clinical setting, and new advances in simulation-based ultrasound training as well as other computer-based instruction and online learning resources. Finally, we offer practical tips for the trainer that can be adopted in daily clinical and educational practice.

Developing Ultrasound Skills

Ultrasonography is a skill that requires a complex interplay of motor skills and visual-cognitive skills [3,4]. The *motor skills* required during ultrasound examinations include hand-eye coordination and follow well-described patterns of skills acquisition [3,11,12]: trainees initially demonstrate flawed, slow, and inconsistent performances, but with training they show increasing levels of automaticity, speed, consistency, and accuracy in movements [3]. *Visual-cognitive skills* are needed to perceive and interpret the ultrasound images that are produced. Moreover, visual-cognitive skills are needed to translate a two-dimensional ultrasound image into a three-dimensional mental model of the organ being examined. Experts are thought to display a two-step process during image interpretation: an initial global impression is followed by a focal search for pathology and key landmarks [5–7]. However, strategies aiming to improve novices' diagnostic accuracy by promoting expert search patterns and diagnostic reasoning have to date shown depressing results [8,9]. Hence, the strategies that are used by experts are not solely responsible for the experts' improved diagnostic accuracy. Instead, experts have through years of dedicated practice established a repertoire of thousands of ultrasound images and patient presentations that they may use for mental comparison when coming across similar new cases—a process known as *illness script theory* [10]. Hence, at least two sets of skills—motor skills and visual-cognitive skills—need to be practiced and refined to attain expert performance in ultrasound [26–29].

Current Methods for Ultrasound Training

Traditionally, ultrasound skills have been taught through apprenticeship learning, where trainees observe senior clinicians and practice under their supervision until they acquire the skills necessary to commence independent practice. For intimate examinations such as transvaginal ultrasound, this may be associated

260

with specific challenges because of the need to have several persons present in the room during the scan and the potential additional discomfort due to unskilled probe handling when the scan is being performed by inexperienced trainees.

There are also considerable personnel costs in terms of the additional time required from both trainees and their supervisors in addition to the need for repeated examinations due to diagnostic uncertainty during early phases of independent practice. In a large survey of Scandinavian obstetrician/gynecologist trainees, it took more than 24 months of clinical practice before trainees performed ultrasound examinations independently, although less time if they received dedicated training in a fetal medicine unit first [11,12]. Despite the high degree of supervised practice, trainees in the Tolsgaard et al. survey reported substantial gaps in the type of ultrasound examinations that they were expected to perform and the examinations that they felt adequately equipped to perform. These results are echoed in a subsequent study, in which trainees failed to demonstrate sufficient skills to independently practice transvaginal ultrasound for early pregnancy complications after 2 months of clinical practice and an average of nearly 50 supervised scans [13,14]. In a recent and large French study, sonologists attending an annual ultrasound licensing exam were asked to perform five scans on a transvaginal ultrasound simulator (Scantrainer, Medaphor; Cardiff, United Kingdom). The average diagnostic accuracy across these five cases was only 72% and 71% for sonologists, who had completed more than 300 and 1000 transvaginal scans, respectively. However, none of the sonologists with less than 100 scans reached a diagnostic accuracy of 100% [15]. Hence, clinical practice is a necessary but not sufficient factor to ensure a high diagnostic accuracy, and even senior clinicians may fail to demonstrate the skills expected based on the extent of their past ultrasound experience.

In another study, the behaviors of fetal medicine consultants were compared to those of fertility medicine consultants, when they performed transabdominal and transvaginal ultrasound examinations, respectively. In this study, fertility medicine consultants demonstrated significantly lower performance scores for image optimization than fetal medicine consultants [11,12]. This may indicate that image optimization was not as essential for fertility medicine consultants to arrive at a diagnosis because of low complexity of the cases scanned (e.g., follicle count). In contrast, the behaviors of fetal medicine consultants may reflect the fact that they must rely more on image optimization to achieve high-quality images for high-complexity scans (e.g., anomaly scans). Finally, the finding may suggest that for nonultrasound specialists, there are significant gaps between best practice and actual practice, even for highly experienced clinicians.

Simulation-Based Ultrasound Training

Because of all the limitations associated with clinical training as mentioned earlier, educators have been searching for alternative methods for training new trainees in ultrasound. In other areas of medical practice, the use of simulation-based training has shown promising results in terms of moderate effects on patient outcomes and large effects on trainee behavior in the clinical setting [16]. These large effects have led some scientists to call simulation-based medical education an "ethical imperative." Over the past decade, increasingly sophisticated simulators designed for ultrasound in obstetrics and gynecology have been developed. These simulators can broadly be divided into physical mannequins and virtual reality simulators.

The physical mannequins are often silicon dummies that enable learners to discover basic anatomical and pathological findings using real ultrasound equipment. The benefits of these simulators include their relatively low cost and the opportunity for trainees to work with their own local ultrasound equipment. The technical aspect of the ultrasound examination is an area that often needs improvement, as lack of knowledge about how to operate the equipment prevents proper image optimization and thereby impairs image interpretation [11–14]. However, the case complexity is limited due to the low fidelity of the physical mannequins, and they often only include one case per mannequin. Ultrasound requires visual-cognitive skills that may only be improved through practicing with multiple different cases, as the case-to-case transfer of skills is often very limited [10,17]. Finally, training with physical mannequins is limited by the fact that there is no automated feedback to the learner or any instructions as to how to perform the scan; therefore, a supervisor is needed to guide and assess the trainee during his or her practice.

The virtual reality simulators include various systems that usually rely on haptic devices or physical mannequins that record probe movements during transabdominal or transvaginal scans. These systems combine probe movements with computer-animated or real ultrasound images. During training, the simulators often provide instructions to the learner, and some systems even provide automated feedback that can be used to track learning and to determine when trainees have attained expert levels of performance. However, some studies have demonstrated that only one-third of the in-built feedback metrics on commercially available virtual reality simulators can be used to distinguish between different levels of operator competence [18] (Madsen et al. 2013), which may question their use for both formative as well as summative assessment purposes [19]. As such, the validity of the automated feedback must be examined before these measures can be used for assessment purposes. Other benefits of the virtual reality simulators include that they contain multiple cases as well as pathology, allowing trainees to be exposed to a large variety of different clinical and ultrasonic presentations. The main drawback is the price, as most of these systems cost between 10,000 and 70,000 GBP (USD 13,100 to 91,000, please note that these prices may vary substantially between manufacturers as well as over time). Finally, the virtual reality simulators may provide instructions and feedback on image optimization, but there is often little resemblance to actual ultrasound machines, making "knobology" training difficult without using real ultrasound equipment.

Evidence Supporting Use of Simulation-Based Ultrasound Training

Several studies have examined the effects of simulation-based ultrasound training. Compared to no hands-on training, simulation-based ultrasound training has demonstrated positive effects on performance in controlled [20] and simulated settings [21] (Figure 20.1). When comparing transvaginal ultrasound training to training on real women on a 1:1 basis, one study demonstrated that simulation-based training led to *inferior* performances on subsequent scans performed on real women (Moak et al. 2015). However, when examining the effects of actual clinical training versus initial simulation-based training followed by clinical training, there were large effects associated with simulation-based training, when assessing trainees' clinical performances after 2 months of clinical practice [13,14]. This indicates that although practicing on standardized patients (real women) may be more realistic and result in superior learning compared with training on a simulator, the clinical reality does not allow us to use patients as we use simulators. During clinical training, trainees may receive supervision from senior clinicians, but they are not allowed to experiment freely or to explore what happens if they commit an error, and they may not receive high-quality feedback during an intimate examination. In a study comparing two different methods for obstetric ultrasound training, one group was instructed to make as many errors as possible and to experiment freely, whereas the other group was instructed to complete the simulation-based training with as few errors as possible. A subsequent transfer test on real women demonstrated superior diagnostic accuracy of the trainees, who had been instructed to experiment freely and encouraged to make errors during their training, compared with the error-avoidance group [18].

A large randomized multicenter trial demonstrated that initial simulation-based transvaginal ultrasound training led to significantly less patient discomfort compared with trainees, who only received clinical training, over the first 6 months of their training. Moreover, the need for supervised practice was reduced over time in the group that received initial simulation-based training, and these trainees also used 20% less time to complete their examinations [22].

The cost-effectiveness of simulation-based ultrasound training has not received much attention. In one study, authors explored the cost-effectiveness of introducing a cervical scan training program using multiple components, including simulation-based training, and demonstrated the cost-effectiveness of reducing waiting time for patients presenting with symptoms of premature onset of labor [13,14]. To date, it remains unclear whether simulation-based training as an adjunct to clinical training is cost-effective or not. The answer to this question may be difficult to obtain as the time dedicated to ultrasound training varies significantly between different institutions and countries, and because outcomes such as improvements in diagnostic accuracy are difficult to measure in a clinical setting, in which patients are seen by multiple different health-care professionals rather than just a single trainee. Whereas the learning outcomes have been shown to vary little between virtual reality simulators and physical mannequins, their cost differs significantly. For example, the cost of a silicone mannequin ranges between 5,000 and 10,000 GBP (USD 30,000 to 60,000), whereas the costs of virtual reality simulators often start around 40,000 GBP (USD 250,000).

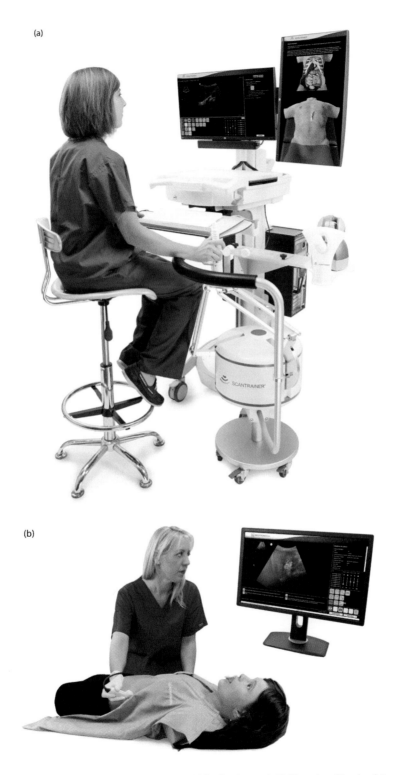

FIGURE 20.1 Examples of different commercially available simulators. (a,b) Virtual reality simulators may use real ultrasound images such as those used by Scantrainer, Medaphor. In the simulator shown, the haptic devices used for probe manipulations are supplied with force feedback to mimic the resistance that is felt during actual transvaginal or transabdominal scans. ScanTrainer (Transvaginal and Transabdominal simulator on a portable cart); Point of Care Ultrasound (PoCUS) simulator Body Works. *(Continued)*

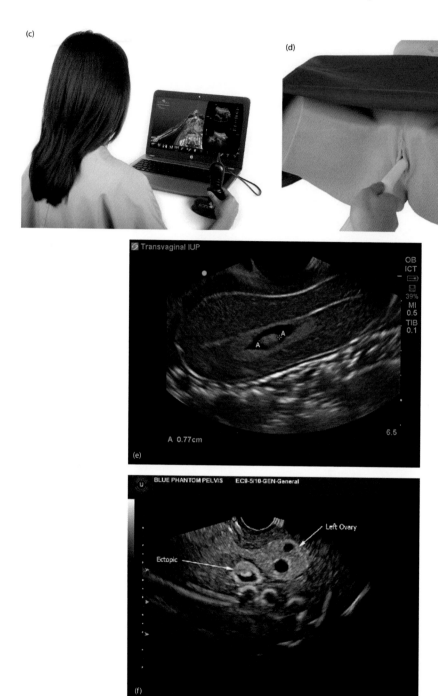

FIGURE 20.1 (Continued) Examples of different commercially available simulators. (c) Several virtual reality simulators offer trainees the possibility to access different types of pathological findings using cloud-based technology. The SonoSim Ultrasound Training Solution shown here provides scanning cases of virtual patients in the SonoSimulator, cloud-based didactic courses, knowledge assessments, performance tracking, and access to real-patient pathology. The advantage is that the simulator is very versatile, but a potential drawback is that the probe movement is limited to tilting in one fixed position. (d,e,f) Some virtual reality simulators make use of computer-generated images. The advantage of these models is that they can produce an endless number of different types of pathology, and they allow moving parts (a whole fetus or the fetal heart) to be visualized a number of different ways. Shown here is the Blue Phantom Female Pelvis Intrauterine Pregnancy Transvaginal Ultrasound Training Model. ([a,b] By permission of Medaphor Group PLC, Cardiff, United Kingdom; [c] Courtesy of SonoSim, Inc., Santa Monica, California; [d,e,f] By permission of CAE Blue Phantom, Redmond, Washington.)

E-Learning, Image Banks, and Assessment of Ultrasound Competence

Over the past decade, the use of massive online open courses (MOOC) have been increasingly used to improve trainees' knowledge. These courses consist of freely available learning materials that trainees can access online. However, the quality of these learning resources may vary, just as there may be large differences in the representativeness and usability of different image banks that are available online. Some of the more promising initiatives include the ISUOG-driven [1] VISUOG that aims to include ultrasound presentations of a large variety of anomalies and different pathology. A large meta-analysis of the effectiveness of e-learning has shown that e-learning can be as effective as traditional learning methods [23]. The drawback of e-learning interventions is, however, that they rely on high levels of user adherence and compliance. Moreover, e-learning programs may help trainees acquire knowledge and image recognition but are not suitable for training technical aspects of a procedure, such as the hand-eye coordination required for practicing ultrasound.

Test-enhanced learning is a well-established method to ensure that trainees have acquired the knowledge needed before entering supervised clinical practice. The use of tests helps identify knowledge gaps, but multiple studies have demonstrated that taking tests also improves trainees' learning. In fact, test-enhanced learning results in better learning outcomes than re-studying written material or attending lectures on the issue to be learned. That said, the validity of the tests used is an issue that needs to be established before any test can be adopted for the use of feedback (formative assessment) or licensing (summative assessment). Yet, validation studies require substantial effort, and clinical educators may therefore save time using tests, for which the validity evidence has already been established, rather than developing tests on their own [24].

For intimate ultrasound examinations such as transvaginal ultrasound, it may not be ethical or feasible to assess trainees' practical skills in the clinical setting [4]. Instead, ultrasound simulators may be used to test trainees' diagnostic accuracy using a number of predefined cases and standardized assessment instruments [15], such as the *Objective Structured Assessment of Ultrasound Skills* (OSAUS) instrument [11,12].

Practical Advice for Clinical Trainers in Assisted Reproduction and Early Pregnancy

There is evidence for the effectiveness of several general principles for learning. These include the use of test-enhanced learning as well as the use of simulation-based training as described earlier. Other established methods that have been proven to improve learning include retrieval practice, distributed learning, elaboration, and the use of mnemonics [25]. These concepts are briefly explained in Box 20.1.

BOX 20.1 WELL-ESTABLISHED METHODS FOR EFFECTIVE LEARNING

Retrieval practice is the deliberate effort of trainees to retrieve the information that has been read or practiced. Retrieving information helps consolidate the neural connections—also called encoding—that learning depends on.

Distributed learning is characterized by distributing the learning sessions over time rather than relying on courses in which the content material is massed into a single session.

Elaboration is the use of multiple pieces of information that can be connected to the same construct that trainees attempt to learn. Adding case information to ultrasound images as well as elaborate clinical presentations helps the learners strengthen the encoding of the information to be learned.

Mnemonics are powerful instruments that help learners add meaning to new information that is difficult to remember. For example, remembering the ways an ultrasound image may be optimized by adding vivid images to each function may improve learning. Other methods include the method of loci, in which learners are instructed to walk through well-known physical locations and to place the content to be learned across these places.

In Box 20.2, practical recommendations to clinical trainers are listed. These pieces of advice are not all evidence-based but are developed based on the principles for learning described in section "Simulation-Based Ultrasound Training."

BOX 20.2 PRACTICAL TIPS THAT MAY BE HANDED DOWN FROM CLINICAL TRAINERS TO TRAINEES

ASSISTED REPRODUCTION SCAN

- Before scanning make sure you know the cycle day, medication (if anti-estrogen treatment— thin endometrium), previously described pathology, or operations (e.g., oophorectomy).
- Make sure the patient has an empty bladder.
- Scan systematically every time, cervix, uterus in two planes, right ovary, left ovary, and pouch of Douglas.
- Uterus pathology of importance for fertility, fibroids, polyps, or septate uterus? Thickness of endometrium, layered or luteinized.
- Hydrosalpinx?
- Ovaries—endometriomas? Cysts?
- Measurements of follicles, not too much pressure, make sure the follicle you measure is as round as possible, follicle diameter is the mean of two perpendicular diameters.

EARLY PREGNANCY SCAN

- Before scanning be sure you know the patient's history of gynecological disease and in particular fertility history: previous pregnancies and outcomes, previous gynecological surgery, last period, cycle length, irregular cycle, presence of symptoms like bleeding and pain, and type of pain and location, in order to do a focused examination.
- Positioning of the patient with legs up in a gynecological examination chair/bed and buttocks to the edge of the bed—in order to be able to move the vaginal transducer as freely as possible—and downward, too.
- Rotate probe and picture in the same way always so that every transvaginal scan is initiated by a midsagittal approach, and the vaginal walls are visualized during probe insertion where urethra can be visualized in full length, too.
- Systematical examination of internal genitals—first in sagittal views from side to side and then by rotating 90° to go through the transverse plane (i.e., up/down).
- It is important that the orientation of the image on the screen and that of the probe are maintained in the same direction throughout training and subsequent practice.
- Full view of cervix and uterus—including fundus and interstitial part of the tubes— reassure uterine cavity is in line with the cervical canal. If uterus cannot be visualized in total using a transvaginal approach, then an abdominal scan is mandatory.
- Evaluate the presence of free fluid—amount and echogenicity.
- Both ovaries must be visualized—if not possible, the examination must be supplemented by a transabdominal approach.
- Uterine corners and adnexa surrounding the ovaries must be evaluated too—look for pathology such as hydrosalpinx or interstitial pregnancy.

- Location of the gestational sac according to usual criteria—be aware that a blurred "sac" located centrally in the uterus might be blood or fluid. The location of the early gestational sac is always embedded in the endometrium in the cavity in normal pregnancies. If corner near location, look for relation to endometrium by gaining up and down, which may help if in doubt.
- If uterus is anteflexed or there is a long distance to gestational sac and in doubt of viability, the abdominal approach may be helpful in reducing the distance to the sac and improving resolution.
- Locating and evaluating ectopic pregnancies is difficult and needs an experienced examiner. In most ectopic gestations, the chorionic tissue can be visualized—often as a homogenic rounded mass of echogenic tissue and often with a small central, well-defined cyst (gestational sac).
- The location of ectopic pregnancies is defined by the surroundings. For example, if the ectopic pregnancy is interstitial, then the myometrium is seen surrounding the sac but might be deforming the surface of the uterine corner.
- When teaching to examine transvaginal sonography—preparation and a systematic approach are the route to success.

Conclusion

Ultrasound training relies on motor skills and visual-cognitive skills. These skills can be trained in the clinical setting as well as in the simulated setting or using e-learning programs. Clinical training does not automatically result in expert performance, but a certain volume of scans is needed. Simulation-based training is an effective method to improve trainees' clinical skills before entering supervised practice. Other effects include decreased patient discomfort, shorter examination time, reduced need for supervised practice, and improved patient satisfaction. E-learning programs are just as effective as traditional lectures for knowledge acquisition, but these programs and the use of test-based learning and assessment require substantial quality assurance and validation efforts, respectively.

REFERENCES

1. ISUOG Education Committee recommendations for basic training in obstetric and gynecological ultrasound. *Ultrasound Obstet Gynecol.* 2014;43:113–6.
2. EFSUMB. European Federation of Societies for Ultrasound in Medicine and Biology. Minimum training recommendations for the practice of medical ultrasound. Appendix 3: Gynaecological ultrasound. Education and Practical Standards Committee. *Ultraschall Med.* 2006;27:79–105.
3. Tolsgaard MG. A multiple-perspective approach for the assessment and learning of ultrasound skills. *Perspect Med Educ.* 2018;7(3):211–3.
4. Tolsgaard MG, and Chalouhi GE. Use of ultrasound simulators for assessment of trainee competence: Trendy toys or valuable instruments? *Ultrasound Obstet Gynecol.* 2018;52(4):424–6.
5. Krupinski EA. The role of perception in imaging: Past and future. *Semin Nucl Med.* 2011;41:392–400.
6. Crowley RS, Naus GJ, Stewart J 3rd, and Friedman CP. Development of visual diagnostic expertise in pathology—An information-processing study. *J Am Med Inform Assoc.* 2003;10:39–51.
7. Kundel HL, and Nodine CF. Interpreting chest radiographs without visual search. *Radiology.* 1975;116:527–32.
8. Boutis K, Pecaric M, Shiau M et al. A hinting strategy for online learning of radiograph interpretation by medical students. *Med Educ.* 2013;47:877–87.
9. Monteiro SM, and Norman G. Diagnostic reasoning: Where we've been, where we're going. *Teach Learn Med.* 2013;25:S26–32.

10. Norman GR, Coblentz CL, Brooks LR, and Babcook CJ. Expertise in visual diagnosis: A review of the literature. *Acad Med*. 1992;67:S78–83.

11. Tolsgaard MG, Rasmussen MB, Tappert C et al. Which factors are associated with trainees' confidence in performing obstetric and gynecological ultrasound examinations? *Ultrasound Obstet Gynecol*. 2014;43:444–51.

12. Tolsgaard MG, Ringsted C, Dreisler E et al. Reliable and valid assessment of ultrasound operator competence in obstetrics and gynecology. *Ultrasound Obstet Gynecol*. 2014;43:437–43.

13. Tolsgaard MG, Ringsted C, Dreisler E et al. Sustained effect of simulation-based ultrasound training on clinical performance: A randomized trial. *Ultrasound Obstet Gynecol*. 2015;46:312–8.

14. Tolsgaard MG, Tabor A, Madsen ME et al. Linking quality of care and training costs: Cost-effectiveness in health professions education. *Med Educ*. 2015;49:1263–71.

15. Tolsgaard M, Veluppilla C, Gueneuc A et al. When are trainees ready to perform transvaginal ultrasound? An observational study. *Ultraschall Med*. 2019;40(3):366–73.

16. Cook DA, Hatala R, Brydges R et al. Technology-enhanced simulation for health professions education: A systematic review and meta-analysis. *JAMA*. 2011;306:978–88.

17. Bjerrum F, Sorensen JL, Konge L et al. Randomized trial to examine procedure-to-procedure transfer in laparoscopic simulator training. *Br J Surg*. 2016;103(1):44–50.

18. Dyre L, Tabor A, Ringsted C, and Tolsgaard MG. Imperfect practice makes perfect: Error management training improves transfer of learning. *Med Educ*. 2017;51(2):196–206.

19. Borgersen NJ, Naur TMH, Sørensen SMD et al. Gathering validity evidence for surgical simulation: A systematic review. *Ann Surg*. 2018;267(6):1063–8.

20. Akoma UN, Shumard KM, Street L, Brost BC, and Nitsche JF. Impact of an inexpensive anatomy-based fetal pig simulator on obstetric ultrasound training. *J Ultrasound Med*. 2015;34(10):1793–9.

21. Chao C, Chalouhi GE, Bouhanna P, Ville Y, and Dommergues M. Randomized clinical trial of virtual reality simulation training for transvaginal gynecologic ultrasound skills. *J Ultrasound Med*. 2015;34(9):1663–7.

22. Tolsgaard MG, Ringsted C, Rosthøj S et al. The effects of simulation-based transvaginal ultrasound training on quality and efficiency of care: A multicenter single-blind randomized trial. *Ann Surg*. 2017;265:630–7.

23. Cook DA, Levinson AJ, Garside S, Dupras DM, Erwin PJ, and Montori VM. Internet-based learning in the health professions: A meta-analysis. *JAMA*. 2008;300(10):1181–96.

24. Hillerup NE, Tabor A, Konge L, Savran MM, and Tolsgaard MG. Validity of ISUOG basic training test. *Ultrasound Obstet Gynecol*. 2018;52(2):279–80.

25. Brown PC, Roediger HL, III, and McDaniel MA. *Make It Stick: The Science of Successful Learning*. Cambridge, MA; 2014.

26. Dyre L, Nørgaard LN, Tabor A et al. Collecting validity evidence for the assessment of mastery learning in simulation-based ultrasound training. *Ultraschall Med*. 2016;37(4):386–92.

27. Fitts PM, and Posner MI. *Human Performance*. Belmont, CA: Brooks/Cole; 1967.

28. Madsen ME, Konge L, Nørgaard LN et al. Assessment of performance measures and learning curves for use of a virtual-reality ultrasound simulator in transvaginal ultrasound examination. *Ultrasound Obstet Gynecol*. 2014;44:693–9.

29. Moak JH, Larese SR, Riordan JP, Sudhir A, and Yan G. Training in transvaginal sonography using pelvic ultrasound simulators versus live models: A randomized controlled trial. *Acad Med*. 2014;89(7):1063–8.

21

Training and Certification

Nazar N. Amso, Arianna D'Angelo, and Costas Panayotidis

Introduction

Ultrasound (US) is now embedded in gynecological and assisted reproduction practice worldwide. Diagnostic errors lead to incorrect management with all its medicolegal consequences and, most importantly, suboptimal patient care [1].

Many organizations have published requirements and guidelines for US practice in general and more specifically in gynecology. There are clearly defined skills and attributes that must be fulfilled for competent practice. However, implementation and standards of training vary considerably worldwide in spite of major efforts by professional societies and organizations. This is not unexpected, as training in the clinical environment is very often dependent on opportunistic acquisition of US skills, along with the availability and quality of the trainer.

The introduction of ultrasound simulation as a training tool has opened new avenues for standardization of training. The systems' increasing sophistication and the spectrum of case scenarios available in them meant that embedding this training tool in the curriculum coupled with timely interventions based on educational pedagogy provide an opportunity to harmonize training, expedite the acquisition of skills, and reduce pressures on clinical resources. Should simulation-based assessment prove to be equally successful, the impact of higher standards of training on improved clinical practice will be realized globally.

Quality Assurance in Ultrasound Practice: Why?

The importance and need for a robust quality assurance program in ultrasound practice stems from the fact that mistakes can lead to litigation and great patient discomfort. Shortfalls in practice may be institutional failings such as inappropriate local protocols, poor quality assurance, and/or governance policies or human error. Often, it is a combination of the aforementioned. In one recent incident [2], a dating scan incorrectly diagnosed a "silent miscarriage" and had the woman not had a further scan at another hospital, which confirmed ongoing pregnancy, she would have inadvertently undergone a "termination of pregnancy." An ombudsman inquiry identified several shortcomings relating to institutional and health-care professional practices. These included failure of the institution to implement national professional guidelines designed to prevent the misdiagnosis of early pregnancy loss, substandard practice in the conduct of the ultrasound scan, and failure of the health-care professionals to consider relevant medical history of the pregnant woman. In this book, Soave and Marci [3] address institutional measures to ensure high quality of service to safeguard patients, which include up-to-date standard operating procedures and key performance indicators to ensure quality of service and uniformity of performance.

It is well recognized that health-care professionals undertaking ultrasound scans vary in their practice, and both inter- and intraobserver variations could lead to errors in measurements [4]. In this book, D'Angelo highlights operator-dependent factors such as ultrasound image optimization and magnification skills and incorrect placement of calipers, adversely impacting measurement accuracy of endometrial thickness and follicular diameters [5]. The literature reviewed in the chapter provides ample evidence of a significant positive correlation between image quality and measurements accuracy. Years of ultrasound practice is not an indicator of image quality or accuracy of measurements. Hence, the role of regular audit of practice cannot be overemphasized. But perhaps the most significant study that highlighted the need to establish an external quality assurance scheme in assisted reproduction treatments (ARTs) was that by Driscoll and colleagues in 1997 [6]. The authors demonstrated a large variation in measuring fixed objects ranging between 10 and 32 mm in diameter embedded in an ultrasound phantom. Given the pivotal role of ultrasound in ART, it becomes clear that a robust training scheme with clear objectives and competency-based assessments is essential for high-quality service and safe practice.

Regrettably, many health-care professionals worldwide undertake ultrasound scanning without having evidence of completing a robust training scheme. Equally, in some institutions or countries, including in the United Kingdom, there is minimal or nonexistent communication between health-care professionals, who undertake the scans, and clinicians, who do not possess ultrasound skills, resulting in false-positive and false-negative ultrasound findings not being communicated and opportunities to improve ultrasound practice wasted [7].

Requirements and Guidelines for Ultrasound Practice

Ultrasound practice in subfertility and reproductive medicine has evolved over time since the early 1980s. As in other fields in gynecology, there were no set standards for practice or training in transvaginal ultrasound (TVS) at the outset. Many of the skills had been acquired from transabdominal scanning and applied to TVS. Several ad hoc short training courses were set up to train gynecologists and fertility practitioners in the art of TVS from the late 1980s. A World Health Organization (WHO) Study Group in 1998 indicated that ultrasound training needs may be defined according to equipment availability, and suggested three levels of training requirement in diagnostic ultrasound [8]. In 2000, the European Federation of Societies for Ultrasound in Medicine and Biology (EFSUMB) established that, in Europe, there was no standardization of training requirements for ultrasound practitioners, either between different countries or between different medical disciplines [9]. Soon afterward, in 2002, the EFSUMB published their landmark document "Minimum Training Requirements for the Practice of Medical Ultrasound in Europe" [10]. In the United Kingdom, the Royal College of Radiologists (RCR) first published its ultrasound training recommendations for medical and surgical specialties in 1997, followed by the Royal College of Obstetricians and Gynaecologists (RCOG) in introducing core and advanced training skills modules in ultrasound since 2001 for specialty trainees, and for subfertility and assisted reproduction trainees in collaboration with the British Fertility Society. The RCR and RCOG training programs have been updated and refined since their introduction but generally follow the original principles.

Unlike the RCOG, the EFSUMB and RCR determined three levels of minimum training requirements and abilities to practice ultrasound [10,11]. For each level of practice, a syllabus and comprehensive recommendations for the necessary practical experience were conceived, and recommendations were made for the evaluation of theoretical knowledge and practical technical and interpretive skills.

Level 1 practice requires a practitioner to do the following:

- Perform common examinations safely and accurately
- Recognize and differentiate normal anatomy and pathology
- Diagnose common abnormalities within certain organ systems
- Recognize when referral for a second opinion is indicated

It was judged that at this level, training would be acquired during conventional postgraduate specialist training programs.

Level 2 practice would require spending a period of subspeciality training and the ability to do the following:

- Accept and manage referrals from level 1 practitioners
- Recognize and correctly diagnose almost all pathology within the relevant organ system

- Perform basic, noncomplex ultrasound-guided invasive procedures
- Teach ultrasound to trainees and to level 1 practitioners
- Conduct some research in ultrasound

At level 3, a practitioner would practice at an expert level, performing complex examinations and ultrasound-guided interventions as well as being involved in teaching and research in ultrasound.

In 2014, the American Institute of Ultrasound in Medicine (AIUM) published "Training Guidelines for Physicians Who Evaluate and Interpret Diagnostic Ultrasound Examinations of the Female Pelvis" [12]. It recommended that trainees would need to present evidence of being involved with the performance, evaluation, interpretation, and reporting of at least 300 diagnostic ultrasound examinations of the female pelvis and a minimum of 170 diagnostic gynecologic ultrasound examinations per year to maintain the physician's skills. In ART, the AIUM guidelines for standards of practice in 2008 required physicians to perform 20 follicular aspirations under direct supervision prior to independent practice, although the revised 2017 version seems to have dropped this requirement [13]. A systematic review of the literature and a Delphi survey of 15 expert s\pecialists in oocyte pickup (OPU) recommended that at least 30 OPUs should be done under supervision per year and at least 50 procedures performed independently before qualification in reproductive medicine [14]. The experts considered that a qualified operator in OPU should undertake 50 procedures per year to maintain competence.

In 2019, the European Society of Human Reproduction and Embryology (ESHRE) published recommendations of its working group on ultrasound in ART [15]. It recognized that "in relation to training and competence in ultrasound guided oocyte pick-up, there are currently no accepted minimal requirements for OPU training" and recommended that for safety reasons, and whenever feasible, simulation could be the initial part of a structured training for novices who want to perform OPU. It further recommended that a minimum of 30 procedures should be undertaken under supervision to reach the minimum criteria for competency, echoing the earlier Delphi survey conclusions.

Acquisition of Ultrasound Skills

Traditionally, individuals seeking to develop their ultrasound skills attended lecture-based meetings and short hands-on training courses. While a short instructional hands-on course helps learners to develop their basic skills when pre- and post-testing are undertaken, carrying this effect to the clinical environment and its long-term impact have not been determined. In this book, Tolsgaard et al. correctly argue that e-learning and image library are just as effective as traditional lectures in developing a learner's cognitive skills [16]. They also elegantly provide evidence that simulation-based training is an effective method to improve a trainee's clinical skills before embarking on supervised practice.

Worldwide, ultrasound education programs emphasize primarily the acquisition of the skill (craft) and professionalism rather than purely knowledge-based education. Hence, competency is prized, and evidence of this competency is sought using Miller's pyramid (Figure 21.1) [17]. In this chapter, we address in brief detail the methods and practices of teaching a skill and where in that continuous process timely interventions could enhance and expedite the development of ultrasound skills as well as reduce the demand on trainers' time and impact on clinical services.

Learners can participate in the learning environment and construct their knowledge in ways that are meaningful to them and facilitate their progression, a philosophy known as "Constructivism." Developing a skill or craft, in this instance ultrasound, encompasses mental action or the process of acquiring knowledge and understanding through thought, experience, and the senses (i.e., to recognize or conceptualize, an approach referred to as "Cognitive Apprenticeship" as described by Collins [18]). When applied in a technologically rich environment, learners construct their knowledge and skills through accurate and realistic practices considerably faster than in a conventional opportunistic environment. The "observation" of an expert is replaced with e-learning and exemplars of lesson plans and video clips of simulated ultrasound scans undertaken by clinical experts often referred to as "modeling"; hints and recommendations extend learners' competencies, referred to as "scaffolding"; while feedback and

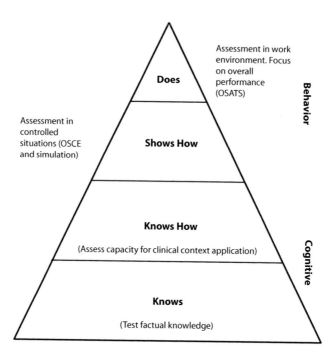

FIGURE 21.1 Miller's pyramid outlining the progressive development of cognitive and behavioral attributes and the appropriate assessments at each stage. (From Miller GE. *Acad Med [Supplement]*. 1990;65: S63–7.)

guidance improve practices, known as "coaching." These learning steps assist them to articulate their knowledge ("articulation"), enable them to be critical of their own performance ("reflection"), and finally drive them into a mode of problem-solving of their own ("exploration").

Progression in the early stages of learning is made possible with modern educational technology (e.g., e-learning, image library, and simulation with built-in feedback), which facilitates acquisition of knowledge and core skills in a controlled environment, "knows how," and "shows how." In the clinical environment, feedback at different stages of the process by a trainer or through reflective portfolio will enhance the student's learning environment and will ensure that he or she is inducted into a community of practice in keeping with an apprenticeship model and the development of professionalism.

Simulators that are curriculum based will help learners develop their skills along the Dreyfus "novice to expert" model published in the mid-1980s [19].

In this model, learners can progress from novice to advanced beginner and benefit from being able to endlessly repeat key procedural tasks with increasing complexity, on a simulator in a safe environment, and when feedback is available are likely to develop their skills to competency at a faster pace than in an "opportunistic" clinical environment. Both competency and proficiency refer to "knowing a skill," but there is value difference between them. Competency can refer to the bare minimum required for acceptability, while proficiency carries with it a level of mastery that is above the minimum. One can be competent without being spectacular, but continuing to grow in his or her proficiency. Attributes related to each stage are outlined in Table 21.1.

Assessments: Why, How, Where, and When?

While professional societies and organizations' programs outline the curriculum and syllabus for various specialties, and describe the minimum competence level and quality of performance required for independent practice, problems remain in that substantial variations persist in the implementation of training standards between individuals, within and between institutions and countries [4]. There is also the

TABLE 21.1

Novice to Expert Attributes

Stage	Attribute
Novice	• Rules and routines: "rigid adherence to taught rules or plans" • No leeway for "discretionary judgment"
Advanced beginner	• Limited "situational perception" • All aspects of work and skill are treated separately with equal importance
Competent	• "Coping with information overload"; multiple activities and accumulated tasks and knowledge • Limited perception of actions in relation to the ultimate goals • Deliberate planning • Begins to formulate and implement routines
Proficient	• Develops a holistic view of the overall situation: "sees the big picture" • Prioritizes tasks • Perceives and recognizes deviations from the normal pattern • Employs principles and rules of conduct for guidance • Adapts to the situation at hand
Expert	• Transcends reliance on rules, guidelines, and rules of conduct • Intuitively grasps situations based on in-depth understanding • Develops a "vision for what is possible" • Adopts an "analytical approach" in unexpected situations

Source: Adapted from Dreyfus HL, and Dreyfus SE. In: Dreyfus HL, and Dreyfus SE (eds.) *Mind Over Machine: The Power of Human Intuition and Expertise in the Era of the Computer.* New York, NY: Free Press; 1986. pp. 1–18.

division between those who advocate completion of a number of procedures before independent practice and others who contend that competency is achieved at varying speeds and is dependent on the innate ability of the individual to develop the complex psychomotor skills required for the practice of ultrasound. In one recent study, the number of completed US scans and the years of training were a poor predictor of the trainees' diagnostic accuracy [20]. In many instances, professional organizations require regular appraisal and assessment of technical skills during the training period culminating in an institutional peer-led competency assessment at the end of training, a process that is both time and resource intensive [11,21]. The concept of a non-credit-bearing approach for acquiring skills was introduced by the RCOG in 2012 and was called "credentialing." It was defined as: "a process that provides formal accreditation of attainment of competencies (which include knowledge, skills and performance) in a defined area of practice, at a level that provides confidence that the individual is fit to practice in that area in the context of effective clinical governance and supervision as appropriate to the credentialed level of practice" [22]. However, the authors are not aware of any active schemes, and the RCOG "Advanced Training in Obstetrics and Gynaecology" curriculum published in 2019 has no reference to credentialing [23]. Ultrasound is viewed as an integral part of obstetric and gynecological practice, and the RCOG's ultrasound training program is competency based and designed to ensure that trainees develop the skills they need to use and understand ultrasound in clinical practice. A module "Intermediate ultrasound in gynaecology" fulfills the requirements for Capabilities in Practice (CiPs), high-level statements setting out what a doctor should be able to do at the end of training. Acquisition and progression of skills are monitored by different types of workplace-based assessments (WPBAs) that include objective structured assessment of technical skill (OSATS), mini clinical evaluation exercise (Mini-CEX), and case-based discussion (CbD). They aim to link teaching, learning, and assessment in a structured way and are not necessarily used to demonstrate competency in a procedure but rather to identify strengths and weaknesses that are discussed during routine appraisals with supervisors. In the adapted Dreyfus model outlined in Figure 21.2, learners having acquired core ultrasound skills using simulation undertake directly supervised practice in the clinical environment to contextualize their learned skills on the simulator and demonstrate their path to competency by undertaking formative OSATS, Mini-CEX, and CbD prior to assessment. In the RCOG curriculum, summative OSATS are designed for assessments of learning and to allow a trainee to demonstrate competence in a given

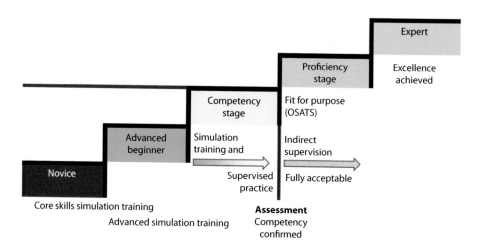

FIGURE 21.2 Dreyfus model of skills acquisition adapted for ultrasound training. (From Dreyfus HL, and Dreyfus SE. In: Dreyfus HL, and Dreyfus SE [eds.] *Mind Over Machine: The Power of Human Intuition and Expertise in the Era of the Computer.* New York, NY: Free Press; 1986. pp. 1–18.)

clinical situation or technical competency (e.g., ultrasound). The ultrasound curriculum sets five key ultrasound assessments in gynecology where a trainee must demonstrate competency in a minimum of three procedures per core assessment. Competency in the observed procedure was generally defined as an expectation to demonstrate an ability to perform all aspects of the procedure safely and competently with no or minimal need for help, or in the context of an unexpectedly difficult case, may have needed more assistance for the more difficult aspects of the procedure.

Interestingly, the curriculum permits other methodologies (e.g., simulation, e-learning, and case-based discussion) to sign-off the early stage of skill acquisition, if direct experience of the procedure or clinical problem has not been possible.

In assisted reproduction, new assessment tools have been explored recently. For OPU, a statistical tool, the "Learning Curve—Cumulative Summation Test" (LC-CUSUM), was developed in an attempt to determine when the learning curve for a procedure is complete by indicating when a predefined level of performance is achieved [24]. Using this model, Dessolle et al. demonstrated in a small study of three trainees that on average, the number of oocytes collected by the trainees did not differ from that of the senior operator, and the number of oocyte retrievals required for a trainee to learn the procedure depended on the trainee [25]. By contrast, Goldman et al., in a study of four trainees only, concluded that irrespective of the trainee's previous experience, there was no statistical difference in their learning curves to achieve proficiency in OPU [26]. When 20 procedures or more have been performed under supervision, the subsequent projection of trainees' learning curves did not change significantly; thus, the authors proposed a minimum of 20 OPUs to attain proficiency. The ensuing debate as to what is the definition of OPU proficiency, what criteria must be satisfied to achieve proficiency, and the multitude of criteria to consider highlighted the complexity of determining a precise definition of proficiency and probably the authors' tendency to mix proficiency stage in skill acquisition with the definition of an expert in OPU [27,28].

An alternative approach for ultrasound education has been pursued by higher education institutions (HEIs) that requires a robust and transparent process for monitoring and assessment of a student's or trainee's skills acquisition in the workplace and competence. These credit-bearing programs are overwhelmingly structured at master's level, and their successful completion through *formal* knowledge and practical assessments leads to academic postgraduate qualification at certificate, diploma, or master's level [29]. Unlike professional bodies, assessment of practical skills is undertaken by the academic institute's faculty at the end of the course, is independent of the student's local mentor, and although it follows a robust procedure, is laborious, involves human volunteers, and is costly. However, it is important to emphasize that both professional and academic educational standards are designed to ensure patient safety and maintain professional standards.

Simulation is widely accepted as having an important role in US training [16]. Its role in assessment is under evaluation and yet to be fully ascertained. A number of questions pose themselves; what is the purpose of the assessment; what skills to assess; what to use for skills assessment, human volunteers and/ or simulation; validity and reliability of the assessment itself; pass/fail skills; consequences of failure; and finally at what stage of the learning process should the assessment take place?

Answering the final question first may determine the answers to the previous ones. In Miller's pyramid and the Dreyfus and Dreyfus model, "Show How" and "Competence," respectively, refer to the ability to demonstrate bare minimum standard required for acceptability [17,19]. This concept is well accepted in undergraduate medical education, where assessment of skills takes place in a controlled situation or a simulated environment. Hence, it is logical that such a simulation-based ultrasound assessment is undertaken at the end of the competency stage.

Returning to the other questions posed earlier, if it is accepted that the purpose of the assessment is to demonstrate competence, then it should be regarded as a high-stakes test. Tolsgaard and Chalouhi correctly argue that using human volunteers for intimate TVS assessments is neither feasible nor ethical and equally correctly, cast doubts about the value of simulator-based metrics in such assessments, as many of these metrics are not discriminatory [30]. These metrics, however, were primarily intended as rigid rules and routines for novices to adhere to in the early stages of training. A more appropriate format is direct observation of performance using a validated standardized assessment score sheet or a similar tool with key skills assigned to pass or fail [16]. The concept of pass/fail for key skills is commonly applied in UK HEI courses accredited by the Consortium of Accreditation for Sonography Education (CASE). A simulation-based exam may include full examination of one or two case scenarios where key skills must be demonstrated competently, and this would be pass/fail, and a number of "short" cases representing varied pathologies that require the student to identify and describe the structure(s) being examined, analyze and provide a reasoned differential diagnosis, and where applicable, propose a treatment plan. Such a combination will allow testing the depth and breadth of skills and applied knowledge in one setting and is based on standardized cases, which is not possible in the clinical environment.

It can be argued that successful completion of such a robust simulation-based assessment could be the entry point to practice in the clinical environment, but with a level of supervision and feedback that will be far less intensive than that required at earlier stages of training and will expeditiously lead to "proficiency" and intuitive practice. Should a learner be unsuccessful in the assessment, then a further period of simulation and supervised training is required. It is also conceivable that in the future, competent but not proficient practitioners will be assisted by new ultrasound or software technology such as artificial intelligence, as this may provide real-time guidance and monitor and audit performance, thereby providing a layer of quality assurance to ensure optimal delivery of patient care [4,31].

Conclusion

Current training schemes and their diverse assessments are not always at the same standard, leading to suboptimal practice and errors. Understanding the learning process and embedding a technology-enhanced environment supplemented by "robust and standardized" simulation-based assessments might be the answer to streamlining the current heterogeneity. Clinical practice would then be to achieve proficiency and ultimately mastery of the skill. Furthermore, health-care professionals must maintain their skills through a continuing professional program and regular audit of one's practice. Professional bodies and learned societies should ensure that guidelines are in place to uphold high standards of ultrasound practice.

REFERENCES

1. Panayotidis C. Legal aspect of gynaecological ultrasound in UK practice. *EC Gynaecol*. 2019;8(2):224–31.
2. Public Services Ombudsman for Wales. *The investigation of a complaint by Ms D against Cardiff and Vale University Local Health Board*. Investigation Report Case: 201202432. 2013. Accessed October 25, 2019. https://www.ombudsman.wales/reports/cardiff-vale-university-health-board-201202432/

3. Soave I, and Marci R. Quality aspects of ultrasound. In: D'Angelo A, and Amso NN (eds.) *Ultrasound in Assisted Reproduction and Early Pregnancy*. Boca Raton, FL: CRC Press; 2020. pp. 242–9.
4. Benacerraf BR, Minton K, Benson C et al. Proceedings: Beyond ultrasound first forum on improving the quality of ultrasound imaging in obstetrics and gynecology. *J Ultrasound Med*. 2018:7–18.
5. D'Angelo A. Ultrasonographic monitoring of follicle growth in controlled ovarian hyperstimulation (COS). In: D'Angelo A, and Amso NN (eds.) *Ultrasound in Assisted Reproduction and Early Pregnancy*. Boca Raton, FL: CRC Press; 2020. pp. 87–101.
6. Driscoll G, Tyler J, and Carpenter D. Variation in the determination of follicular diameter: An inter-unit pilot study using an ultrasonic phantom. *Hum Reprod*. 1997;12(11):2465–8.
7. Torrington J. Are sonographers advanced practitioners? A survey of sonographers' opinions on their level of practice analysed against the Society of Radiographers Advanced Practitioner. *MSc Dissertation*. Cardiff University. 2017.
8. World Health Organization. *Training in Diagnostic Ultrasound: Essentials, Principles and Standards: Report of WHO Study Group 1998*. WHO technical report series: 875. 1998.
9. European Federation of Societies for Ultrasound in Medicine and Biology. Training and accreditation: A report from the EFSUMB Education and Professional Standards Committee. *EFSUMB Newsletter*. 2000;14:20.
10. European Federation of Societies for Ultrasound in Medicine and Biology. Minimum Training Requirements for the Practice of Medical Ultrasound in Europe: A report from the EFSUMB Education and Professional Standards Committee. *EFSUMB Newsletter*. 2002.
11. The Royal College of Radiologists. Ultrasound training recommendations for medical and surgical specialties. 2017. Accessed October 12, 2019. https://www.rcr.ac.uk/publication/ultrasound-training-recommendations-medical-and-surgical-specialties-third-edition
12. American Institute of Ultrasound in Medicine. Training guidelines for physicians who evaluate and interpret diagnostic ultrasound examinations of the female pelvis. 2014. Accessed March 1, 2020. https://www.aium.org/resources/viewStatement.aspx?id=58
13. American Institute of Ultrasound in Medicine. Guideline: AIUM practice parameter for ultrasonography in reproductive medicine and infertility. 2017. Accessed January 14, 2017. http://www.aium.org/resources/guidelines/reproductivemed.pdf
14. Panayotidis C. Interventional ultrasound: Standardisation of oocyte retrieval in assisted reproduction treatments. 2017. Accessed September 5, 2018. https://www.researchgate.net/publication/327142563_Interventional_Ultrasound_Standardisation_of_Oocyte_Retrieval_in_Assisted_Reproduction_Treatments
15. The ESHRE Working Group on Ultrasound in ART. Recommendations for good practice in ultrasound: Oocyte pick-up. 2019. Accessed March 1, 2020. https://www.eshre.eu/Guidelines-and-Legal/Guidelines/USS-practice-in-ART
16. Tolsgaard MG, Sundberg K, and Nielsen HS. Ultrasound training in assisted reproduction and early pregnancy. In: D'Angelo A, and Amso NN (eds.) *Ultrasound in Assisted Reproduction and Early Pregnancy*. Boca Raton, FL: CRC Press; 2020. pp. 258–66.
17. Miller GE. The assessment of clinical skills/competence/performance. *Acad Med (Supplement)*. 1990;65: S63–7.
18. Collins A, Brown J, and Newman S. Cognitive apprenticeship: Teaching the crafts of reading, writing and mathematics. In: Resnick LB (ed.) *Knowing. Learning and Instruction: Essays in Honor of Robert Glaser*. Mahweh, NJ: Lawrence Erlbaum Associates; 1989. pp. 453–94.
19. Dreyfus HL, and Dreyfus SE. The five-stage model of adult skill acquisition. In: Dreyfus HL, and Dreyfus SE (eds.) *Mind Over Machine: The Power of Human Intuition and Expertise in the Era of the Computer*. New York, NY: Free Press; 1986. pp. 1–18.
20. Tolsgaard M, Veluppillai C, Gueneuc A et al. When are trainees ready to perform transvaginal ultrasound? An observational study. *Ultraschall in Med*. 2019;40(03):366–73.
21. Royal College of Obstetricians and Gynaecologists. US training. Accessed January 10, 2020. https://www.rcog.org.uk/en/careers-training/specialty-training-curriculum/ultrasound-training/
22. Royal College of Obstetricians and Gynaecologists. Tomorrow's specialist. 2012. Accessed December 20, 2019. https://www.rcog.org.uk/globalassets/documents/guidelines/tomorrows-specialist_fullreport.pdf

23. Royal College of Obstetricians and Gynaecologists. 2019. Advanced training in obstetrics and gynaecology. 2019. Accessed March 24, 2020. https://www.rcog.org.uk/en/careers-training/specialty-training-curriculum/atsms/

24. Biau DJ, and Porcher, R. A method for monitoring a process from an out of control to an in-control state: Application to the learning curve. *Stat Med.* 2010;29(18):1900–9.

25. Dessolle L, Leperlier F, Biau DJ et al. Proficiency in oocyte retrieval assessed by the learning curve cumulative summation test. *Reprod Biomed Online.* 2014;29:187–92.

26. Goldman KN, Moon KS, Yauger BJ et al. Proficiency in oocyte retrieval: How many procedures are necessary for training? *Fertil Steril.* 2011;95(7):2279–82.

27. Siristatidis C, Lykakis A, and Chrelias C. Proficiency in oocyte retrieval: Plausible steps before perfection. *Letter to Editor. Fertil Steril.* 2011;96(5):161.

28. Stegmann BJ, Goldman KN, and Moon KN. Reply of the authors. *Fertil Steril.* 2011;96(5):162.

29. National qualifications frameworks in the United Kingdom. Accessed March 12, 2020. https://en.wikipedia.org/wiki/National_qualifications_frameworks_in_the_United_Kingdom

30. Tolsgaard M, and Chalouhi G. Use of ultrasound simulators for assessment of trainee competence: Trendy toys or valuable instruments? *Ultrasound Obstet Gynecol.* 2018;52:424–6.

31. Han CS, and Datkhaeva I. Artificial intelligence in OB/GYN ultrasound. *Contemporary OB/GYN.* 2019;64(10). Accessed March 15, 2020. https://www.contemporaryobgyn.net/obstetrics/artificial-intelligence-obgyn-ultrasound

Index